Frontiers in Anti-infective Agents

(Volume 2)

Anti-infective Research and Development:
Updates on Infection Mechanisms and Treatments

Edited by

Gloria G. Guerrero Manriquez

University Autonome of Zacatecas
Unit of Biological Sciences
Zacatecas
México

Frontiers in Anti-Infective Agents

Volume # 2

Anti-infective Research and Development: Updates on Infection Mechanisms and Treatment

Editor: Gloria G. Guerrero Manriquez

ISSN (Online): 2705-1080

ISSN (Print): 2705-1072

ISBN (Online): 978-981-14-6958-9

ISBN (Print): 978-981-14-6956-5

ISBN (Paperback): 978-981-14-6957-2

Published by Bentham Science Publishers Pte. Ltd. Singapore. All Rights Reserved.

need for a court order if at any point you breach any terms of this License Agreement. In no event will any delay or failure by Bentham Science Publishers in enforcing your compliance with this License Agreement constitute a waiver of any of its rights.

3. You acknowledge that you have read this License Agreement, and agree to be bound by its terms and conditions. To the extent that any other terms and conditions presented on any website of Bentham Science Publishers conflict with, or are inconsistent with, the terms and conditions set out in this License Agreement, you acknowledge that the terms and conditions set out in this License Agreement shall prevail.

Bentham Science Publishers Pte. Ltd.
80 Robinson Road #02-00
Singapore 068898
Singapore
Email: subscriptions@benthamscience.net

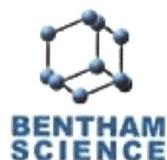

BENTHAM SCIENCE

CONTENTS

PREFACE

A plethora of anti-infective agents is found in nature. Their properties and the mechanism of action are also diverse for treatment and vaccination against intracellular microorganisms (J.M. Favela-Hernandez and G.G. Guerrero). In the last decades, there was an increase in the emergence and reemergence of multi-drug resistant strains. Unfortunately, despite intense efforts, for most of these infectious diseases, there are no safe and effective treatments that are affordable for people in developed countries. Moreover, the pathogens have developed a successful evasion mechanism to survive the host selection pressure at the molecular and neuro-immunological level (A. Montoya Rosales and Noe Macias-Segura). In recent years, it has become evident that there is a connection between the nervous, endocrine and immunologic system that play a key role in the homeostatic control in the presence of different environment stimuli and infectious diseases caused by a virus, bacteria, fungus, and parasites (A. Montoya Rosales and Noe Macias-Segura). For this reason, it is pivotal to continue the search for novel and effective natural products showing an action against tuberculosis to decrease the incidence and prevalence of this pathogen (S. Guzman Beltran, F. Hernandez-Sanchez, and M.O. Barrientos). The innate and cellular immune response to *M. tuberculosis* infection is characterized, addressing specifically the innate components in the up-respiratory tract (URT), cytokines, antimicrobial peptides' induction and activation of T cellular responses to promote the clearance of the *M. tuberculosis* (M.A. Moncada and M.A. Herrera-Barrios). Interestingly the induction of the antimicrobial peptides (AMPs) such as Cathelicidins (LL-37) and β-defensins (HBD-2), represents one of the most promising approach, along with the reactive oxygen species (ROS), to kill intracellular bacteria. Furthermore, the induction of AMPs in response to bacterial stimuli can be enhanced by vitamin D and IFN-γ in several infections (E.L. Carreto-Binaghi and Y. Gonzalez). The deleterious effect of the reactive oxygen species (ROS) can be ameliorated by vitamin D, which at the same time, can regulate nitric oxide (NO), leading to cell integrity protection and an antimicrobial mechanism by the induction of AMPS and autophagy. As a lysosome-based degradation pathway and recycling mechanism of cellular components, autophagy has been proposed as an immunological response to circumvent the escape of bacteria. If this can be approached therapeutically with autophagy inducers (natural products, drugs), is an issue that deserves further clinical consideration (A. Ruiz and E. Juarez).

On the other hand, gastric and peptic ulcers caused by *Helicobacter pylori* represent a serious health problem due to the increasing evidence that suggests that this gram-negative spiral bacteria predispose to gastric cancer and anemia. The enormous iron requirements of this bacteria can be fulfilled by different human sources. How can this be accomplished? And how this allows the bacteria to survive? Are the subjects of intense research for the clinic and therapeutic implications (T.J. Olivares and J. Mosqueda).

Finally, genomic studies have allowed a step forward in the identification of new genes as candidates vaccines with therapeutic potential against parasites such Apicomplexa protozoan, *e.g. Babesia bigemina*) of animal organisms, including humans. The understanding and elucidation of the cellular and molecular mechanisms that trigger a protective, immune response, play a key role in eliminating this type of pathogen and, thereby, are fundamental for clinical translation (J. Mosqueda, S. Mejia-Lopez. and U.M.A. Mercado).

In the present book, we aimed to update key aspects of the development and research of anti-infective agents in terms of how they can influence the host response at the pharmacological and immunological level against microbial and parasites infections. Thus, I hope this book can be helpful for readers of different disciplines to get updates on these main aspects.

Gloria G. Guerrero Manriquez
University Autonome of Zacatecas
Unit of Biological Sciences
Zacatecas
México

List of Contributors

Andy Ruiz
Departamento de Inmunología Integrativa, Instituto Nacional de Enfermedades RespiratoriasIsmael Cosío Villegas, Ciudad de México, México
Posgrado en Ciencias Biológicas, UNAM, México

Angélica Moncada Morales
Microbiology Department, National Institute of Respiratory Diseases Ismael Cosío Villegas, México City, México

Esmeralda Juárez
Departamento de Investigación en Microbiología, Instituto Nacional de EnfermedadesRespiratorias Ismael Cosío Villegas, Ciudad de México, México

Fernando Hernández-Sánchez
Departamento de Investigación en Microbiología, Instituto Nacional de EnfermedadesRespiratorias Ismael Cosío Villegas, CDMX, Mexico

Gloria G. Guerrero Manriquez
University Autonome of Zacatecas, Unit of Biological Sciences, Zacatecas, México

José de Jesús Olivares Trejo
Universidad Autónoma de la Ciudad de México, Posgrado en Ciencias Genómicas San Lorenzo 290, C.P. 03100, Ciudad de México, México

Juan Mosqueda
Facultad de Ciencias Naturales, Universidad Autónoma de Querétaro, 76230 Juriquilla, Qro., Mexico
Immunology and Vaccines Laboratory, Natural Sciences College, Autonomous University of Queretaro, Queretaro, Qro, Mexico

Juan Manuel Favela-Hernández
Institute Mulitdisciplinary of Sciences, AVICENA, Campus Torreón Coahuila, México

Laura E. Carreto-Binaghi
Departamento de Investigación en Microbiología, Instituto Nacional de EnfermedadesRespiratorias Ismael Cosío Villegas, CDMX, Mexico

Macías-Segura Noé
Laboratorio de Neuroimunoendocrinología, Departamento de Fisiología y Farmacología, Centrode Ciencias Básicas, Universidad Autónoma de Aguascalientes, 20130 Aguascalientes, Ags., Mexico

María Teresa Herrera Barrios
Microbiology Department, National Institute of Respiratory Diseases Ismael Cosío Villegas, México City, México

Montoya-Rosales Alejandra
Laboratorio de Neuroimunoendocrinología, Departamento de Fisiología y Farmacología, Centrode Ciencias Básicas, Universidad Autónoma de Aguascalientes, 20130 Aguascalientes, Ags., Mexico

Miguel Angel Mercado-Uriostegui
Immunology and Vaccines Laboratory, Natural Sciences College, Autonomous University of Queretaro, Queretaro, Qro, Mexico
Doctorado en Ciencias Biológicas, Natural Sciences College, Autonomous University of Queretaro, Queretaro, Qro, Mexico

Omar M. Barrientos
Departamento de Investigación en Microbiología, Instituto Nacional de EnfermedadesRespiratorias Ismael Cosío Villegas, CDMX, Mexico

Silvia Guzmán-Beltrán
Departamento de Investigación en Microbiología, Instituto Nacional de EnfermedadesRespiratorias Ismael Cosío Villegas, CDMX, Mexico

Susana Mejia-López   Immunology and Vaccines Laboratory, Natural Sciences College, Autonomous University of Queretaro, Queretaro, Qro, Mexico
Doctorado en Ciencias Biológicas, Natural Sciences College, Autonomous University of Queretaro, Queretaro, Qro, Mexico

Yolanda Gonzalez   Departamento de Investigación en Microbiología, Instituto Nacional de EnfermedadesRespiratorias Ismael Cosío Villegas, CDMX, Mexico

CHAPTER 1

The Anti-Infective Agents

Juan Manuel Favela-Hernández[1] and **Gloria G. Guerrero Manriquez**[2,*]

[1] *Institute Mulitdisciplinary of Sciences. AVICENA. Campus Torreón Coahuila. México*

[2] *University Autonome of Zacatecas. Unit of Biological Sciences. Zacatecas, México*

Abstract: Anti-infective agents are secondary metabolites produced and obtained from a different sources (plants, bacteria, virus, fungi, and marine oceans) with antibacterial or antiviral properties. The mechanism of action of these compounds is also broad and extensive as well. Anti-infective agents (antibacterial or antiviral) possess either a bactericidal/virucidal or bacteriostatic /virustatic ability against microbes and viruses. To impact as safer alternatives for the treatment of emergent and reemergent infectious diseases, it is neccesary to have a better knowledge of the more recent advances in phytomedicine, etnopharmacology, and omics technologies that might lead to therapies a based on natural formulations of adjuvants and/or of different combinations of compounds (*e.g.* secondary metabolites+antimicrobial peptides) with complementary properties (immunological, pharmacological), that are a promised strategy to curb multidrug resistance strains (MDR) and/or super drug resistance bacteria (XDR). Therefore, the aim of the present chapter is to outline the world of anti- infective agents, along with their mechanism of action.

Keywords: Anti-Infective Agents, Gram(+), Gram(-) Bacteria, Intracelular, Viruses.

INTRODUCTION

The emergent and reemergent resurgence of old infectious diseases (measles, tuberculosis, leprosy) represents a threat to human beings in developed countries [1]. First second and third-generation antibiotics have been the alternative as a treatment against infectious diseases. However, the recent uprising of Multi-drug resistant (MDR), and Extensively-drug resistant (XDR) such as Super Bug resistant (SBR) strains of *Staphylococcus aureus*. (*S. aureus*) has curbed the functions of antibiotics used for the treatment of infectious diseases (bacterial/viral) nowadays (Fig. **1**).

To overcome the MDR, it has been proposed to use a combination or a mixture of

* **Corresponding author Gloria G. Guerrero Manriquez:** Biological Sciences Unit, University Autonome of Zacatecas Campus II, Av Preparatoria S/N Col Agronomicas ZP 98066, Zcatecas, México; Tel: +52 4921564376; E-mail: gloriaguillermina@uaz.edu.mx

different compounds with different properties that can be given as additives to make a synergy that potentiates the pharmacological as well as the immunological effects (*e.g.* drugs and antimicrobial peptides). More recent work has suggested virustatic agents that can be repurposed to virucidal agents using high throughput technologies [2 - 9].

In the present chapter, we revisited the anti-infective agents from natural sources by highlighting their mechanism of action and at the same time, we outlined the mechanisms of resistance. We think that host-pathogen interaction analysis in conjunction with the more recent advances in phytomedicine, ethnopharmacology, and omics technologies may lead to a better understanding and development of natural effective therapies as well as innovative technologies in clinical immuno-pharrmacology research.

SOURCE OF THE ANTI-INFECTIVE AGENTS

A plethora of anti-infective agents (either antimicrobial and/or anti-viral) are secondary metabolites, isolated and extracted from different natural sources (plants, bacteria, fungi, virus and marine oceans) [10 - 13] but they can also be chemically synthesized. The mechanism of action of anti-infective agents in general can be direct and irreversible (bactericidal/virucidal) or indirect and reversible (bacteriostatic/virustatic) depending on the intrinsic properties of the anti-infective agent [14 - 18].

The bactericidal agents can exert their action toward Gram(+)[*Staphylococcus aureus, Streptococcus pneumonia, Clostridium perfrrngerns, Clostridium tetanic; Listeria monocytogenes, Mycobacterium tuberculosis*]. Whereas the bacteriostatic agents can act against to Gram (-) bacterias, (*Pseudomonas aeruginosa, Campylobacter jejuni, Salmonella tiphi, Vibrio cholera, Escherichia coli, Helicobacter pylori, Haemophilus influenza*) and DNA viruses (Parvovirus, Papovavirus, Adenovirus, Iridovirus, Poxvirus, Herpes, Hepadnaviruses) or RNA viruses (Rabdovirus, Togavirus, Bunyavirus, Coronavirus, Arenavirus, Retrovirus, Paramyxovirus), see viruses section [14 - 18].

GRAM POSITIVE BACTERIA	INFECTIOUS DISEASE	GRAM NEGATIVE BACTERIA
(*Streptococcus pneumoniae; Streptococcus agalactiae; Listeria monocytogenes*)	Bacterial meningitis	(*Haemophilus influenzae; Neisseria meningitidis*)
(*Streptococcus pyogenes*)	Upper respiratoy tract infection	(*Haemophilus influenzae; Moraxella catarrhalis*)
(*Staphylococcus aureus Streptococcus pneumoniae;* **ATYPICAL:** *Mycobacterium tuberculosis*)	Pneumonia	(*Haemophilus influenzae; Chlamydia pneumoniae; Legionella pneumophilia*); *Acinetobacter spp*
(*Streptococcus pneumoniae*)	Otitis Media	
(*Streptococcus pneumoniae*)	Sinusitis	(*Haemenophilus influenzae*)
(*Staphylococcus aureus*)	Eye infection	(*Chlamydia trachomatis; Neisseria gonorrhoeae*)
	Gastrointestinal tract infection	(*Escherichia coli and other Enterobacteriaceae members ; Vibrio cholerae*)
	Gastritis	(*Helycobacter pylori*)
(*Staphylococcus aprophyticus; Enterococcus faecalis*)	Urinary tract infection	(*Escherichia coli and other Enterobacteriaceae ; Pseudomonas aeruginosa ; Proteus spp*)
Staphylococcus aureus; Enterococcus spp	Endocarditis, Peritonitis	*Chlamydia trachomatis, Haemophilus ducreyl; Neisseria gonorrheaee*)
(*Staphylococcus aureus; Streptococcus pyogenes*)	Skin infection	(*Pseudomonas aeruginosa*)
(*Staphylococcus aureus, Clostiridium spp*)	Food poisoning	*Enterobacteria; -Campylobacter*

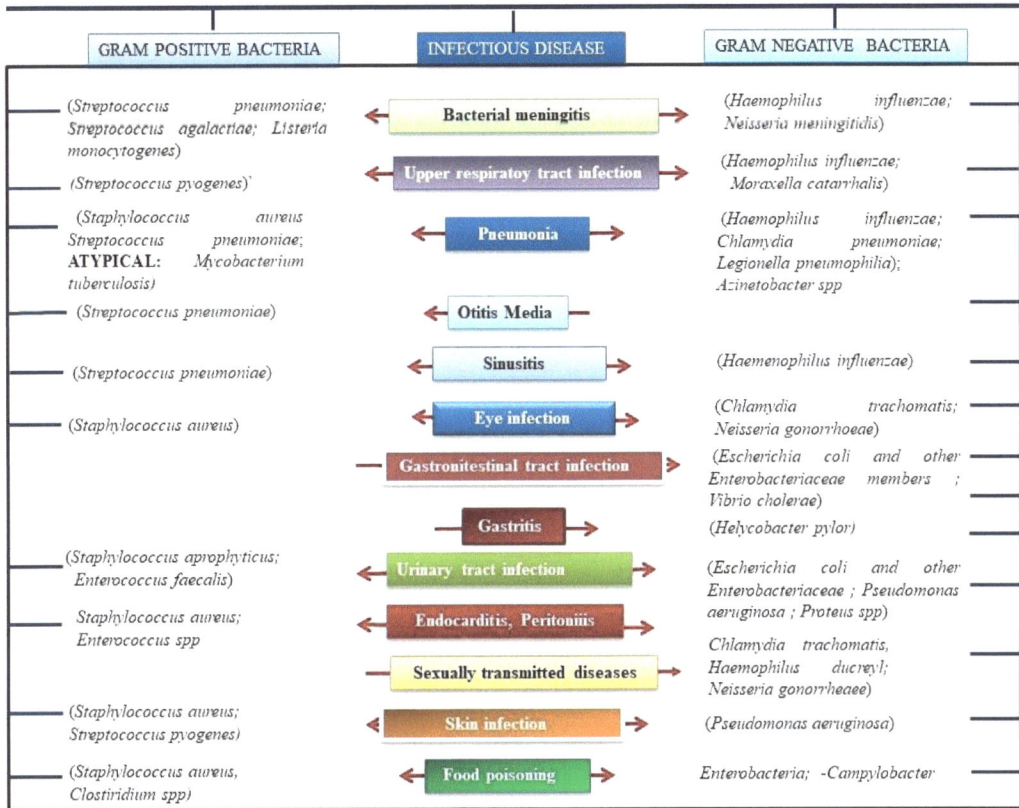

Fig. (1). A-Scheme of the main human infectious diseases caused by gram postive (+) and gram negative (-) bacteria. Some of them are shared eihter by both types of bacteria. Some of them are still a serious health problema worldwide due to appearnce of multidrug resistance strains (MDR) and/or super drug resistance bacteria (XDR). (*e.g. Staphylococcus aureus, Salmonella typhimurium; Mycobacteirum tuberculosis*). Other infectious diseases like those caused by *Helyobacter pylori* constitute a major risk for cáncer development. Bacterial toxins produced by the genus *Clostridium, Bacillus, Vibrio cholerae, E. coli* enteropathogenic, comprise a powerful virulence factor in the interaction host-pathogen) and potential target; quórum sensing and biofiilm foramtion by *P aeruginosa* as well.

Plant-Derived Anti-bacterial Agents

Plant-derived secondary metabolites possess a variety of biological properties. Pharmacological or toxicological and recent studies indicate that glucosides triterpenes are potential adjuvants in cáncer and other inflammatory diseases [19 - 22]. Phenols and phenolic acids ((PCs) (flavonoids and nonflavonoids), tannins, anthocyanins, stilbenes, coumarins, tannins, lignans and lignins) are one of the most potential antimicrobial agents derived from diverse natural sources such as from fruits, vegetables, seeds, vegetables, tea, wine and honey. Around 400 products have been described with these properties [23, 24], whose chemical structure can neutralize reactive species of oxygen (ROS) (anti-oxidant activity) and can interact positively with gut microbiota. The hydroxyl group in the molecules of the PCs has been associated with the inhibitory effect exerted by PC on target bacteria.

The fruit rich in PCs (taxifolin, myricetin and quercetin) is blueberry, active against L. *monocytogenes* and *Salmonella enteritidis* [23, 24]. In addition, PCs such as as caffeic acid have antibacterial activities *to Escherichia. coli* (*E. coli*) and *Staphylococcus aureus* (*S. aureus*). Whereas, gallic acid is active against *Enterococcus faecalis* (*E. faecalis*) and also against *Pseudomonas aeruginosa (P. aeruginosa), Staphylococcus aureus (S. aureus), Moraxella catarrhalis* (*M. catarrhalis*) *Streptococcus agalactiae* (*S. agalactiae*) and *Streptococcus pneumonia* (*S. pneumoniae*), C*ampyloba*cter jejuni *(C. jejuni)* and *Helicobacter pylori* (*H. pylori*). Moreover, gallic acid has also shown bactericidal activity and immunomodulatory properties against *Campylobacter coli (C. coli) and Listeria monocytogenes (L. monocytogenes)* [25]. Besides, phenolic compounds (PC) as drug candidates for Tuberculosis therapy have also been effective [26].

Potentilla species were found to be rich in hyperoxide, (+) catechin, caffeic acid, ferulic acid, rutin, and ellagic acid, which were tested for their antibacterial activities. Potentilla fruticosa has the highest effect against *S. aureus, S pneumonia* (Gram-positive bacteria); *P aeruginosa, P. mirabils (Gram-negative bacteria*) (Fig. **1**) and/or toward the fungus *Candida albicans.*(*C. albicans)* [27]. Other phenolic compounds such as hydroquinone, thymol, carvacrol, butylated hydroxyanisole and octyl gallate were assayed against *S. aureus* [28].

Panduratin A, a natural chalcone compound, extracted from Kaempferia pandurata ROxb, had potent activity against *S. aureus* [27]. Zheng *et al.,* 2014 [29] reported around 100 natural products with inhibitory activities against *Mycobacterium tuberculosis (M.tuberculosis, MTb)* proteasome [29]. Among them, 22 are phenolic compounds; flavonoids, coumarins, phenol and lignans. These include baicalein, pectrolinari, quercetin, hispidulin, myricetin, Isoliquiritigenin icariin, kaempferol, curcumin, and baicalin. The main target of phenolic compounds, particularly lignans (dihydrocubebin, hinokinin, ethoxycubebin) are the biosynthesis of mycolic acids of *M. tuberculosis* (Gram-positive mycobacteria) (Fig. **1**) [29, 30].

Triterpenes, the sesquiterpenoids, whcih are a class of terpenoids composed of three isoprenes units (15 carbons), as antiinfective agents, have antioxidative and anti-inflammatory properties and can function as neuropeptides A clear example is *Quillaga saponaria* or QS-21 [27] which has been shown to be promising in some assays as a vaccine in terms of efficacy and toxicity [27]. Riccardi, a natural product of liverwort and 6,6'dihydrothiobinupharidine (from the crude drug

Senkotsu [31] can also be found in volatile oils obtained from different parts of plants like flowers, leaves, seeds, stems, roots and wood [32, 33]. They are characterized by a strong smell and by variable mixtures of bioactive compounds mainly terpenoids (monoterpenes and sesquiterpenes). Some of them also contain nonterpenic compounds by the phenylpropanoid pathway., *e.g.* Eugenol, Cinnamaldehyde and Safrole [34]. These compounds exhibit antibacterial properties against Gram-positive bacteria (*S. aureus*) and Gram-negative bacteria *(Salmonella enteritidis, Pseudomonas aeruginosa, Yersinia enterocolitica*) [34].

Alkaloids represent another type of natural products isolated from plants, animals, bacteria and fungi. They are considered as healing secondary metabolites. In general, most of the alkaloids are bactericidal rather than bacteriostatic. Thus, for example, Squalamine showed higher bactericidal activity than bacteriostatic [35]. Other alkaloids with antimicrobial, antiviral and anticancer activities are the dehydrocavidine, coptivine, dehydrospocavidine and tetrahydroscoulerine of Yanhuanglian extracted from *Corydalis Saxicola Butning* [35].

Plant-Derived Antiviral Agents

Around 40 compounds of this type have been observed that possess antiviral activity (virucidal). Leurocristine, periformyline, perivine and vincaleucoblastine are natural alkaloids that have been obtained from *Catharanthus roseus* (L) and lanceusPih (Apycycaceae). Leurocristine is active against poliovirus, vaccinia, and influenza viruses [36]. Periformyline inhibits poliovirus replication [36]. Perivine exhibits activity against vaccinia, and vinaleucoblastine possesses virucidal activity against poliovirus vaccinia and influenza virus [36]. The michellamines naphthylisoquinoline alkaloids obtained from the tropical liana *Ancistrodalus korupensis* have demonstrated HIV-inhibitory activities [37]. A series of isoquinoline alkaloids such as lycorine, lycoridicine, narcidasine, and cis.dihydronarciclasine, obtained from *Narcissu poeticus* (Amaryllidaceae) have shown significant *in vitro* activity against flaviviruses and bunyaviruses (Fig. **2**) [38, 39].

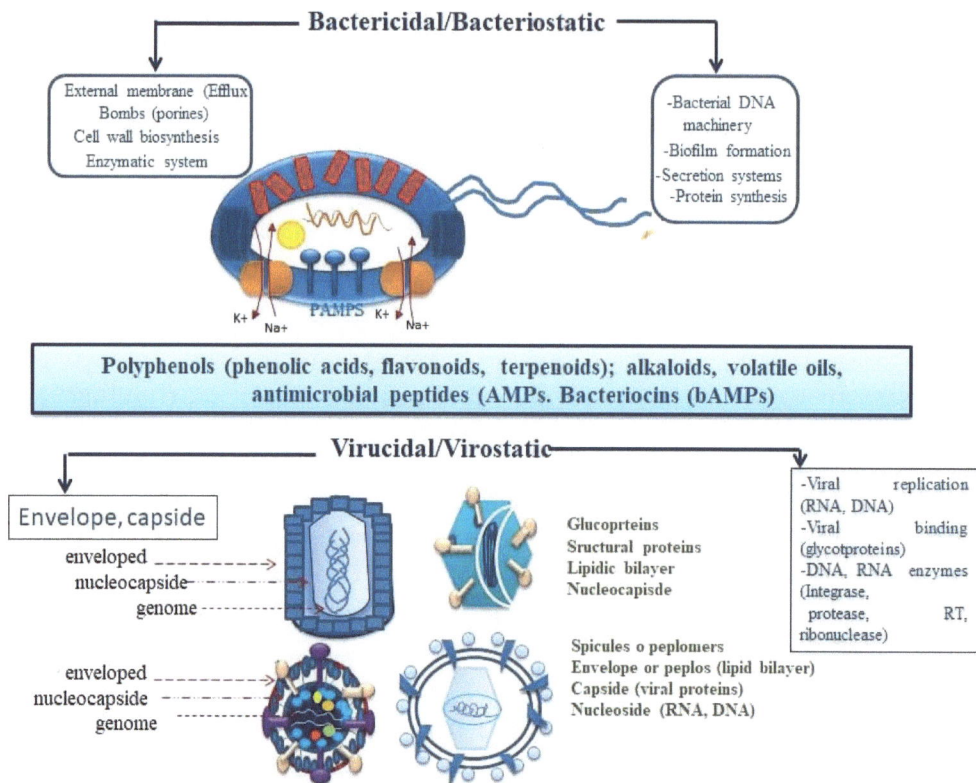

Fig. (2). The antiinfective agents are compounds that are obtained from different sources, In general are derived from either, the nature (plants, bacteria, fungi, marine oceans, animals) or chemically synthesized. The most common plant derived compounds are the alkaloids (chalcone), phenolic acid (flavaonoids, terpenoids), which exert their activity directly (bactericidal) or indirectly (bacteriostatic) leading to a loss of cellular integrity or disruption of any processes (cell growth, cell viability, protein biosynthesis, DNA replication) or structure (membrane integrity). In a similar concepts is applied for viruses.

OTHER SOURCES OF ANTI-INFECTIVE AGENTS

The bacterium *Chromobacterium violaceum*, is a Gram-negative bacteria that produce violacein considered as a bioactive metabolite involved in quórum sensing. This is one of the thousands of possibilities that can be explored from pathogens and the unveiled interaction between host-pathogen components [40]. Another bacteria that produce beta-lactamase (inhibitor of cell wall biosynthesis) belong to the *Streptomyces genus* [41]. By other hand, wild polish mushrooms, containing protocatechuic acid, 4-hydroxybenzoic acid, vanillic acid, syringic acid, caffeic acids, p-coumaric and ferulic acids, show antibacterial activities against a range of Gram (-) and Gram (+) bacteria [42] while the effect is stronger against Gram(+) microorganisms. Methyl gallate is effective against enterobacteria such as *S. typhi, E. coli and S. flexneri* [42]. Interestingly, marine-derived anti-infective agents have also been described particularly with their antimycobacterial activity [43, 44].

MECHANISM OF ACTION OF THE ANTI-INFECTIVE AGENTS (BACTERIAL/VIRAL)

In general, the anti-infective agents (antibiotics natural and synthetic, secondary metabolites) target key áreas in the bacterial life such as protein synthesis, folate pathway, DNA replication, cell wall biosynthesis, and also structures such as the external membrane. Of note is the action of the antiviral compound whose main action is viral binding, viral replication and blockade of the DNA enzymes (Fig. 3).

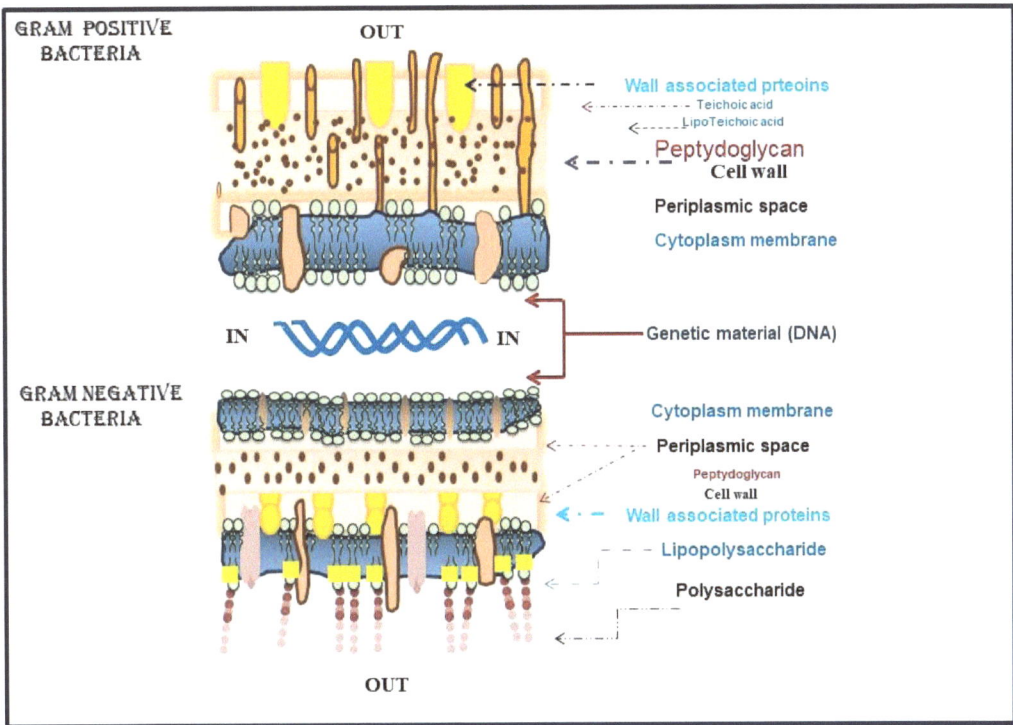

Fig. (3). The cell envelope of Gram positive and Gram negative bacteria is a complex barrier characterized by a thick layer of peptidoglycan (PG) immersed in the periplasmic space and connected to the internal cytoplasmic membrane. In Gram negative bacteria, is comprised by two membranes, an intersticial or the periplasmic space in which is inmersed a thin layer of peptidoglycan (PG). The cell Wall polymeric structure is comprised by glycan strands covalently linked to each other (in a perpendicular fashion with respect to the length of the glycan strands) by an interconnecting peptide stalk attached to an alternating saccharide of the glycan strands.. In Gram negative bacteria, the full length stalk structure is the peptapeptide L-Ala-γ-D-Glu-meso-diaminopimelate-D-Ala.D-Ala(lysine replaces the diaminopimelate in many Gram positive cell walls. The chemical composition in either cell envelope of Gram positive and Gram negative is based on membrane binding proteins (BNPs), polysaccharides polymers, phospholipids, and teichoic acids.

Bactericidal Anti-infective Agents

A bactericidal anti-infective agent is a compound that can damage and disrupte the external membrane or the cell wall biosynthesis, causes an irreversible change, affecting bacterial viability and a leaky memabrane either from Gram positive or Gram negative bacteria as outlined in Fig. (**2**) [45 - 50], *e.g.* Ethambutanol [51]; Ethionamide [52 - 54]; and Cephalosporins [55, 56] are able to block Gram-positive cell wall biosynthesis (Fig. **3**).

-Ethambutanol (EMB) (a first-line antibiotic for Tb treatment), has a cell wall acting as an antibiotic that targets enzymes that are part of the mycolic acid synthesis machinery [51], thus limiting the apical growth (mycolic acid synthesis) and inhibiting arabinogalactan, a component of the cellular membrane of *M. tuberculosis* [27].

-EMB remains as the most effective against mycobacteria, which requires an mAGP layer for viability. Furthermore, EMB is also the drug of choice for treating various infections caused by non-tuberculous mycobacteria (NTM) [51]. To note EMB also has an effect on *Corynebacterium glutamicum* (*C. glutanicum*) growth [50].

-Ethionamide and prothionamide are prodrugs that are activated by EThA and inhibit the synthesis of mycolic acid [49 - 51], whereas cycloserine antibiotics also inhibit the peptidoglycan synthesis, another major component of *M. tuberculosis* cellular membrane [52 - 54].

-Ceftazidime and apigenin damage the cytoplasmic membrane of ceftazidime-resistant *Enterobacter cloacae* and cause subsequent leakage of intracellular components and inhibition of bacterial energy metabolism [55, 56].

-Isoniazid is a prodrug that is activated by the *Mtb* catalase-peroxidase (KatG) and inhibits the synthesis of *M. tuberculosis* mycolic acid [57, 58].

Bactericidal Plant Derived- Secondary Metabolites

Phenolic compounds (flavonoids, non-flavonids, triterpenes, butyric actidcin-namic acid and thymol) can damage and irreversibly alter bacterial cell membrane accompanied by changes in permeability, polarization as well as the interruption of flux activtiy. Polyphenols constitute a promising weapon against nosocomial infections if *S aureus* strains are present [59 - 62]. Tannins, which is one of the most representative phenolic compounds [subclassified into condensed tannins (proanthocyanidins orcatechins) and hydrolyzable tannins (gallotannins and ellagitannins) [59 - 61] are able to penétrate and interact with lipid bilayers and can cause a membrane fusion, a process that results in the leakage of intramembranous materials and aggregation [59 - 61]. Triterpenes like *Quillaja Saponaria* or QS induce a membrane leakage and 6,6'dihydrothiobiparidine-inhibited DNA topoisomerase IV exerts a synergistic effect either with drugs against multiresistant strains of *S. aureus* (MRSA) or with vancomycin against resistant bacteria of the genus *Streptococcus* [63, 64]. Squalamine (s polyamine alkaloid class) acts by disturbing the bacterial membrane integrity [65]. Sanguinarine (a benzo phenanthridine alkaloid) obtained from the root of *S. canadensis I.,* acts through the release of autolytic enzymes, and destroys tissues when applied to the skin (Fig. **3**) [66].

Antimicrobial peptides are one of the best examples of this type of anti-bacterial agent is the cationic peptides (AMPs), a stretch of +2 - 11 aminoacids and even more +34 aminoacids (a.a.) are promising and potential antibiotics that can interfere with microorganism virulence [67 - 69]. Cationic peptides can easily cause a leaky membrane due to their amphipathic nature and secondary structure. AMPs are considered one of the most promising antiinfective agents able to trigger host innate immune response [70 - 72]. Examples can be listed, colistin, melittin, indolicidin, risin, CAMA, defensins, protegrins, magainins, *etc* [67 - 69], which have been reported as bactericidal or haemolytic molecules (Fig. **3**) [73, 74].

Bacteriostatic Anti-Infective Agents

They are capable of inhibiting or limiting bacterial growth by blocking protein biosynthesis, DNA *i.e.,* drugs, extracted from natural sources or chemically synthesized, perform in a bacteriostatic mode of action against some variant colonies of *S. aureus. e.g.,* daunorubicin, ketoconazole, rifapentine and sitafloxacin [49, 50].

Drugs

Tetracycline derivatives, as well as sulphonamides, are bacteriostatic drugs. Tetracyclines have a high affinity to form chelates with polyvalent metallic cations such as iron (Fe^{3+}, Fe^{2+}), aluminum (Al^{3+}), magnesium (Mg^{2+}) and calcium (Ca^{2+}) [75], while sulphonamides inhibit folic acid metabolism pathway [76]. 4-aminosalicylic acid (PAS) (a second-line anti-TB drug) was initially used as a first-line anti-TB drug before the discovery of rifampicin and pyrazinamide. Although the mode of action of PAS is unclear, it is thought to act by inhibiting dihydrofolate reductase (DHFR) in the folate pathway of *M. tuberculosis* [77].

Aminoglycosides such as kanamycin and amikacin and the cyclic peptide, Capreomycin, act by protein synthesis inhibition [78]. Fluoroquinolones such as ciprofloxacin, levofloxacin, and moxifloxacin show anti-TB activity through the inhibition of DNA gyrase [79, 80]. Rifampin acts by inhibiting RNA synthesis through binding to the DNA-dependent RNA polymerase of *M. tuberculosis* [81]. Pyrazinamide is a prodrug that is activated in its acidic form by pyrazinamide of *M. tb* and inhibits mycobacterial growth [82].

Bacteriostatic Activity of Bacteria-derived Secondary Metabolites

Piericidin A and Glucopiericidin A are two potential inhibitors of the quórum sensing (QS) system produced by the *Streptomyces Xanthocidicus (S. xanthocidicus)* KPP01532 strain against plant pathogens (and applied for the control of potato soft rot caused by *erwinia carotovora* subsp. atroseptica [83].

Bacteriostatic Activity of Plant-derived Secondary Metabolites

Secondary metabolites that are plant-derived act by the inhibition of biofilms [84]; a different system of *M. tuberculosis* such as [85 - 87] the inhibition of virus replication, inhibition of viruses binding, and inhibition of DNA enzymes (Fig. **2**) [88, 89].

Phenols can act through interaction with sulfhydryl groups in microbial enzymes, leading to inhibition of those enzymes through non-specific protein interactions. Phenolic compounds (flavonoids, nonflavonoids, triterpenes, butyric actid cinnamic acid and thymol) are able to inhibit virulence factors such as enzymes and toxins and suppress the bacterial biofilm formation (Fig. **2**) [90].

Flavonoids are able to form a complex with cell wall components and consequently inhibit further adhesions and, therefore, limiting microbial growth. Flavan-3-ol, isofalvons and flavanoid compounds inhibit nucleic acid synthesis through the inhibition of topoisomerases and dihydrofolate reductases and alter cytoplasmic membrane function, (posibly by generating hydrogen peroxide) (Fig. **3**) [91]. Furthermore, flavonoids with antimycobacterial activity have the ability to inhibit proteasome inhibition and mycolic acid biosynthesis [85 - 87]. Other secondary metabolites with antimycobacterial activity are plant-derived from *Byttneria herbacea,* which have also exhibited a potential activity of inhibition of glutamine synthetase and have activity either in growing and/or dormant *Mycobacterium*. In a similar way, the herbal composition PHY906 consisting of *Scutellaria baicalensis, Ziziphus jujuba, Glycyrrhiza uralensis* and *Paeonia lactifloa* and extracts of aerial portions of *Leucas stelligera* contains di-terpenes and flavones that have antimycobacterial activity [85 - 87].

Phenolic rich fruit extracts or individual fruit-related PCs act against bacterial cells. Modifications occurring in the regulation of genes associated with certain virulence features in the microorganism include hydrophobicity, adhesión, motility, invasión, and inhibition of porins (integral membrane proteins) [92 - 94]. **Phenolic acids** like gallic, vanillic, syringic, p-coumaric, ellagic and protocatechuic acid are able to make changes in the fatty acid membrane composition to different ranges of concentration and thus, have the capacity to dampen bacterial spread dissemination of *S. aureus, E. coli* [16, 24 - 26]. **Epigallocatechin gallate** (EGCg) limits bacterial growth and invasión observed at suboptimal doses against species of *Staphylococcus* by the inhibition of the Tet(K) efflux pump. In addition, gallic acid is well known for antimicrobial and immunomodulating properties [94, 95].

Alkaloids are most of the secondary metabolites derived from alkaloids are able to inhibit the bacterial enzyme dihydrofolate reductase, thereby inhibiting nucleic acid synthesis [96, 97]. The alkaloid quinolones, is also able to inhibit key enzymes in the bacterial metabolism, while the alkaloid Agelasines, inhibits dioxygenase enzyme BCG 3185c, causing a disturbance in the bacterial homeostasis [98].

Volatile oils (EOS) obtained from different parts of a plant have the ability to interfere in bacterial physiological and biochemical processes during their development and multiplication. Cinnamon oil is amongst the most effective EOSs against foodborne pathogens. The effect of these EOSs depends on either Gram (+) (*S. aureus, S. pneumniae, M. tuberculosis, L. monocytogenes, C. diphteriae, C. perfringes*) or Gram (-) (*B. melintensis, B. aboruts, P. aeruginosa, N. gonorrhea, H. influenzae, H. pylori, V. cholerae, S. typhi, E. coli* enteropathogenic) (Fig. **1**), since the lipopolysaccharide (LPS) layer in gram-negative bacteria acts as a barrier for macromolecules and hydrophobic compounds such as those present in volatile oils (EOs) (Fig. **3**) [99].

Interestingly, these compounds have shown immunomodulatory effects of EO on the secretion of important cytokines in stimulated cell culture with LPS as well as in the inflammatory pathways such as nuclear factor-kappa light-chain-enhancer of activated B cells (NF-kB). At low concentrations, EOs can induce cytotoxic effects [99].

MECHANISM OF BACTERIAL RESISTANCE

1. Modification of protein targets of antibiotics.
2. Production of enzymes which can degrade or modify the antibiotic structure rendering unsuccessful and ineffective treatment.
3. The use of pumping systems to expel antibiotic molecules.

Modification of Protein Targets of Antibiotics

Resistance-modificative agents (RMAs) such as polyphenols and phenolic acids as well as other anti-infective agents, can be more plausible to develop using *in silico* EBSCO bioinformatic studies. Phenolic compounds can diminish antibiotic resistance of *S. aureus* clinical strains [101, 102]. The green tea (*Camellia sinensis*) rich in catechins has the capacity to reverse methicillin resistance in MRSA isolates at lower concentrations than those needed for the inhibition of bacterial growth [102]. Catechin has a modulatory effect on bacterial drug resistance. One mechanism of resistance that some charged molecules like antibiotics develop is the interaction on the cell surface, which reduces or decreases the interaction of cationic peptides with the bacterium. Among other mechanisms that lead to resistance to AMPs could be the decrease in the permeability toward the cells, secretion of proteases reléase of AMP degrading enzymes, downregulation of host responses, active efflux, and alteration of membrane physiology [103].

Production of Enzymes which can Degrade or Modify the Antibiotic Structure

MTb proteosome plays a crucial role in providing intrinsic resistance against deleterious effects of reactive nitrogen intermediate (RNI) such as nitric oxide (NO) and radical NO_2 that are produced by the inducible nitric oxide synthase (iNOs) in activated macrophages, all of which inflict nitrosative stress to *MTb*. NO may also combine with superoxide from bacterial metabolism to form peroxynitrite that inflicts oxydative damage to *MTB* [103, 104].

The intrinsic resistance can be attributed to cell wall permeability and system efflux pumps that mediate only selected solutes, be it hydrophilic or hydrophobic to enter into the bacteria and extracting foreign compounds out from the bacteria. Mutations in the chromosome in the gene encoding drugs target drug activating enzymes. This results in the alteration of the structure of the target proteins, hence reducing the susceptibility of the bacteria to a particular drug [105, 106].

The Use of the Pumping Systems to Expel Antibiotic Molecules

Regulatory genes controlling multidrug resistance by the expression of efflux pump and bacterial biofilm formation also show important roles in antibacterial resistance. Nowadays, several diverse strategies are being designed and employed against MDR. Among them, the new generation of antibiotics, combination therapy *via* natural antibacterial substances and also use of drug delivery systems represent important advances in the field [105].

HOW ENVIRONMENTAL STRESS IN BIOFILMS CONTRIBUTES TO THE BACTERIAL RESISTANCE MECHANISM

Biofilms formation by a microorganism is like a matrix composed of polysaccharides, proteins and extracellular released nucleic acids. One of the main functions of the bacterial biofilms is that they decrease the penetration of antimicrobial agents [100, 105]. *S. auresu* and *Staphylococci* and/*or S.* mutants can capture positively charged molecules through the extracellular polymeric biofilm matrix, but it can also concéntrate the bacterial enzymes which inactivate antibiotics. Biofilm formation can be viewed as a bacterial resistance mechanism and defense against several environmental stresses that can limit bacterial survival. Gradients of nutrients, metabolites, oxygen, pH, redox potential or antibiotics can penétrate the biofilm and cause the expression of an inducible resistance mechanism, increased mutability rate and bacterial adaptive phenotype changes [106]. These changes lead to metabolic suppression of bacteria, which causes increased ability to survive the exposure to antibiotics and an increasing rate of persistence cell formation. The epigallocatechin gallate (EGCg) inhibition of *S. aureus* biofilm formation at subinhibitory concentrations, has been shown to decrease slime layer production [106, 107].

HOW NATURE APPROACHES THE MICROBIAL RESISTANCE

The paucity of infections in wild plants supports the role of the innate defense system in plants. Most of the researchers focus on how the anti-infective agents (either anti-bacterial or antiviral) can target mainly bacterial resistance mechanism. A promising alternative *versus* antibiotics that has been proposed to able to overcome bacterial resistance mechanism, is the secondary metabolites derived from natural extracts. In addition, a therapy based on the combination of plant extracts, antibiotics and antimicrobial peptides can also be considered a suitable option [106 - 108]. Furthermore, phenols and phenolic acids could serve as good and potential candidates as natural anti-bacterial arsenals as well as good adjuvants of antibiotics. A clear example is the combination of:

(a) Phenols compounds such as catechols or resorcinols and pyrogallol, which showed a higher potent activity rather than individual compounds [2, 29] against a number of microbial complexes as causal agents of periodontitis. One complex (so-called "red complex") is comprised of Gram-negative bacteria (*Porphyromonas gingivalis, Treponema denticola, and Tannerella forsythia*) [109, 110]. The second complex consists of Gram-positive bacteria (*Peptostreptococcus micros. Eubacterium nodatu and Streptococcus constellatus*) [111, 112] as well as Gram-negative bacteria (*Campylobacter rectus, Campylobacter showae, and Campylobacter gracilis*). A third complex formed mostly of Gram positive bacteria *S. sanguis, S. oralis, S. mitis, S. gordonii* and *S. intermedius* (Figs. **1** and **2**) [112 - 114]. A fourth complex comprised of Gram-negative bacteria such as *Campylobacter concisus, Eikenella corrodens* and *Actinobacillus actinomycetemcomitans* serotype a [115 - 117] and a fifth complex consisted of *Veillonella parvula* and *Actinomyces odontolyticus* (*Actinomuces odontolycus*); *Aggregatibacter. Actinomycetemcomitans* serotype b, *Selenomonas noxia* and *Actinomyces naeslundii* genospecies 2 (*Actinomuces viscosus*) (Figs. **1** and **2**) [116 - 118].

(b) Pyrogallol-based compounds are more potent than others such as catechol or resorcinol, gallic acid and hydroxycinnamic acid (ferolic acid) to destroy bacterial cell wall of *S. aureus* (Gram positive bacteria); *E. coli* and *P. aeruginosa (*Gram negative bacteria*)* leading to leakage of cellular contents. These compounds have exerted strong activity against Gram (+) microorganisms (Figs. **1** and **3**) and some of them showed good synergism with antibiotics.

(c) Pentagalloylglucopyranose, combined with penicillin G, was active against methicillin-resistant *S. aureus*.

(d) The combination of epicatechin gallate and oxacillin reduced around 500 times the minimal inhibitory concentration by the addition of epicatechin gallate to the antibiotic (Figs. **1** and **3**) [119].

Antibiotics synergy is also an important strategy to control drug resistance by targeting more than one site of action which increases the bioavailability and/or modify the resistance mechanism induction [69, 89]. In the study on multidrug-resistant bacteria, antimicrobial peptides (colistin, melittin, indolicidin, risin, CAMA, defensins, protegrins, magainins, etc) with bactericidal activity that work throughout detergent-like mechanisms against *P. aeruginosa* [37, 82, 120 - 123], constitute one of the most promising alternatives against MDR bacteria. Another property that indolicidin (isolated from bovine neutrophils) possesses is the haemolytic activity. How the AMPs avoid the resistance developed by microbials is that its action is so fast that the bacteria do not get the chance to mutate or express resistance genes and/or prepare their defense [40 - 45, 103, 112].

CONCLUDING REMARKS

Plant-derived metabolites or compounds with antibacterial activity (leaves or roots) form healthy specimens; however, there is evidence that key components of plant defenses against phytopathogens are induced by infection. Plants respond to microbial attack through a highly coordinated repertoire of molecular, cellular and tissue-based defensive barriers to colonization and invasión. PCs that are fruit-derived can be explored for innovative therapies against pathogenic microorganisms in human, veterinary medicine, and agro-food industry. For the design and development of innovative therapies for medical use, anti-infective agents should be able to modulate some important virulence factors of bacteria, such as adhesivity, biofilm formation and the phenomenon of bacterial persistence.

As highlighted from medicine advances, antibiotics are considered one of the most important contributions against infectious diseases. The challenge of the natural products derived from diverse natural sources lies in the translation of research from *in vitro* to *in vivo* studies, and hence to human clinical trials that will lead to the development of new phytochemicals. Different programs have been proposed as alternatives or strategies to face multidrug-resistant viruses and bacteria (WHO). The first thing is the use of antimicrobial peptides that have a bactericidal action and a role as an immunomodulator of the innate host response. The use of natural products (secondary metabolites) in conjunction with antibiotics in an appropriate dose and route of administration and different targets might be a weapon to tackle microbial resistance mechanisms. Therefore, the knowledge and understanding of the mode of action of pathogens (bacterial or viral) concurrent with the advances in innovative technologies might allow the development of more effective and safe treatments in developed countries.

CONSENT FOR PUBLICATION

Not applicable.

CONFLICT OF INTEREST

The authors confirm that the content of this chapter have no conflict of interest.

ACKNOWLEDGEMENTS.

The authors are grateful for the financial support of SEP (PERFIL PRODEP 2019-2022 - GGGM) and CONACYT (FHM and GGGM).

REFERENCES

[1]   World Health Organization World Tuberculosis report World Health Organization(fecha de consulta (2012-2016) www.who.int/tb/publications/global_report/2008/pdf/annex3_amr.pdf

[2]   Zhang HM, Yaqin ZY. N Niluhol, Shen M, Kebebew E. Quantitative high-throughput drug screening identifies novel classes of drugs with anticancer activity in thyroid cancer cells: Opportunities for repurposing. J Clin Endocrinol Metab 2012; 97: 319-28.
[http://dx.doi.org/10.1210/jc.2011-2671]

[3]   Xu M, Lee EM, Wen Z, *et al*. Identification of small-molecule inhibitors of Zika virus infection and induced neural cell death *via* a drug repurposing screen. Nat Med 2016; 22(10): 1101-7.
[http://dx.doi.org/10.1038/nm.4184] [PMID: 27571349]

[4]   Feng J, Wang T, Shi W, *et al*. Identification of novel activity against *Borrelia burgdorferi* persisters using an FDA approved drug library. Emerg Microbes Infect 2014; 3(7): e49.
[PMID: 26038747]

[5]   Barrows NJ, Campos RK, Powell ST, *et al*. A Screen of fda-approved drugs for inhibitors of zika virus infection. Cell Host Microbe 2016; 20(2): 259-70.
[http://dx.doi.org/10.1016/j.chom.2016.07.004] [PMID: 27476412]

[6]   Johansen LM, DeWald LE, Shoemaker CJ, *et al*. A screen of approved drugs and molecular probes identifies therapeutics with anti-Ebola virus activity. Sci Transl Med 2015; 7(290): 290ra89.
[http://dx.doi.org/10.1126/scitranslmed.aaa5597] [PMID: 26041706]

[7]   He S, Lin B, Chu V, *et al*. Repurposing of the antihistamine chlorcyclizine and related compounds for treatment of hepatitis C virus infection. Sci Transl Med 2015; 7(282): 282ra49.
[http://dx.doi.org/10.1126/scitranslmed.3010286] [PMID: 25855495]

[8]   He S, Jain P, Lin B, *et al*. High-throughput screening, discovery, and optimization to develop a benzofuran class of hepatitis c virus inhibitors. ACS Comb Sci 2015; 17(10): 641-52.
[http://dx.doi.org/10.1021/acscombsci.5b00101] [PMID: 26332742]

[9]   Trombetta RP, Dunman PM, Schwarz EM, Kates SL, Awad HA-A. High-throughput screeing in approach to repurpose fda-approved drugs for bactericidal applications against *Staphylococcus aureus* small-colony variants. MSphere 2018; 3(5): 1-13.
[http://dx.doi.org/10.1128/mSphere.00422-18] [PMID: 30381352]

[10]   Menéndez-Arias L, Gago F. Antiviral agents: Structural basis of action and rational design. Subcell Biochem 2013; 68: 599-630.
[http://dx.doi.org/10.1007/978-94-007-6552-8_20] [PMID: 23737066]

[11]   Raju RM, Goldberg AL, Rubin EJ. Bacterial proteolytic complexes as therapeutic targets. Nat Rev Drug Discov 2012; 11(10): 777-89.
[http://dx.doi.org/10.1038/nrd3846] [PMID: 23023677]

[12]   Xue H, Jiang Y, Zhao H, *et al*. Characterization of composition and antifungal properties of leaf secondary metabolites from thirteen cultivars of *chrysanthemum morifolium* ramat. Molecules 2019; 24(23): 4202.
[http://dx.doi.org/10.3390/molecules24234202] [PMID: 31756889]

[13]   Kang HK, Seo CHH, Park Y. Marine peptides and their anti-infective activities. Mar Drugs (2915) 13(1): 618-54.
[http://dx.doi.org/10.3390/md13010618]

[14]   Bechinger B, Lohner K. Detergent-like actions of linear amphipathic cationic antimicrobial peptides. Biochim Biophys Acta 2006; 1758(9): 1529-39.
[http://dx.doi.org/10.1016/j.bbamem.2006.07.001] [PMID: 16928357]

[15]   Roy R, Tiwari M, Donelli G, Tiwari V. Strategies for combating bacterial biofilms: A focus on anti-biofilm agents and their mechanisms of action. Virulence 2018; 9(1): 522-54.
[http://dx.doi.org/10.1080/21505594.2017.1313372] [PMID: 28362216]

[16]   Campbell EA, Korzheva N, Mustaev A, *et al.* Structural mechanism for rifampicin inhibition of bacterial rna polymerase. Cell 2001; 104(6): 901-12.
[http://dx.doi.org/10.1016/S0092-8674(01)00286-0] [PMID: 11290327]

[17]   Paik S, Kim JK, Chung C, Jo EK. Autophagy: A new strategy for host-directed therapy of tuberculosis. Virulence 2019; 10(1): 448-59.
[http://dx.doi.org/10.1080/21505594.2018.1536598] [PMID: 30322337]

[18]   Chamni S, De-Eknamkul W. Recent progress and challenges in the discovery of new neuraminidase inhibitors. Expert Opin Ther Pat 2013; 23(4): 409-23.
[http://dx.doi.org/10.1517/13543776.2013.765861] [PMID: 23369206]

[19]   Wang S, Yao J, Zhou B, *et al.* Bacteriostatic effect of quercetin as an antibiotic alternative *in vivo* and its antibacterial mechanism *in vitro* . J Food Prot 2018; 81(1): 68-78.
[http://dx.doi.org/10.4315/0362-028X.JFP-17-214] [PMID: 29271686]

[20]   David J. Newman, Gordon M Cragg. natural products as sources of new drugs from 2014. J Nat Prod 2016; 79: 629-61.
[PMID: 26852623]

[21]   Lima MC, Paiva de Sousa C, Fernandez-Prada C, Harel J, Dubreuil JD, de Souza EL. A review of the current evidence of fruit phenolic compounds as potential antimicrobials against pathogenic bacteria. Microb Pathog 2019; 130: 259-70.
[http://dx.doi.org/10.1016/j.micpath.2019.03.025] [PMID: 30917922]

[22]   Aldulaimi OA. General overview of phenolics from plant to laboratory, good antibacterials or not. Pharmacogn Rev 2017; 11(22): 123-7.
[http://dx.doi.org/10.4103/phrev.phrev_43_16] [PMID: 28989246]

[23]   Cushnie TP, Lamb AJ. Recent advances in understanding the antibacterial properties of flavonoids. Int J Antimicrob Agents 2011; 38(2): 99-107.
[http://dx.doi.org/10.1016/j.ijantimicag.2011.02.014] [PMID: 21514796]

[24]   Farhadi F, Khameneh B, Iranshahi M, Iranshahy M. Antibacterial activity of flavonoids and their structure-activity relationship: An update review. Phytother Res 2019; 33(1): 13-40.
[http://dx.doi.org/10.1002/ptr.6208] [PMID: 30346068]

[25]   Kuroda T, Ogawa W. Search for novel antibacterial compounds and targets. Yakugaku Zasshi 2017; 137(4): 383-8.
[http://dx.doi.org/10.1248/yakushi.16-00235-3] [PMID: 28381710]

[26]   Mazlun MH, Sabran SF, Mohamed M, Abu Bakar MF, Abdullah Z. Phenolic compounds as promising drug candidates in tuberculosis therapy. Molecules 2019; 24(13): 1-16.
[http://dx.doi.org/10.3390/molecules24132449] [PMID: 31277371]

[27]   Lacaille-Dubois MA, Wagner H. New perspectives for natural triterpene glycosides as potential adjuvants. Phytomedicine 2017; 37: 49-57.
[http://dx.doi.org/10.1016/j.phymed.2017.10.019] [PMID: 29239784]

[28]   Miklasińska-Majdanik M, Kępa M, Wojtyczka RD, Idzik D, Wąsik TJ. Phenolic compounds diminish antibiotic resistance of *Staphylococcus aureus* clinical strains. Int J Environ Res Public Health 2018; 15(10): 2321-38.
[http://dx.doi.org/10.3390/ijerph15102321] [PMID: 30360435]

[29]   Zheng Y, Jiang X, Gao F, *et al.* Identification of plant-derived natural products as potential inhibitors of the *Mycobacterium tuberculosis* proteasome. BMC Complement Altern Med 2014; 14: 400.
[http://dx.doi.org/10.1186/1472-6882-14-400] [PMID: 25315519]

[30]   Baquero E, Quiñones W, Ribon W, Caldas ML. Effect of an oxadiazoline and a lignan on mycolic acid biosynthesis and ultrastructural changes of *Mycobacterium tuberculosis*. Tuberc Res Treat 2011; 1-6.
[PMID: 986409]

[31]   Fu JJ, Qin JJ, Zeng Q, Huang Y, Zhang WD, Jin HZ. Two new monoterpene alkaloid derivatives from the roots of Incarvillea arguta. Arch Pharm Res 2011; 34(2): 199-202.
[http://dx.doi.org/10.1007/s12272-011-0203-3] [PMID: 21380801]

[32]   Mahapatra DK, Bharti SK, Asati V. Chalcone scaffolds as anti-infective agents: Structural and molecular target perspectives. Eur J Med Chem 2015; 101: 496-524.
[http://dx.doi.org/10.1016/j.ejmech.2015.06.052] [PMID: 26188621]

[33]   Thawabteh A, Juma S, Bader M, *et al.* The biological activity of natural alkaloids against herbivores, cancerous cells and pathogens. Toxins (Basel) 2019; 11(11): 656.
[http://dx.doi.org/10.3390/toxins11110656] [PMID: 31717922]

[34]   Nina N, Quispe C, Jiménez-Aspee F, *et al.* Antibacterial activity, antioxidant effect and chemical composition of propolis from the región del Maule, Central Chile. Molecules 2015; 20(10): 18144-67.
[http://dx.doi.org/10.3390/molecules201018144] [PMID: 26457694]

[35]   Li H, Zhang WD, Zhang CH, *et al.* Chen. CHL. Bioavailabilty and pharmacokinetics of four active alkaloids of traditional chinese medicine yanhuanglian in rats following intravenous and oral administration. J Pharm Biomed Anal 2016; 41: 1342-6.
[http://dx.doi.org/10.1016/j.jpba.2006.03.029] [PMID: 16644173]

[36]   Grienke U, Mair CE, Kirchmair J, Schmidtke M, Rollinger JM. Discovery of bioactive natural products for the treatment of acute respiratory infections-an integrated approach. Planta Med 2018; 84(9-10): 684-95.
[http://dx.doi.org/10.1055/a-0590-5153] [PMID: 29554706]

[37]   Zakaryan H, Arabyan E, Oo A, Zandi K. Flavonoids: Promising natural compounds against viral infections. Arch Virol 2017; 162(9): 2539-51.
[http://dx.doi.org/10.1007/s00705-017-3417-y] [PMID: 28547385]

[38]   Mazzucco MB, Talarico LB, Vatansever S, *et al.* Antiviral activity of an N-allyl acridone against dengue virus. J Biomed Sci 2015; 22: 29.
[http://dx.doi.org/10.1186/s12929-015-0134-2] [PMID: 25908170]

[39]   Kumar D, Judge V, Narang R, *et al.* Benzylidene/2-chlorobenzylidene hydrazides: Synthesis, antimicrobial activity, QSAR studies and antiviral evaluation. Eur J Med Chem 2010; 45(7): 2806-16.
[http://dx.doi.org/10.1016/j.ejmech.2010.03.002] [PMID: 20347509]

[40]   Kothari V, Sharma S, Padia D. Recent research advances on *Chromobacterium violaceum*. Asian Pac J Trop Med 2017; 10(8): 744-52.
[http://dx.doi.org/10.1016/j.apjtm.2017.07.022] [PMID: 28942822]

[41]   Livermore DM, Warner M, Mushtaq S. Evaluation of the chromogenic Cica-beta-Test for detecting extended-spectrum, AmpC and metallo-beta-lactamases. J Antimicrob Chemother 2007; 60(6): 1375-9.
[http://dx.doi.org/10.1093/jac/dkm374] [PMID: 17913719]

[42]   Xue H, Jiang Y, Zhao H, *et al.* Characterization of composition and antifungal properties of leaf secondary metabolites from thirteen cultivars of *Chrysanthemum morifolium* ramat. Molecules 2019; 24(23): 4202.
[http://dx.doi.org/10.3390/molecules24234202] [PMID: 31756889]

[43]   Hou XM, Wang CY, Gerwick WH, Shao CL. Marine natural products as potential anti-tubercular agents. Eur J Med Chem 2019; 165(165): 273-92.
[http://dx.doi.org/10.1016/j.ejmech.2019.01.026] [PMID: 30685527]

[44]   Khan MT, Kaushik AC, Bhatti AI, *et al.* Marine natural products and drug resistance in latent tuberculosis. Mar Drugs 2019; 17(10): 1-13.
[http://dx.doi.org/10.3390/md17100549] [PMID: 31561525]

[45]   Ladram A, Nicolas P. Antimicrobial peptides from frog skin: biodiversity and therapeutic promises. Front Biosci 2016; 21: 1341-71.

[http://dx.doi.org/10.2741/4461] [PMID: 27100511]

[46] Patel S, Akhtar N. Antimicrobial peptides (AMPs): The quintessential 'offense and defense' molecules are more than antimicrobials. Biomed Pharmacother 2017; 95: 1276-83.
[http://dx.doi.org/10.1016/j.biopha.2017.09.042] [PMID: 28938518]

[47] Sumi CD, Yang BW, Yeo IC, Hahm YT. Antimicrobial peptides of the genus Bacillus: a new era for antibiotics. Can J Microbiol 2015; 61(2): 93-103.
[http://dx.doi.org/10.1139/cjm-2014-0613] [PMID: 25629960]

[48] Klöckner A, Bühl H, Viollier P, Henrichfreise B. Deconstructing the chlamydial cell wall. Curr Top Microbiol Immunol 2018; 412: 1-33.
[PMID: 27726004]

[49] Swietnicki W, Czarny A, Urbanska N, Drab M. Identification of small molecule compounds active against *Staphylococcus aureus* and Proteus mirabilis. Biochem Biophys Res Commun 2018; 506(4): 1047-51.
[http://dx.doi.org/10.1016/j.bbrc.2018.10.189] [PMID: 30409430]

[50] Garcia LG, Lemaire S, Kahl BC, *et al.* Antibiotic activity against small-colony variants of *Staphylococcus aureus*: review of *In Vitro*, animal and clinical data. J Antimicrob Chemother 2013; 68(7): 1455-64.
[http://dx.doi.org/10.1093/jac/dkt072] [PMID: 23485724]

[51] Schubert K, Sieger B, Meyer F, *et al.* The antituberculosis drug ethambutol selectively block aplical growth in CMN group bacteria. MBio 2017; 8(1): 1-21.
[http://dx.doi.org/10.1128/mBio.02213-16] [PMID: 28174310]

[52] Vale N, Gomes P, Santos HA. Metabolism of the antituberculosis drug ethionamide. Curr Drug Metab 2013; 14(1): 151-8.
[http://dx.doi.org/10.2174/138920013804545151] [PMID: 23215813]

[53] Thee S, Garcia-Prats AJ, Donald PR, Hesseling AC, Schaaf HS. A review of the use of ethionamide and prothionamide in childhood tuberculosis. Tuberculosis (Edinb) 2016; 97: 126-36.
[http://dx.doi.org/10.1016/j.tube.2015.09.007] [PMID: 26586647]

[54] Momin MAM, Sinha S, Tucker IG, Das SC. Carrier-free combination dry powder inhaler formulation of ethionamide and moxifloxacin for treating drug-resistant tuberculosis. Drug Dev Ind Pharm 2019; 45(8): 1321-31.
[http://dx.doi.org/10.1080/03639045.2019.1609494] [PMID: 31014129]

[55] George G. Zhanel, Christopher D Lawson, Heather Adam, Frank Schweizer, Sheryl Zelenitsky, Philippe R S Lagacé-Wiens, Andrew Denisuik, Ethan Rubinstein, Alfred S Gin, Daryl J Hoban, Joseph P Lynch 3rd, James A Karlowsky. Ceftazidime-avibactam: A Novel Cephalosporin/β-Lactamase Inhibitor Combination. Drugs 2013; 73: 159-77.

[56] Evan J. Zasowski, Jeffrey M Rybak, Michael J Rybak. The β-Lactams Strike Back: Ceftazidime-Avibactam. Pharmacotherapy 2015; 35: 755-70.
[http://dx.doi.org/10.1002/phar.1622]

[57] Lei B, Wei CJ, Tu SC. Action mechanism of antitubercular isoniazid. Activation by *Mycobacterium tuberculosis* KatG, isolation, and characterization of inha inhibitor. J Biol Chem 2000; 275(4): 2520-6.
[http://dx.doi.org/10.1074/jbc.275.4.2520] [PMID: 10644708]

[58] Vosátka R, Krátký M, Švarcová M, *et al.* New lipophilic isoniazid derivatives and their 1,3,4-oxadiazole analogues: Synthesis, antimycobacterial activity and investigation of their mechanism of action. Eur J Med Chem 2018; 151: 824-35.
[http://dx.doi.org/10.1016/j.ejmech.2018.04.017] [PMID: 29679902]

[59] Khameneh B, Iranshahy M, Soheili V, Fazly Bazzaz BS. Review on plant antimicrobials: a mechanistic viewpoint. Antimicrob Resist Infect Control 2019; 8: 118.
[http://dx.doi.org/10.1186/s13756-019-0559-6] [PMID: 31346459]

[60] Sadowska B, Laskowski D, Bernat P, *et al*. Molecular mechanisms of *Leonurus cardiaca* L. extract activity in prevention of staphylococcal endocarditis-study on *in vitro* and *ex vivo* models. Molecules 2019; 24(18): 1-15.
[http://dx.doi.org/10.3390/molecules24183318] [PMID: 31547303]

[61] Marín L. MIguelez EM, Villar CL, Lombó F. Bioavailability of dietary polyphenols and gut microbiota metabolism: Antimicrobial properties. BioMed Res Int 2015; 2015: 1-18.
[http://dx.doi.org/10.1155/2015/905215]

[62] Agrawal M. Natural polyphenols based new therapeutic avenues for advanced biomedical applications. Drug Metab Rev 2015; 47(4): 420-30.
[http://dx.doi.org/10.3109/03602532.2015.1102933] [PMID: 26526493]

[63] Smułek W, Zdarta A, Pacholak A, *et al*. Saponaria officinalis L. extract: Surface active properties and impact on environmental bacterial strains. Colloids Surf B Biointerfaces 2017; 150: 209-15.
[http://dx.doi.org/10.1016/j.colsurfb.2016.11.035] [PMID: 27918965]

[64] Sewlikar S, D'Souza DH. antimicrobial effects of quillaja saponaria extract against *Escherichia coli* O157:H7 and the emerging non-O157 shiga toxin-producing *E. coli*. J Food Sci 2017; 82(5): 1171-7.
[http://dx.doi.org/10.1111/1750-3841.13697] [PMID: 28452110]

[65] Nicol M, Mlouka MAB, Berthe T, *et al*. Anti-persister activity of squalamine against Acinetobacter baumannii. Int J Antimicrob Agents 2019; 53(3): 337-42.
[http://dx.doi.org/10.1016/j.ijantimicag.2018.11.004] [PMID: 30423343]

[66] Och A, Zalewski D, Komsta L, Kołodziej P, Kocki J, Bogucka-Kocka A. Cytotoxic and proapoptotic activity of sanguinarine, berberine, and extracts of *Chelidonium majus* l. and berberis thunbergii DC. Toward hematopoietic cancer cell lines. Toxins 2019; 11: 1-19. 635

[67] Kang HK, Kim C, Seo CH, Park Y. The therapeutic applications of antimicrobial peptides (AMPs): a patent review. J Microbiol 2017; 55(1): 1-12.
[http://dx.doi.org/10.1007/s12275-017-6452-1] [PMID: 28035594]

[68] Döşler S. Antimicrobial peptides: Coming to the end of antibiotic era, the most promising agents. Istanbul J Pharm 2017; 47(2): 72-6.
[http://dx.doi.org/10.5152/IstanbulJPharm.2017.0012]

[69] Rončević T, Puizina J, Tossi A. Antimicrobial peptides as anti-infective agents in pre-post-antibiotic era? Int J Mol Sci 2019; 20(22): E5713.
[http://dx.doi.org/10.3390/ijms20225713] [PMID: 31739573]

[70] Wilmes M, Sahl HG. Defensin-based anti-infective strategies. Int J Med Microbiol 2014; 304(1): 93-9.
[http://dx.doi.org/10.1016/j.ijmm.2013.08.007] [PMID: 24119539]

[71] Ageitos JM, Sánchez-Pérez A, Calo-Mata P, Villa TG. Antimicrobial peptides (AMPs): Ancient compounds that represent novel weapons in the fight against bacteria. Biochem Pharmacol 2017; 133: 117-38.
[http://dx.doi.org/10.1016/j.bcp.2016.09.018] [PMID: 27663838]

[72] Verdon J, Falge M, Maier E, *et al*. Detergent-like activity and alpha-helical structure of warnericin RK, an anti-Legionella peptide. Biophys J 2009; 97(7): 1933-40.
[http://dx.doi.org/10.1016/j.bpj.2009.06.053] [PMID: 19804724]

[73] Lee J, Lee DG. Antimicrobial peptides (AMPs) with dual mechanisms: Membrane disruption and apoptosis. J Microbiol Biotechnol 2015; 25(6): 759-64.
[http://dx.doi.org/10.4014/jmb.1411.11058] [PMID: 25537721]

[74] Wilmes M, Sahl HG. Determination of bacterial membrane impairment by antimicrobial agents. Methods Mol Biol 2017; 1520: 133-43.
[http://dx.doi.org/10.1007/978-1-4939-6634-9_8] [PMID: 27873250]

[75] Alikhan A, Kurek L, Feldman SR. The role of tetracyclines in rosacea. Am J Clin Dermatol 2010;

11(2): 79-87.
[http://dx.doi.org/10.2165/11530200-000000000-00000] [PMID: 20141228]

[76] Jain P, Saravanan C, Singh SK. Sulphonamides: Deserving class as MMP inhibitors? Eur J Med Chem 2013; 60: 89-100.
[http://dx.doi.org/10.1016/j.ejmech.2012.10.016] [PMID: 23287054]

[77] Marverti G, Ligabue A, Lombardi P, Ferrari S, Monti MG, Frassineti C. Maria paola costi modulation of the expression of folate cycle enzymes and polyamine metabolism by berberine in cisplatin-sensitive and -resistant 663 human ovarian cancer cells. Int J Oncol 2013; 43: 1269-80.
[http://dx.doi.org/10.3892/ijo.2013.2045] [PMID: 23903781]

[78] Dijkstra JA, van der Laan T, Akkerman OW, *et al. In Vitro* susceptibility of *Mycobacterium tuberculosis* to amikacin, kanamycin, and capreomycin. Antimicrob Agents Chemother 2018; 62(3): 62.
[http://dx.doi.org/10.1128/AAC.01724-17] [PMID: 29311078]

[79] Kim Hyun-Joo, Seol Min-Jeong, Park Hee-Soo, *et al.* Antimicrobial activity of DW-224a, a new fluoroquinolone, against streptococcus pneumoniae. J Antimicrob Chemother 2006; 57: 1256-8.
[http://dx.doi.org/10.1093/jac/dkl144]

[80] Durcik M, Lovison D, Skok Ž, *et al.* New N-phenylpyrrolamide DNA gyrase B inhibitors: Optimization of efficacy and antibacterial activity. Eur J Med Chem 2018; 154: 117-32.
[http://dx.doi.org/10.1016/j.ejmech.2018.05.011] [PMID: 29778894]

[81] Peek J, Lilic M, Montiel D, *et al.* Rifamycin congeners kanglemycins are active against 681 rifampicin-resistant bacteria *via* a distinct mechanism. Nat Commun 2018; 9: 4147.
[http://dx.doi.org/10.1038/s41467-018-06587-2] [PMID: 30297823]

[82] Lamont EA, Baughn AD. Impact of the host environment on the antitubercular action of pyrazinamide. EBioMedicine 2019; 49: 374-80.
[http://dx.doi.org/10.1016/j.ebiom.2019.10.014] [PMID: 31669220]

[83] Kang JE, Han JW, Jeon BJ, Kim BS. Efficacies of quorum sensing inhibitors, piericidin A and glucopiericidin A, produced by Streptomyces xanthocidicus KPP01532 for the control of potato soft rot caused by Erwinia carotovora subsp. atroseptica. Microbiol Res 2016; 184: 32-41.
[http://dx.doi.org/10.1016/j.micres.2015.12.005] [PMID: 26856451]

[84] Slobodníková L, Fialová S, Rendeková K, Kováč J, Mučaji P. Antibiofilm activity of plant polyphenols. Molecules 2016; 21(12): 1717-27.
[http://dx.doi.org/10.3390/molecules21121717] [PMID: 27983597]

[85] Lee H, Suh JW. Anti-tuberculosis lead molecules from natural products targeting *Mycobacterium tuberculosis* ClpC1. J Ind Microbiol Biotechnol 2016; 43: 12.83-205.

[86] Vasudevan D, Rao SP, Noble CG. Structural basis of mycobacterial inhibition by cyclomarin A. J Biol Chem 2013; 288(43): 30883-91.
[http://dx.doi.org/10.1074/jbc.M113.493767] [PMID: 24022489]

[87] Sasikumar K. Antimycobacterial potentials of quercetin and rutin against *Mycobacterium tuberculosis* H37Rv. Biotech 2018; 8: 1-6.

[88] Pendergrass HA, May AE. Natural product type III secretion system inhibitors. Antibiotics (Basel) 2019; 8(4): 1-14.
[http://dx.doi.org/10.3390/antibiotics8040162] [PMID: 31554164]

[89] Müller B, Kräusslich HG. Antiviral strategies. Handb Exp Pharmacol 2009; 189(189): 1-24.
[PMID: 19048195]

[90] Chen X, Mukwaya E, Wong MS, Zhang Y. A systematic review on biological activities of prenylated flavonoids. Pharm Biol 2014; 52(5): 655-60.
[http://dx.doi.org/10.3109/13880209.2013.853809] [PMID: 24256182]

[91] Euba B, López-López N, Rodríguez-Arce I, *et al.* Resveratrol therapeutics combines both antimicrobial and immunomodulatory properties against respiratory infection by nontypeable Haemophilus influenzae. Sci Rep 2017; 7(1): 12860-7.
[http://dx.doi.org/10.1038/s41598-017-13034-7] [PMID: 29038519]

[92] Daglia M, Di Lorenzo A, Nabavi SF, Talas ZS, Nabavi SM. Polyphenols: well beyond the antioxidant capacity: gallic acid and related compounds as neuroprotective agents: you are what you eat! Curr Pharm Biotechnol 2014; 15(4): 362-72.
[http://dx.doi.org/10.2174/138920101504140825120737] [PMID: 24938889]

[93] Lu Z, Nie G, Belton PS, Tang H, Zhao B. Structure-activity relationship analysis of antioxidant ability and neuroprotective effect of gallic acid derivatives. Neurochem Int 2006; 48(4): 263-74.
[http://dx.doi.org/10.1016/j.neuint.2005.10.010] [PMID: 16343693]

[94] Lu J, Wang Z, Ren M, *et al.* Antibacterial effect of gallic acid against aeromonas hydrophila and aeromonas sobria through damaging membrane integrity. Curr Pharm Biotechnol 2016; 17(13): 1153-8.
[http://dx.doi.org/10.2174/1389201017666161022235759] [PMID: 27774889]

[95] Choubey S, Varughese LR, Kumar V, Beniwal V. Medicinal importance of gallic acid and its ester derivatives: a patent review. Pharm Pat Anal 2015; 4(4): 305-15.
[http://dx.doi.org/10.4155/ppa.15.14] [PMID: 26174568]

[96] Pacholak A, Simlat J, Zgoła-Grześkowiak A, Kaczorek E. Biodegradation of clotrimazole and modification of cell properties after metabolic stress and upon addition of saponins. Ecotoxicol Environ Saf 2018; 161: 676-82.
[http://dx.doi.org/10.1016/j.ecoenv.2018.06.050] [PMID: 29935432]

[97] Shao B, Liu Z, Zhong H, *et al.* Effects of rhamnolipids on microorganism characteristics and applications in composting: A review. Microbiol Res 2017; 200: 33-44.
[http://dx.doi.org/10.1016/j.micres.2017.04.005] [PMID: 28527762]

[98] Hertiani T, Edrada-Ebel R, Ortlepp S, *et al.* From anti-fouling to biofilm inhibition: new cytotoxic secondary metabolites from two Indonesian Agelas sponges. Bioorg Med Chem 2010; 18(3): 1297-311.
[http://dx.doi.org/10.1016/j.bmc.2009.12.028] [PMID: 20061160]

[99] Valdivieso-Ugarte M, Gomez-Llorente C, Plaza-Díaz J, Gil Á. Antimicrobial, antioxidant, and immunomodulatory properties of essential oils: a systematic review. Nutrients 2019; 11(11): 1-29.
[http://dx.doi.org/10.3390/nu11112786] [PMID: 31731683]

[100] Panesso D, Planet PJ, Diaz L, *et al.* Methicillin-susceptible, vancomycin-resistant *Staphylococcus aureus*, Brazil. Emerg Infect Dis 2015; 21(10): 1844-8.
[http://dx.doi.org/10.3201/eid2110.141914] [PMID: 26402569]

[101] Kong C, Neoh HM, Nathan S. Targeting *Staphylococcus aureus* toxins: A potential form of anti-virulence therapy. Toxins (Basel) 2016; 8(3): 1-21.
[http://dx.doi.org/10.3390/toxins8030072] [PMID: 26999200]

[102] Hanif E, Hassan SA. Evaluation of antibiotic resistance pattern in clinical isolates of *Staphylococcus aureus*. Pak J Pharm Sci 2019; 32(3 (Supplementary)): 1219-23.
[PMID: 31303594]

[103] Sato T, Kawamura M, Furukawa E, Fujimura S. Screening method for trimethoprim/sulfamethoxazole-resistant small colony variants of *Staphylococcus aureus*. J Glob Antimicrob Resist 2018; 15: 1-5.
[http://dx.doi.org/10.1016/j.jgar.2018.05.008] [PMID: 29857058]

[104] Prasanth MI, Sivamaruthi BS, Chaiyasut C, Tencomnao T. A Review of the role of green tea (*Camellia sinensis*) in antiphotoaging, stress resistance, neuroprotection, and autophagy. Nutrients 2019; 11(2): 1-24.

[http://dx.doi.org/10.3390/nu11020474] [PMID: 30813433]

[105] Khameneh B, Diab R, Ghazvini K, Fazly Bazzaz BS, Bazzaz F. Breakthroughs in bacterial resistance mechanisms and the potential ways to combat them. Microb Pathog 2016; 95: 32-42.
[http://dx.doi.org/10.1016/j.micpath.2016.02.009] [PMID: 26911646]

[106] Sousa V, Luís Â, Oleastro M, Domingues F, Ferreira S. Polyphenols as resistance modulators in Arcobacter butzleri. Folia Microbiol (Praha) 2019; 64(4): 547-54.
[http://dx.doi.org/10.1007/s12223-019-00678-3] [PMID: 30637574]

[107] Stavri M, Paton A, Skelton BW, Gibbons S. Antibacterial diterpenes from Plectranthus ernstii. J Nat Prod 2009; 72(6): 1191-4.
[http://dx.doi.org/10.1021/np800581s] [PMID: 19445517]

[108] Sharma S, Hameed S, Fatima Z. Natural compounds for overcoming multidrug resistance in mycobacteria. Recent Pat Biotechnol 2016; 10(2): 167-74.
[http://dx.doi.org/10.2174/1872208310666160919122629] [PMID: 27652611]

[109] Socransky SS, Haffajee AD, Cugini MA, Smith C, Kent RL Jr. Microbial complexes in subgingival plaque. J Clin Periodontol 1998; 25(2): 134-44.
[http://dx.doi.org/10.1111/j.1600-051X.1998.tb02419.x] [PMID: 9495612]

[110] Clais S, Boulet G, Kerstens M, *et al.* Importance of biofilm formation and dipeptidyl peptidase IV for the pathogenicity of clinical Porphyromonas gingivalis isolates. Pathog Dis 2014; 70(3): 408-13.
[http://dx.doi.org/10.1111/2049-632X.12156] [PMID: 24532232]

[111] Bodet C, Chandad F, Grenier D. Pathogenic potential of *Porphyromonas gingivalis*, Treponema denticola and Tannerella forsythia, the red bacterial complex associated with periodontitis. Pathol Biol (Paris) 2007; 55(3-4): 154-62.
[http://dx.doi.org/10.1016/j.patbio.2006.07.045] [PMID: 17049750]

[112] Severin AI, Kokeguchi S, Kato K. Chemical composition of *Eubacterium nodatum* cell wall peptidoglycan. Arch Microbiol 1989; 151(4): 353-8.
[http://dx.doi.org/10.1007/BF00406564] [PMID: 2742451]

[113] Jakubovics NS, Gill SR, Iobst SE, Vickerman MM, Kolenbrander PE. Regulation of gene expression in a mixed-genus community: stabilized arginine biosynthesis in *Streptococcus gordonii* by coaggregation with *Actinomyces naeslundii*. J Bacteriol 2008; 190(10): 3646-57.
[http://dx.doi.org/10.1128/JB.00088-08] [PMID: 18359813]

[114] Kim AR, Ahn KB, Kim HY, *et al. Streptococcus gordonii* lipoproteins induce IL-8 in human periodontal ligament cells. Mol Immunol 2017; 91: 218-24.
[http://dx.doi.org/10.1016/j.molimm.2017.09.009] [PMID: 28963931]

[115] Im J, Baik JE, Kim KW, *et al. Enterococcus faecalis* lipoteichoic acid suppresses Aggregatibacter actinomycetemcomitans lipopolysaccharide-induced IL-8 expression in human periodontal ligament cells. Int Immunol 2015; 27(8): 381-91.
[http://dx.doi.org/10.1093/intimm/dxv016] [PMID: 25840438]

[116] Cheng YA, C Chen. Integration and expression of the aggregatibacter actinomycetemcomitans catalase gene in aggregatibacter aphrophilus. Arch Oral Biol 2018; 86: 116-22.

[117] Uchida-Fujii E, Niwa H, Kinoshita Y, Nukada T. Actinobacillus species isolated from Japanese Thoroughbred racehorses in the last two decades. J Vet Med Sci 2019; 81(9): 1234-7.
[http://dx.doi.org/10.1292/jvms.19-0192] [PMID: 31292334]

[118] Takiguchi Y, Terano T, Hirai A. Lung abscess caused by Actinomyces odontolyticus. Intern Med 2003; 42(8): 723-5.
[http://dx.doi.org/10.2169/internalmedicine.42.723] [PMID: 12924500]

[119] Gandhi NR, Nunn P, Dheda K, *et al.* Multidrug-resistant and extensively drug-resistant tuberculosis: a threat to global control of tuberculosis. Lancet 2010; 375(9728): 1830-43.
[http://dx.doi.org/10.1016/S0140-6736(10)60410-2] [PMID: 20488523]

[120] Christaki E, Marcou M, Tofarides A. Antimicrobial resistance in bacteria: mechanisms, evolution, and persistence. J Mol Evol 2020; 88(1): 26-40.
[http://dx.doi.org/10.1007/s00239-019-09914-3] [PMID: 31659373]

[121] Gilabert-Oriol R, Thakur M, Haussmann K, *et al.* Saponins from *Saponaria officinalis* L. augment the efficacy of a rituximab-immunotoxin. Planta Med 2016; 82(18): 1525-31.
[http://dx.doi.org/10.1055/s-0042-110495] [PMID: 27392242]

[122] Sbaraglini ML, Talevi A. Hybrid compounds as anti-infective agents. Curr Top Med Chem 2017; 17(9): 1080-95.
[http://dx.doi.org/10.2174/1568026616666160927160912] [PMID: 27697047]

[123] Bechinger B, Gorr SU. Antimicrobial peptides: mechanisms of action and resistance. J Dent Res 2017; 96(3): 254-60.
[http://dx.doi.org/10.1177/0022034516679973] [PMID: 27872334]

CHAPTER 2

Natural Products with Antimicrobial Activity for *Mycobacterium tuberculosis*

Silvia Guzmán-Beltrán*, Fernando Hernández-Sánchez and Omar M. Barrientos

Departamento de Investigación en Microbiología, Instituto Nacional de Enfermedades Respiratorias Ismael Cosío Villegas, CDMX, Mexico

Abstract: Tuberculosis (TB) is an infectious disease caused by *Mycobacterium tuberculosis*. TB is one of the top ten causes of death in the world and it is highly prevalent, characterized by the constant occurrence of drug-resistant cases, and confounded by the incidence of respiratory diseases caused by nontuberculous mycobacteria (NTM). The anti-TB drugs commonly used are insufficient and have multiple adverse effects. Therefore, a new strategy to eradicate this infectious disease is required. The implementation of new anti-TB drugs together with host-directed therapy (HDT) can decrease the duration of treatment and improve the TB patients' health. It is proposed that natural products are an enormous source of bioactive compounds to treat TB. They can be new anti-TB drugs or agents for HDT.

Keywords: Allicin, Antimycobacterial compounds, Baicalin, α-Mangostin, Host-Directed Therapy (HDT), Nordihydroguaiaretic acid, Pasakbumin A, Tuberculous and nontuberculous mycobacteria, (10-15) Tuberculosis.

INTRODUCTION

TB has become a global health problem. It is estimated that one-third of the population in the world is infected with latent *M. tuberculosis,* and only 10% of infected individuals develop an active disease [1]. The TB-patients require long-term antibiotic treatment (6–12 months), and patient non-compliance with the complete therapeutic regime could lead to the emergence of multi- and extensively-drug resistant *M. tuberculosis* strains (MDR and XDR) [2]. MDR and XDR have already become a global health threat requiring extended treatment lengths, and there are increasing numbers of resistant TB cases, coupled with an increase of NTM lung infection cases [3]. There are 10 drugs that are currently

* **Corresponding author Silvia Guzmán-Beltrán:** Departamento de Investigación en Microbiología, Instituto Nacional de Enfermedades Respiratorias Ismael Cosío Villegas, CDMX, Mexico; Tel: 548717005117; E-mail: sguzman@iner.gob.mx

approved for treating TB [4]. The first-line anti-TB drugs are isoniazid (INH), ethambutol (EMB), pyrazinamide (PZA), and rifampicin (RIF). The first three anti-TB drugs are synthetic, while RIF is a semi-synthetic compound, derived from chemical modifications of the rifamycin B, the natural metabolites of *Amycolatopsis mediterranei*, and a soil bacterium [5]. There have been a few anti-TB agents under preclinical and clinical evaluations, and, probably, a combination regimen containing various new drugs with different effects that kill bacteria, leads to the design of successful drug regimens for TB treatment. Most of the promising anti-TB drug candidates in preclinical and clinical trials are synthetic compounds, with a limited spectrum of antimicrobial activity [6]. Additional alternatives are required to treat TB. Host-directed therapy (HDT) is a new strategy that involves directly targeting host factors rather than pathogen components [7]. The ideal HDT is to generate an immune response that promotes the antimicrobial mechanisms in the host cells and decreases the exacerbated inflammation caused during infection without consequences for the host [8]. In the present report, several natural compounds able to directly kill mycobacteria and enhance the immune response are described. These promising compounds could be an HDT alternative to treat TB.

Tuberculosis

TB is one of the major causes of health problems worldwide. According to the World Health Organization, it is estimated that approximately 10 million are affected by this infectious disease and 1.5 million people died in 2018 because of it [9]. *M. tuberculosis* is the causative agent of TB that can spread from person to person through microscopic droplets. The common site of TB infection is the lung (pulmonary TB), but it can also transmit to other parts of the body causing tuberculous meningitis, osteoarticular tuberculosis, and miliary tuberculosis [10]. In recent years, treatments currently available against TB have become inefficient due to the emergence of MDR and XDR strains [9]. Several mechanisms are involved in the development of these resistant TB forms, such as overexpression of drug efflux pumps, alteration in membrane permeability, modification of drug, and alteration of target site [11]. In addition, the frequency of pulmonary disease caused by NTM has increased and most NTM are resistant to different anti-TB drugs.

In the last decade, there has been a renewed focus on the development of drugs to treat TB, and several compounds are being evaluated in clinical trials. While new drugs in development may appear promising, their efficacy and safety for use in humans remain to be validated, which requires cost and time [12]. The current anti-TB drugs are very expensive and cause adverse side effects on the human body and, in certain disease conditions, are inefficient. Therefore, it is necessary to develop novel, effective, and affordable anti-TB drugs [9, 13].

Potential Actions of Natural Compound as Antituberculosis Agents

Nature has been a major source of compounds used in traditional and modern medicine and plants and microbes provide a wide diversity of bioactive molecules. Natural compounds are a better alternative with possibly minor side effects used currently [14]. To evaluate the potential of molecules from natural products, it is fundamental to consider their mode of action (Fig. **1**). For example, compounds should be able to inhibit the mycobacterial envelope. They should inhibit the synthesis of mycolic acids, a specific component of *Mycobacterium*, located at the outer layer of the cell wall, another target is the peptidoglycan synthesis, a principal constituent of the bacterial wall. DNA replication inhibition, DNA gyrase inhibition, and may arrest DNA synthesis and bacterial replication. Transcription and translation inhibition, RNA polymerase inhibition or blocking ribosomes function should also be considered. Other mechanisms are blocking the membrane potential like the loss of proton motive force or by inhibition of ATP synthesis [5]. And the last mechanism efficient is the generation of reactive nitrogen and oxygen species (RNOS), as they provoke damage to macromolecules and then bacterial death [6].

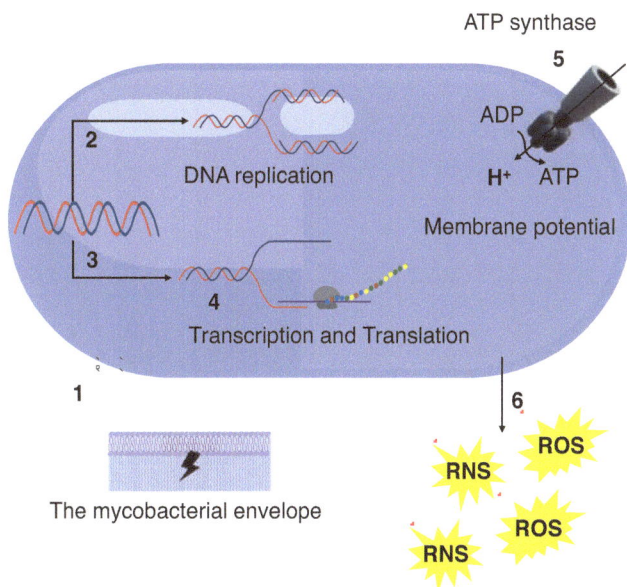

Fig. (1). Mode of action of diverse antituberculosis natural compounds. The compounds able to inhibit: the mycobacterial envelope (**1**), DNA replication (**2**), transcription (**3**), translation (**4**), and membrane potential (**5**). ATP, Adenosine triphosphate; ADP, adenosine diphosphate and H^+, hydrogen ion and production of reactive oxygen species (ROS) and reactive nitrogen species (RNS) (**6**).

Action Against Mycobacterial Cell Surface

The most widely known mode of action of antibacterial agents is the rupture of the cell wall and membrane integrity. Diverse natural compounds affect the peptidoglycan or cell wall lipid biosynthesis: these are the extracts from *Hypericum acmosepalum* and *Warburgia salutaris,* respectively [15, 16]. The *H. acmosepalum* extract inhibits a Mur synthetase (MurE) responsible for the ligation of meso-diaminopimelic acid to the soluble muropeptide, required for the peptidoglycan cross-linking [17]; while in the second, *W. salutaris* extract hampers the activity of an arylamine N-acetyltransferase (NAT), essential for the synthesis of mycolic acids [18]. Other inhibitor extracts of mycobacterial cell wall include *Toxicodendron vernicifluum, Dalbergia odorifera, Camelia sinensis, and Piper nigrum,* among others. Novel compounds that inhibit the same enzymes are (S)-leucoxine and psoromic acid. The first is a benzylisoquinoline, isolated from the Lauraceae tree *Rhodostemonodaphne crenaticupula,* which inhibits MurE. It seems that the key structural motif in (S)-leucoxine is the presence of dissimilar pairs of electrostatically positive patches, caused by the nitrogen atoms and the relative spatial closeness of the methylenedioxy groups. And, the halogens in position 5 of the isoquinoline nucleus increases the enzyme inhibition [19]. The second is a polyphenol isolated from the lichen *Rhizoplaca melanophthalma* [20]. Psoromic acid blocks two critical enzymes UDP-galactopyranose mutase (UGM) and NAT. Furthermore, using molecular docking and structure-activity relationship studies, a molecular interaction of psoromic acid with the active sites of UGM and NAT is observed [21].

Action Against Mycobacterial Nucleic Acids Synthesis

Bacterial genome replication is another attractive target of antibacterial agents. Khusenic acid, isolated from *Vetiveria zizanoides,* is sesquiterpene active against MDR strains, *M. smegmatis,* and shows better bactericidal activity on *M. tuberculosis* H37Rv than nalidixic acid. In an *in silico* analysis, khusenic acid binded with both subunits of DNA gyrase, because it exhibits similar binding affinity with subunits A (2Y3P) and subunit B (1EI1). Furthermore, it is suggested that the antimycobacterial activity may be due to the presence of (+) zizaene skeleton and acidic group [22]. But, more studies about its potential in humans that evaluate its toxicity are necessary.

Chebulinic acid is a phenolic compound obtained from *Terminalia chebula.* An *in silico* analysis predicted its' DNA gyrase inhibitory properties. Chebulinic acid may change the shape of the enzyme, increase the distance from catalytic tyrosine residue at 129 positions to DNA phosphate and bind at DNA attaching site of enzyme creating steric hindrance, leading to the inhibition and consequent failure in DNA replication, and provoking mycobacterial death [23].

Another potential compound is a coumarin, calanolide A, it is an antiviral against HIV and active against replicative and non-replicative mycobacteria [24]. Calanolide A is obtained from *Calophyllum lanigerum*, and binds to viral reverse transcriptase. However, this compound halts replication, transcription, and protein synthesis in *Mycobacterium*, but its exact action mechanism has not been elucidated [25]. Calanolide A is active against rifampicin-resistant strains suggesting that both compounds may affect the same biological event (RNA synthesis) but act on different targets [26].

Action Against Mycobacterial Protein Synthesis

Spectinomycin is a natural product of aminocyclitol, produced by *Streptomyces spectabilis*. This compound belongs to the aminoglycoside family of compounds like kanamycin and amikacin that can block the 30s ribosomal subunit [27]. Lee and col. generated new semi-synthetic compounds derived from spectinomycin called spectinamides, with potent activity against *M. tuberculosis*. The new spectinamides inhibit the protein synthesis and bind to a multidrug efflux pump protein, promoting their accumulation into bacteria [28]. The experimental and computational analysis showed that the spectinomycin core interacts with the 16S ribosome, and the R conformation is required for ribosome binding, and the acetamide provides optimal spacing and orientation of the aryl side chain for this union. 2-N-heteroaryl motif hydrogen bond donor position is relevant for interaction with the mycobacterial efflux pumps [29]. Recently, several research groups have reported the isolation of aminocyclitolic compounds from free-living microbes, as well as from plant endosymbionts, which deserves further investigation.

Action Against Mycobacterial Membrane Potential

Lassomycin is a potent antibiotic obtained from an extract of bacterium *Lentzea kentuckyensis sp*. Lassomycin has a minimum inhibitory concentration (MIC) of 0.8–3 mg/mL and inhibits a variety of *M. tuberculosis* strains, including MDR, XDR, and NTM. Lassomycin is a peptide that inhibits the caseinolytic protease (Clp) [30]. The Clp complex plays a main role in degrading proteins and maintaining mycobacterial integrity. The Clp complex has two components: two proteolytic subunits (ClpP1 and P2) and two regulatory ATPase subunits (ClpC1 and X). The proteins susceptible to proteolysis are recognized by the Clp complex, unfolded using energy from ATP hydrolysis, and directed into the proteolytic cavity where degradation occurs [31]. Lassomycin seems to decouple the ATPase and proteolytic activity, increase ATPase activity, and simultaneously, the loss of proteolytic activity within the Clp complex. Lassomycin is a basic peptide of 16 residues that enters mycobacteria and binds to an acidic N-terminal pocket on ClpC1 and inhibits the Clp complex, thus exerting its bactericidal effect [30].

Reactive Nitrogen and Oxygen Species (RNOS) Generators Against Mycobacteria

The immune cells, such as macrophages and neutrophils, carry out phagocytosis of pathogens and kill them by a combination of RNOS and enzymatic activity [32]. The abrupt production of RNOS or "respiratory burst" occurs when phagocytes engulf mycobacteria, these molecules cause damage and inactivate invading microbial pathogens [33]. It is well documented that different anti-TB drugs, such as rifampicin, kanamycin, and delamanid, induce RNOS *in vivo* and *in vitro* [34, 35]. The RNOS generated from the treatment with these antibiotics modify the bacterial metabolism causing depletion of NADH, destabilization of iron-sulfur, and iron misregulation [36].

Vitamin C or ascorbic acid is a vitamin found in various foods. This compound has effects as an anti-oxidant and as a pro-oxidant [37]. Vitamin C reduces ferric ions to ferrous ions, and generates the reactive oxygen species (ROS) (superoxide, hydrogen peroxide, and hydroxyl radicals) *via* the Harber-Weiss and Fenton reactions. This exacerbated ROS production causes redox unbalance, affects lipid biosynthesis, DNA replication, and finally causes DNA damage. The mycobactericidal activity of vitamin C is dependent on high ferrous ion levels generated, and only 4 mM vitamin C increases three-fold the total ROS production [38].

Imidazole is a natural compound obtained from leguminous plants, such as *Lens culinaris, Adenanthera pavonina,* and others [39]. Currently, some imidazoles, such as econazole, ketoconazole, and miconazole, have antimycobacterial activity *in vitro* and *in vivo*, and against persistent bacteria. It is demonstrated that imidazoles induce RNOS in a concentration-dependent manner, and modify the metabolism leading to kill bacteria, but it is necessary to elucidate whether there is an intracellular target for imidazoles or not [40].

Despite the limitations of obtaining drugs from natural products, there is still scientific interest in drug discovery. Several natural compounds with potential as the mycobacterial activity have been mentioned, and classified based on their mode of action. Table **1** shows the chemical structure of each compound described above, the action mode, and its' evidence about the interaction with their target.

Table 1. Chemical structure of natural compounds as antituberculosis agents.

Natural Compound	Chemical Structure	Action Mode [Ref]	Structure-based Data or Docking Data
Action against mycobacterial cell surface			
S-Leucoxine		Inhibitor of Mur synthetase (MurE) [19]	Yes
Psoromic acid		Inhibitor of enzyme NAT [21]	Yes
Action against mycobacterial nucleic acids synthesis			
Khusenic acid		Inhibitor of DNA gyrase [22]	Yes
Chebulinic acid		Inhibitor of DNA gyrase [23]	Yes
Calanolide A		Inhibitor of RNA synthesis [25, 26]	No
Action against mycobacterial protein synthesis			
Spectinamide		Inhibitor of 30s ribosomal subunit [26, 28]	Yes
Action against mycobacterial membrane potential			

(Table 1) cont.....

Natural Compound	Chemical Structure	Action Mode [Ref]	Structure-based Data or Docking Data
Lassomycin		Inhibitor of ATPase [28, 29]	Yes
	Reactive Nitrogen and Oxygen species (RNOS) generators against Mycobacteria		
Vitamin C		Produces Hydroxyl radical [38]	No
Imidazoles		Produce RNOS [40]	No

Natural Compounds with Potential to Anti-TB Drugs

The compounds or extract obtained from natural sources described above will allow the development of new treatments in the future, but still require a rigorous evaluation of their applicability as therapeutic drugs. The ideal anti-TB drug must display high potency, exceptionally against MDR, XDR, and NTM strains. The new antimycobacterial compounds should possess an adequate safety profile and be active against latent and replicating forms of mycobacteria. The best antimycobacterial compounds should also have limited drug/drug interactions, particularly with antiviral agents or hypoglycemic drugs, considering the common co-morbidities of TB patients: diabetes and HIV.

In recent years, the field of drug discovery has focused on target-based and genetics-driven approaches to identify new antibiotics. However, this strategy has not been successful. The inhibition of the enzymatic activity of a target protein does not often correlate with the killing of whole bacteria or is inactive against intracellular mycobacteria. High-throughput screening (HTS) is a method employed to elucidate ideal molecules in a short time [41]. However, this assay is typically performed using small molecules with restricted diversity. We should have another vision to discover the ideal molecules to treat TB. The anti-TB treatment should be integral using anti TB drugs able to kill bacteria in dormancy or replicative growth and HDT that enhance the immune response in the host to lead to cure patients in less time and with minimal adverse effects [41]. Recently, it was described that some natural compounds, such as NDGA, α-mangostin, allicin, baicalin, and pasakbumin A, could have the potential to treat TB [42 - 45]. In the following paragraphs, the most important characteristics that make them suitable candidates for their use in TB treatment are described.

Nordihydroguaiaretic Acid (NDGA)

NDGA is the most abundant compound in *Larrea tridentata*, it is between 5 and 10% of the total dry weight of the leaves and is the most abundant phenol resin (> 80%) [46, 47]. *L. tridentata* is a Mexican plant used to treat tuberculosis in the indigenous peoples. The ethanolic extract from this plant has a mycobactericidal effect *in vitro* [48]. *L. tridentata* is an extraordinary source of bioactive compounds. Several bioactive molecules, reported as glycosylated flavonoids, sapogenins, essential oils, waxes, and alkaloids, have been isolated from this plant.

Extensive studies have shown that NDGA presents beneficial properties, including anti-oxidant, antitumor, antiviral, antibacterial, and anti-inflammatory activity [49]. NDGA selectively inhibits arachidonic acid 5-lipoxygenase activity, which, in turn, reduces leukotriene and prostaglandin synthesis, thus leading to a reduction of inflammatory activity. NDGA reduces cytokine production, such as IL-4, IL-5, IL-13, and TNFα, in human cell lines and murine models [50].

It has been demonstrated that NDGA reduces bacterial growth *in vitro* at concentrations ranging from 8 to 125 µg/mL, having MIC of 250 µg/mL. This activity may be related to the structural similarity of other flavonoids, such as butein and isoliquiritigenin. These compounds show complex structures that destabilize the bacterial cell wall and inhibit the synthesis of fatty acids and mycolic acids [51, 52]. Furthermore, it has been reported that similar phenols, such as masoprocol, can inhibit the alpha subunit of coenzyme A transferase, which is involved in the carbon metabolism of *M. tuberculosis*, and might potentially prevent bacterial growth *in vitro* [53].

It has also been demonstrated that NDGA, at a low concentration (7 µg/mL), significantly decreased the intracellular growth of *M. tuberculosis* without any adverse effect on macrophages viability. The NDGA activity was explained by two mechanisms: induced autophagy and reduced TNFα decreasing the inflammatory process. The NDGA treatment with autophagy inhibitors, such as wortmannin (PI3K inhibitor) and SB (p38 inhibitor), caused an increase in bacterial load and a significant decrease of LC3-II puncta formation. NDGA may induce autophagy through the PI3K/AKT/mTOR pathway in human macrophages and provoke bacterial death [54]. Moreover, it has been reported that NDGA induces the nuclear translocation of nuclear factor erythroid-2-related factor 2 (Nrf2) and consequently, the release of Kelch-like ECH-associated protein 1 (Keap1) [55, 56], and the interaction of the polyubiquitin-binding protein p62 with Keap1also increases the autophagic flux [57].

Regarding NDGA toxicity in humans, this compound has been tested for prostate cancer therapy; the daily and continuous administration of NDGA ($\leq$ 2250 mg) for 28 days was well tolerated, and only some patients presented fatigue, diarrhea, nausea, dizziness, and headache. In contrast, the continuous administration of NDGA for more than 18 weeks was slightly toxic, 60% of patients showed high transaminase levels, a marker of liver damage [58]. Additional studies are required to determine the optimum concentration to obtain the desirable immunomodulatory effects in TB treatment without the possible adverse effects.

NDGA is symmetric dimethyl butyl benzene, which is identical to masoprocol, an approved lipoxygenase inhibitor that interferes with arachidonic acid metabolism. Masoprocol also inhibits formyltetrahydrofolate synthetase, carboxylesterase, and cyclooxygenase [59]. Another structural analog is cyclandelate, which is used as a smooth muscle relaxant, and to dilate blood vessels; this drug is approved in various European countries [60].

In summary, NDGA is a potential candidate to treat TB because it is a lipophilic anti-oxidant, it may destabilize the bacterial cell wall, inhibit the synthesis of fatty acids and mycolic acids and even may inhibit the alpha subunit of coenzyme A transferase preventing carbon assimilation and consequently, reduce the bacterial growth. According to the *in silico* analysis in the TDR Targets Database (http://tdrtargets.org) [61], NDGA may have different targets in *M. tuberculosis,* such as enzyme 6-phosphofructokinase (PfkA), inositol-1-monophosphatase (SuhB), aldehyde dehydrogenase, and diverse fatty-acid-CoA synthases, essential enzymes for bacterial growth. Furthermore, NDGA is an immunomodulator because it induces autophagy and reduces inflammation promoting the mycobacterial elimination in the host cell (Fig. **2**).

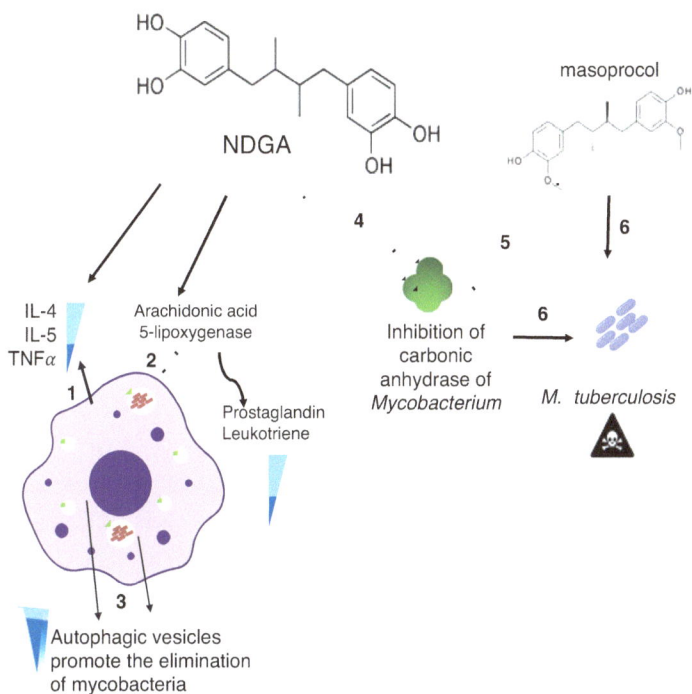

Fig. (2). NDGA possess different ways to combat TB. NDGA decreases inflammatory status in two ways: reduction the pro-inflammatory cytokines production (IL-4, IL-5 and TNFα) **(1)** and arachidonic acid 5-lipoxygenase **(2)**. NDGA activates the autophagic vesicles promoting the mycobacterial elimination in infected macrophages **(3)**. In addition, NDGA probably inhibits carbon anhydrase, involved in carbon metabolism **(4)** like meso-dihydroguaiaretic acid **(5)** and kills the mycobacteria **(6)**. NDGA, nordihydroguaiaretic acid; IL-4 or 5, interleukin 4 or 5; TNFα, tumor necrosis factor alpha.

α-Mangostin

α-Mangostin is the most abundant xanthone of *Garcinia mangostana*; it yields 30–50% from the fruit pericarp [62, 63]. The pericarp of *G. mangostana* has a variety of compounds, such as xanthones, benzophenones, bioflavonoids, and triterpenes [64, 65]. It has been reported that several xanthones isolated from the fruit hull of *G. mangostana*, such as α- and β-mangostins and garcinone B, exert an inhibitory effect against *M. tuberculosis* [66]. Numerous studies have shown that α-mangostin has remarkable anti-oxidant, antitumoral, anti-inflammatory, anti-allergy, antibacterial, antifungal and antiviral biological activities [67].

Previous studies demonstrated that α-mangostin has an anti-inflammatory activity in diverse human cells in response to immunostimulatory agents. α-Mangostin (10-15 μM) treatment of activated THP-1, Caco-2, and HT-29 cells inhibited IL-8 chemokine secretion by 30–40%. Similarly, α-mangostin attenuated TNFα secretion by 22% in cultures of HepG2 cells activated with PMA [68]. Mohan and col. showed that α-mangostin decreases the production of the pro-inflammatory cytokines, prevents the translocation of NFκB, and inhibits the COX-2 enzyme in the RAW 264.7 cells treated with LPS [69]. Recently, it was demonstrated that α-mangostin has a hepatoprotective effect on lipopolysaccharide/d-galactosamine (LPS/D-GalN)-induced acute liver. α-Mangostin decreases the hepatic malondialdehyde (MDA) level, serum alanine aminotransferase (ALT), aspartate transaminase (AST), TNFα, IL-1β, IL-6 levels and increases the hepatic glutathione (GSH), superoxide dismutase (SOD), and catalase (CAT) activities. Possibly, α-mangostin protects against LPS/D-GalN-induced liver failure by activating Nrf2 to induce anti-oxidant defense and to inhibit the TLR4 signaling pathway, then favoring an anti-inflammatory effect [70].

α-Mangostin is a potent antimicrobial agent, which reduces mycobacterial growth at 6.25 to 25 μg/mL [42, 71]. α-Mangostin is also active against *Staphylococcus aureus*, quickly disrupts the bacterial wall, leading to the loss of intracellular components, and may interact directly with the bacterial membrane, provoking membrane disruption and bactericidal action [72]. α-Mangostin also inhibits enzymes involved in glycolysis, such as glyceraldehyde-3-phosphate dehydrogenase (GAPDH), fructose-bisphosphate aldolase (FBA), and lactate dehydrogenase in *Streptococcus mutans* [73]. In this context, α-mangostin may dilute lipophilic substances, such as wall components, and simultaneously inhibit several enzymes in *M. tuberculosis,* avoiding bacterial growth.

It was previously demonstrated that α-mangostin avoids the intracellular growth of *M. tuberculosis* H37Ra in infected human macrophages [42]. In this context, α-mangostin induces autophagy through mTOR pathway and the autophagic vesicle colocalized with mycobacteria promoting bacterial elimination. It has been reported that α-mangostin induces autophagic cell death in mouse intestinal epithelial cells [74], human glioblastoma cells [75], and chronic myeloid leukemia (CML) cell lines [76].

Different parts of *G. mangostana*, commonly fruit hull and barkand roots, have been used by diverse ethnic groups of Southeast Asia as a medicine for a great variety of medical conditions [77]. The pharmacokinetics and bioavailability of α-mangostin in humans has not been explored. Kondo and col. simply showed the use of a mix of α-mangostin with vitamins and Aloe Vera as a nutritional supplement in healthy volunteers. This study was conducted with male and female subjects between 20 and 23 years of age and they demonstrated that the volunteers had a higher degree of anti-oxidant potency [78]. Consequently, more studies about the safe use of α-mangostin in humans are required.

α-Mangostin is an over the counter drug and is not approved by the FDA. It is a member of the class of xanthones with three aromatic rings in a linear arrangement with oxygen in the center ring. It has a similarity with the approved drug propantheline, which is an antimuscarinic agent used to treat urinary incontinence, and spasms of the stomach, intestines, and bladder [79]. α-Mangostin also shares the three-ring structure with other drugs that have a sulfur atom instead of oxygen and used for the treatment of central nervous system disorders, they are flupentixol and tiotixene [80, 81]. Probably, α-mangostin may be a prodrug, because it has the potential to get a tetracycline like structure.

In brief, α-mangostin is another potential candidate to treat TB because it is a lipophilic compound able to disrupt the bacterial wall and interact with the bacterial membrane, provoking membrane disruption. α-Mangostin may inhibit metabolic enzymes avoiding bacterial growth. According to the analysis in TDR, it predicts that α-mangostin may have multiple targets, such as various polyketide synthetases involved in the lipid metabolism. This may limit mycobacterial growth in the host cells. Other possible targets are GAPDH and FBA, essential enzymes in the intermediary metabolism [82]. Additionally, α-mangostin is also a potent immunomodulator because it induces autophagy and reduces inflammation contributing to the mycobacterial elimination (Fig. **3**).

Allicin

Garlic (*Allium sativum*) is a natural plant with widespread biological properties, including antimicrobial, anticancer, anti-oxidant, immunomodulatory, anti-inflammatory, hypoglycemic, and cardioprotection activity [83].

Garlic is one of the established natural remedies for TB, innumerable phytoconstituents from garlic have shown antimycobacterial against tuberculous and NTM species [84]. *In vitro* antimycobacterial activity of different garlic extracts were determined, for example, the allicin-rich extract, ajoene-rich extract, garlic oil, and the garlic extract had a significant antibacterial activity against *M. tuberculosis* [85].

The biological effects of garlic have been attributed to organosulfur compounds [86]. Garlic possesses at least a 100 sulfur-containing bioactive compounds, such as S-allylcysteine, saponins, ajoene, flavonoids, and phenols [87, 88]. Allicin is the most predominant, making up 70% to 80% of all thiosulfates. Allicin is not present in garlic, but only produced when garlic cloves are cut or crushed. Despite this, allicin is the most pharmacologically active compound of raw crushed garlic showing a wide range of effects. It is a thiosulfinate with two allyl groups as carbon chains (diallylthiosulfnate or thio-2-propene-1-sulfinic acid S-allyl ester) and the precursor is the non-proteinogenic amino acid, alliin (S-allyl-L-cysteine sulfoxide) [89].

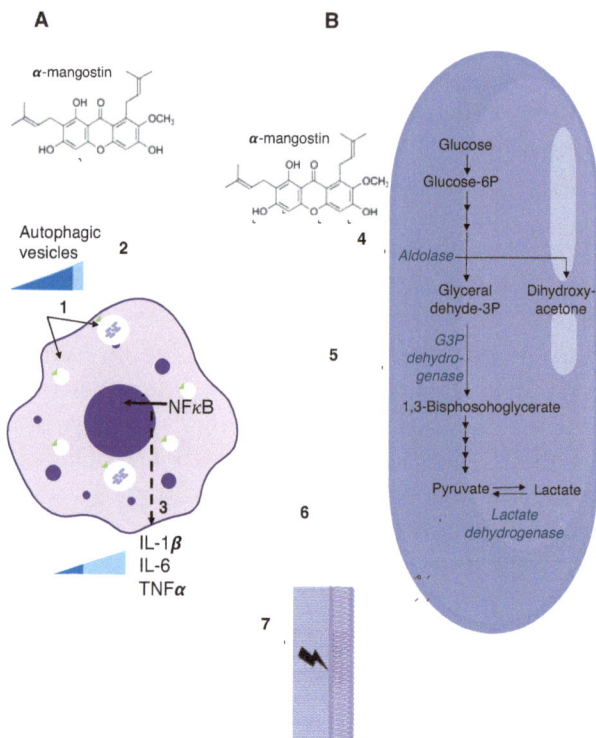

Fig. (3). Bactericidal effect of α-mangostin on infected macrophages (A) and *M. tuberculosis* (B). α-Mangostin activates the autophagic vesicles that promote the mycobacterial elimination in infected macrophages (1), and it prevents the nuclear factor NFκB translocation (2) and probably decreases the production of the pro-inflammatory cytokines (3). In addition, α-mangostin also inhibits some mycobacterial enzymes of glycolysis pathways like aldolase (4), G3P dehydrogenase (5), and lactate dehydrogenase (6). α-Mangostin is highly lipophilic and can interact with the bacterial surface provoking its rupture and mycobacterial killing. NFκB, nuclear factor κB; IL-1β or 6, interleukin 1β or 6; TNFα, tumor necrosis factor alpha.

Allicin is a potent antimicrobial agent that is active against a wider spectrum of microorganisms. It can kill Gram-Positive and Gram-Negative bacteria and even pathogens that are resistant to diverse antibiotics (Fig. **4**). Allicin can cross the bacterial membrane allowing it to rapidly penetrate the cell [90]. Although allicin has lower bactericidal efficacy compared to penicillin, it has a particular mode of action because it reacts with free cysteine residues available of the proteins and low molecular weight thiols. Then, allicin reacts with the sulfhydryl-group of cysteine *via* a disulfide exchange-like by inhibiting the enzymatic activity [91]. Allicin also possesses antifungal activity against some species of *Candida,*

Cryptococcus and *Trichophyton* [92, 93] and is antiparasitic against *Babesia* and *Theileria equi* [94].

Recently, it was demonstrated that allicin reduced mycobacterial growth at a concentration of 8.17 to 33 µg/mL against *M. tuberculosis* drug-sensitive and several MDR and XDR strains *in vitro*. In context to infection, the macrophages, pretreated with allicin, are more resistant to *M. tuberculosis* infection and the macrophages treated post-infection avoid the intracellular growth of *M. tuberculosis* in peritoneal macrophages from C57BL/6 mice. The precise mechanism of allicin against this bacteria is unknown, and it would be of great relevance to know it [43].

Moreover, allicin has immunomodulatory properties, it induces high levels of pro-inflammatory cytokines like IL-1β in infected macrophages, but reduces the levels of TNFα [43, 95] through a blockade of p38 MAPK phosphorylation. Furthermore, allicin induces autophagic cell death in human liver cancer Hep G2 cells [96], this mechanism may be activated in infected macrophages and reduce the intracellular growth of *M. tuberculosis*.

Garlic and its derivatives have been used for centuries because of their numerous health benefits. There are studies of garlic consumption in different presentations like fresh raw bulbs, oils, powder, and even liquid supplements [89]. Regarding allicin, it is known that it is the most active compound of crushed raw garlic cloves. However, its pure form is difficult and expensive. Therefore its consumption is more feasible in supplements forms and garlic foods. Recently, Lawson and Hunsaker (2018) showed the allicin bioavailability in garlic products in healthy individuals. They established that tablet consumption varied from 36–104%, but it was reduced when consumed with a high-protein meal. For example, another presentation in powder tablets, give 80% of bioavailability. Cooked or acidified garlic foods, which have no alliinase activity, gave higher bioavailability than estimated and varied from 16-66% [97]. This information gives the guidelines to determine the type of product that can be taken as a supplement to contribute to improving health in patients with TB.

Allicin is a low molecular weight sulfur-containing compound that is known to functionally modify proteins by thioallylation at cysteine residues. It also has been proposed as a potential inhibitor of enolase, an enzyme considered a cancer therapy target [98]. In that respect, allicin shares some structural similitude with phosphono-acetohydroxamic acid, which also interacts with enolases from *Trypanosoma brucei* and yeasts [99].

In summary, allicin is a potential compound to treat TB because it kills mycobacteria. Allicin may cross the bacterial membrane, then react with free cysteine residues of proteins and inhibit the enzymatic activity. According to the analysis in TDR, allicin does not have any specific druggable targets in *Mycobacterium*. Furthermore, allicin prevents the bacterial internalization and after infection, it promotes the bacterial elimination in macrophages. Also, allicin is a powerful immunomodulator because it induces IL-1b and IL-12 production and inhibits TNFα and IL-10 production, generating a protective response contributing to the mycobacterial elimination (Fig. **4**).

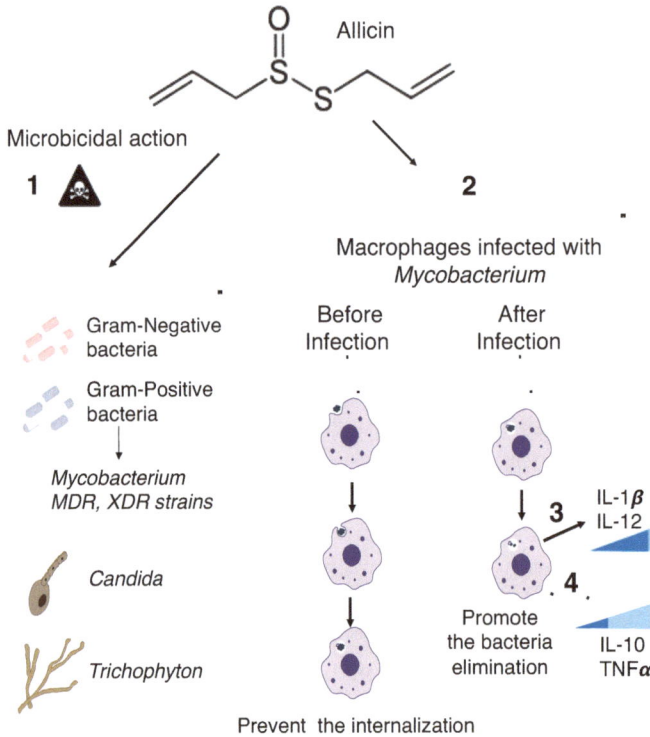

Fig. (4). Microbicidal action of Allicin. This organosulfur compound has a microbicidal effect on Gram-Negative and Gram-Positive bacteria and some fungi, such as *Candida* and *Trichophyton* (1). Allicin is also active against mycobacteria (2). The treatment with allicin before infection of macrophages prevents the bacterial internalization and the treatment after infection of macrophages promotes the bacterial elimination. Allicin selectively inhibits TNFα and IL-10, but IL-1β and IL-12 are moderately elevated. TNFα, tumor necrosis factor alpha; IL1β, IL-10 and IL-12, interleukin 1β or 10, 12.

Baicalin

Scutellaria baicalensis is a plant with extensive medicinal uses in China. The root is commonly used to treat diseases, such as hepatitis, hypertension, respiratory infection and gastric diseases such as gastroenteritis, diarrhea, and others. Besides, this plant has neuroprotective, antiallergic, anti-oxidant, and antitumoral action [100]. *S. baicalensis* has antimicrobial activity, which is effective against

Gram-Positive and Gram-Negative bacteria, such as *Bacillus subtilis, Streptococcus mutans, Enterococcus faecalis, Klebsiella pneumoni*a, and *Salmonella enterica* [101 - 103].

S. baicalensis possesses hundreds of bioactive compounds, such as free flavonoids, glycosylated flavonoids, phenylethanoid glycosides, phenolic compounds, polysaccharides, oils, and alkaloids [104]. Although, *S. baicalensis* has a variety of health benefits, only the most abundant compounds have been isolated, characterized, and evaluated for their biological activity, such as baicalin, baicalein and wogonin [105].

Baicalin is a flavone glucuronide, the most abundant component of *S. baicalensis,* and possesses many biological activities such as antibacterial, anti-inflammatory, antiallergic, antispasmodic, and anticancer activity [106, 107].

It was previously shown that baicalin inhibits bacterial growth at 1 to 4 mg/mL, it disrupts the bacterial wall leading to the loss of intracellular components [108]. Baicalin has shown inhibitory effects on different Gram-Negative bacteria *in vitro*, such as *Escherichia coli*, Pseudomonas aeruginosa, and *Helicobacter pylori* [108 - 110]. Also, baicalin inhibits biofilm formation of *P. aeruginosa* and *S. aureus* in the mouse model [109, 111]. It has been shown that baicalin directly binds virulence factors, such as sortase B (SrtB) in *S. aureus* and decreases the bacterial growth [111].

Baicalin inhibits the intracellular growth of *M. tuberculosis* in macrophages derived from Raw 264.7 cell line. This compound induces autophagy through PI3K/Akt/mTOR signaling pathway and the MAPK pathway. Baicalin also suppresses the activation of NLRP3 inflammasome during mycobacterial infection controlling the exacerbated inflammation [45].

Moreover, baicalin has anti-inflammatory activity in the liver damage model in mice. It prevents LPS/D-GalN-induced liver injury by inhibition of NFκ-β activity to reduce TNFα production and increases HO-1, an anti-oxidant and protective enzyme that avoids cellular damage [112].

Concerning the pharmacokinetics and bioavailability studies of baicalin, very little is known. In rats, it was demonstrated that baicalin is absorbed rapidly into the plasma and accumulated in several tissues [113]. This compound is metabolized and excreted in bile and urine [114, 115]. But, the baicalin administration with other drugs may affect its properties *in vivo* [116]. In human studies showed the use of baicalin in patients with rheumatoid arthritis who have an increased risk of coronary artery disease. This study was conducted with male and female subjects over 45 years of age. The patients received 500 mg baicalin orally every day for 12 weeks. After the baicalin treatment, the patients had reduced blood lipids and inflammation without any apparent adverse effect [117]. Thus, more studies about the safety and efficacy of this compound in humans are necessary.

Baicalein and baicalin are trihydroxy-flavones with a wide range of biological activities. Hydroxy-flavones belong to a diverse family of compounds that have many experimentally tested applications, but none of them are currently approved by the FDA. Apigenin and diosmetin are similar to baicalin and are more promising compounds of the family that could be available in the future for cancer treatment [118, 119].

Baicalin may be a potent drug to treat TB because it kills bacteria in many ways: disrupts the bacterial wall, inhibits biofilm formation, and binds with virulence factors. According to the TDR analysis, baicalin may inhibit the protease II PtrBa, an oligopeptidase (Rv0781) involved in the intermediary metabolism and respiration in mycobacteria and required for survival in primary murine macrophages [82, 120]. Furthermore, baicalin is a potent immunomodulator because it reduces pro-inflammatory effectors and increases autophagy contributing to the mycobacterial elimination (Fig. **5**).

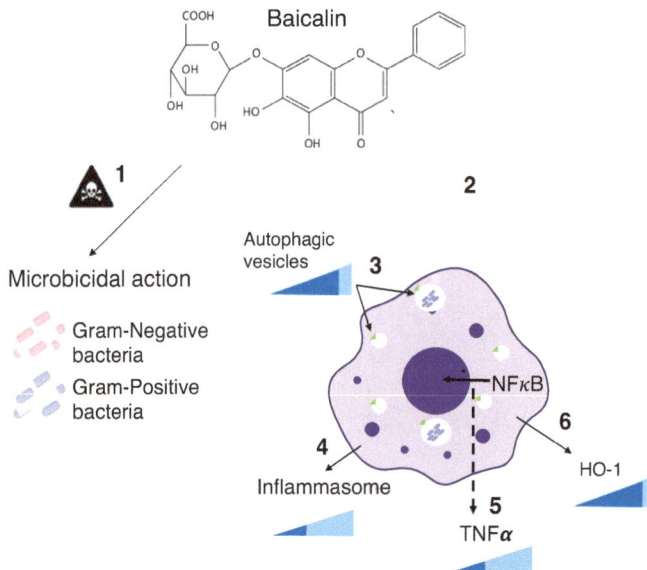

Fig. (5). Bactericidal effect of Baicalin. This compound has a microbicidal effect on Gram-Negative and Gram-Positive bacteria (1). Baicalin is also active against mycobacteria on infected macrophages (2), activates the autophagic vesicles promoting the mycobacterial elimination (3), suppresses the activation of inflammasome (4), prevents the nuclear factor NFκB translocation decreasing TNFα production (5) and induces a protective enzyme with anti-oxidant activity HO-1(6). NFκB, nuclear factor κB; TNFα, tumor necrosis factor alpha and HO-1, hemo-oxigenase-1.

Pasakbumin A

Eurycoma longifolia Jack is a medicinal plant of South- East Asian countries used for its' antimalarial, antidiabetic antimicrobial antipyretic, antiulcer, aphrodisiac, among other, properties [121, 122]. The root is the part traditionally used by indigenous people but leaves and stem have shown pharmacological properties, for example the aqueous extracts of leaves from *E. longifolia* exhibit antibacterial activity against *S. aureus* and *Serratia marscesens* [123].

E. longifolia has a wide range of chemical compounds, such as alkaloids, squalene derivatives, and quassinoids [124]. The quassinoids are the major proportions in the *E. longifolia* in the root, such as pasakbumin -A, -B, -C and -D, eurycomanols, hydroxyklaineanones, eurycomalactones, eurycomadilactones, eurylactones, laurycolactones, longilactones, and hydroxyglaucarubol. The quassinoids have diverse pharmacological activities, for example, pasakbumin-A and -B have antiulcer activity [125] and the pasakbumin-A, -B, -C, and -D are cytotoxic on cancer human cell lines [126].

Pasakbumin A has antibacterial activity against the virulent *M. tuberculosis* H37Rv in Raw 264.7 macrophage cell line and protects the host cells from apoptotic cell death induced by *M. tuberculosis*. Pasakbumin A activates autophagy in infected macrophages through the ERK1/2-mediated signaling pathway. This compound increases nitric oxide and pro-inflammatory cytokine *via* the ERK1/2-and NFκB-mediated signaling pathways in macrophages infected with *M. tuberculosis*. The combination of anti-TB drugs (INH and RIF) with pasakbumin A enhances the reduction of intracellular mycobacterial growth by increasing autophagy and TNFα production [44].

The pharmacokinetics and bioavailability of Pasakbumin A is unknown. There are two clinical studies, where *E. longifolia* root water extract is administered in adults. One group evaluated whether the comprehensive immune functions of volunteers with comparatively lower levels of immunity would be improved by the ingestion of a 200 mg/day dose for 4 weeks. It showed that the extract improves the immunological condition, which results in the improvement of health [127]. The other group evaluated the administration of *E. longifolia* root water extract with propranolol (a non-selective beta-blocker used lipophilic antihypertensive drug). They showed that *E. longifolia* extract interacts with propranolol by reducing its bioavailability rather than interfering with its metabolism [128]. Accordingly, it is necessary for more studies about the bioavailability, efficacy, and safety of *E. longifolia* root water extract and Pasakbumin A.

Pasakbumin A is a triterpene lactone belonging to the quassinoid group of compounds. As such, they are structural analogs of some androgens derivatives like bevirimat, which is currently under investigation as an anti-HIV drug [129]. Pasakbumin A is partially similar to trioxsalen, that is approved for the treatment of skin vitiligo and eczema [130].

In summary, Pasakbumin A does not kill mycobacteria and according to the analysis in TDR, this compound does not have a specific druggable target in *Mycobacterium*. But, Pasakbumin A is a potent immunomodulator because it reduces pro-inflammatory effectors and increases autophagy contributing to the mycobacterial elimination (Fig. **7**).

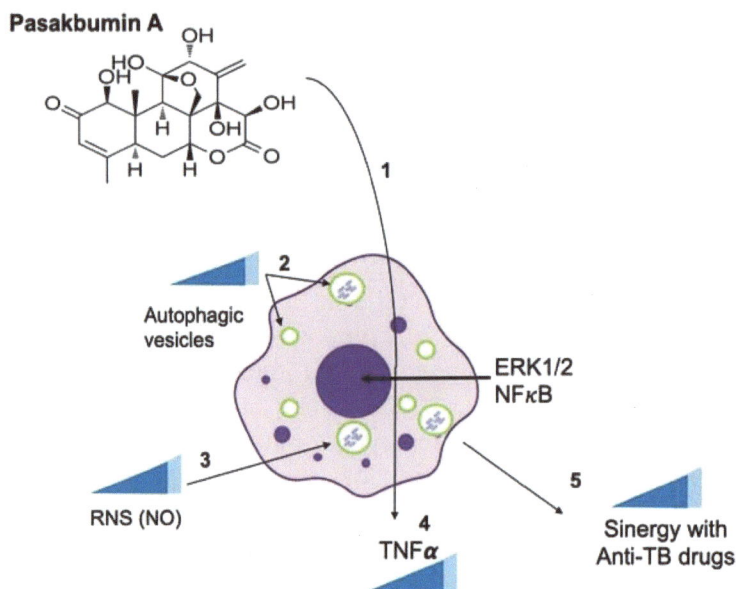

Fig. (6). Mycobactericidal effect of Pasakbumin A on infected macrophages (1). Pasakbumin A induces the autophagic vesicles promoting the mycobacterial elimination (2), activates NO (3) and TNFα (4) production through the ERK1/2 and NFκB signaling pathway. Pasakbumin A synergizes with anti-TB drugs decreasing intracellular mycobacteria (5). RNS, reactive nitrogen species; NO, Nitric Oxide; TNFα, tumor necrosis factor alpha; ERK1/2, extracellular signal-regulated protein kinases 1 and 2; NFκB, nuclear factor κB.

Host-directed Therapies for Tuberculosis (HDT)

Despite the recent increase in the development of anti-TB drugs, antimycobacterial resistance and the lack of broad-spectrum of drugs are still important problems. Additional alternatives to treat TB are urgently needed. HDT is an emerging approach in the field of infectious diseases, this strategy is to interfere with host cell factors that are required by mycobacterial replication or persistence, to enhance the protective immune response against this pathogen, to reduce exacerbated inflammation and to balance immune reactivity at the sites of infection [131].

HDT-TB includes agents that may have microbicidal activity, and may, additively or synergistically, enhance the activity of the anti-TB drugs and modulate host immunity. The immunomodulators have different functions that lead to eradicate TB [7]. These agents may activate the antimicrobial mechanisms, such as antimicrobial peptides induction (cathelicidin LL-37 and the human β-defensin), the respiratory burst, and autophagy activation combating mycobacteria. Also, these agents may attenuate the inflammatory responses in TB leading to host lung damage through the decrease in exacerbated pro-inflammatory chemokines (TNFα, IL-1β, and IL-6) [8, 41]. Diverse studies have demonstrated that host-directed adjunctive therapies can decrease the duration of treatment, reduce transmissibility, and improve the TB patient health. It was also found that innumerable agents could be used in HDT [132], however, many of them are drugs that could interact with anti-TB drugs or have adverse side effects that should be evaluated in clinical trials.

CONCLUDING REMARKS

TB is one of the leading causes of mortality and morbidity around the world. The currently recommended long term treatment regimen with multiple antibiotics is associated with poor patient compliance, which, in turn, may contribute to the emergence of MDR and XDR. It is essential to expand the TB treatment with new effective drugs or compounds useful as adjuvants to decrease the incidence and the prevalence of TB.

The natural products have been an important source of TB therapeutics with a difference in bioactivity. NDGA, α-mangostin, allicin, baicalin, and pasakbumin A are natural compounds that could be new and excellent alternatives as HDT-TB. Hence, the current standard antibiotics for treating TB together with HDT could lead to end this horrendous infectious disease. Although significant advances have been made recently, it is necessary to develop effective models to evaluate the immunomodulatory functions of HDT-compounds with anti-TB drugs and evaluate their safety in clinical trials.

CONSENT FOR PUBLICATION

Not applicable.

CONFLICT OF INTEREST

The authors confirm that this chapter contents have no conflict of interest.

ACKNOWLEDGEMENT

Declared none.

REFERENCES

[1]   MacNeil A, Glaziou P, Sismanidis C, Date A, Maloney S, Floyd K. Global epidemiology of tuberculosis and progress toward meeting global targets - worldwide, 2018. MMWR Morb Mortal Wkly Rep 2020; 69(11): 281-5.
        [http://dx.doi.org/10.15585/mmwr.mm6911a2] [PMID: 32191687]

[2]   Bloom BR, Atun R, Cohen T, Dye C, Fraser H, Gomez GB, *et al.* Disease control priorities. Major Infectious Diseases The World Bank. Third Edition. 2017; 6.
        [http://dx.doi.org/doi:10.1596/978-1-4648-0524-0]

[3]   Drummond WK, Kasperbauer SH. Nontuberculous mycobacteria: Epidemiology and the impact on pulmonary and cardiac disease. Thorac Surg Clin 2019; 29(1): 59-64.
        [http://dx.doi.org/10.1016/j.thorsurg.2018.09.006] [PMID: 30454922]

[4]   Treatment for TB Disease | Treatment | TB | CDC n.d. https://www.cdc.gov/ tb/ topic/ treatment/ tbdisease.htm [(accessed March 30, 2020).];

[5]   Parenti F, Lancini G. Rifamycins Antibiot Chemother. Elsevier 2010; pp. 326-33.
        [http://dx.doi.org/10.1016/B978-0-7020-4064-1.00027-0]

[6]   Pstragowski M, Zbrzezna M, Bujalska-Zadrozny M. Advances in pharmacotherapy of tuberculosis. Acta Pol Pharm 2017; 74(1): 3-11.
        [PMID: 29474756]

[7]   Hawn TR, Matheson AI, Maley SN, Vandal O. Host-directed therapeutics for tuberculosis: Can we harness the host? Microbiol Mol Biol Rev 2013; 77(4): 608-27.
        [http://dx.doi.org/10.1128/MMBR.00032-13] [PMID: 24296574]

[8]   Ahmed S, Raqib R, Guðmundsson GH, Bergman P, Agerberth B, Rekha RS. Host-directed therapy as a novel treatment strategy to overcome tuberculosis: Targeting immune modulation. Antibiotics (Basel) 2020; 9(1): E21.
        [http://dx.doi.org/10.3390/antibiotics9010021] [PMID: 31936156]

[9]   WHO. WHO Global Tuberculosis Report 2018. World Health Organization 2018; Vol. 69.

[10]   Carrol ED, Clark JE, Cant AJ. Non-pulmonary tuberculosis. Paediatr Respir Rev 2001; 2(2): 113-9.
        [http://dx.doi.org/10.1053/prrv.2000.0118] [PMID: 12531057]

[11]   Schön T, Miotto P, Köser CU, Viveiros M, Böttger E, Cambau E. *Mycobacterium tuberculosis* drug-resistance testing: challenges, recent developments and perspectives. Clin Microbiol Infect 2017; 23(3): 154-60.
        [http://dx.doi.org/10.1016/j.cmi.2016.10.022] [PMID: 27810467]

[12]   Bahuguna A, Rawat DS. An overview of new antitubercular drugs, drug candidates, and their targets. Med Res Rev 2020; 40(1): 263-92.
        [http://dx.doi.org/10.1002/med.21602] [PMID: 31254295]

[13]   Prasad R, Singh A, Gupta N. Adverse drug reactions in tuberculosis and management. Indian J Tuberc 2019; 66(4): 520-32.
        [http://dx.doi.org/10.1016/j.ijtb.2019.11.005] [PMID: 31813444]

[14]   Farah SI, Abdelrahman AA, North EJ, Chauhan H. Opportunities and challenges for natural products as novel antituberculosis agents. Assay Drug Dev Technol 2016; 14(1): 29-38.
        [http://dx.doi.org/10.1089/adt.2015.673] [PMID: 26565779]

[15]   Osman K, Evangelopoulos D, Basavannacharya C, *et al.* An antibacterial from Hypericum acmosepalum inhibits ATP-dependent MurE ligase from *Mycobacterium tuberculosis*. Int J

Antimicrob Agents 2012; 39(2): 124-9.
[http://dx.doi.org/10.1016/j.ijantimicag.2011.09.018] [PMID: 22079533]

[16]   Madikane VE, Bhakta S, Russell AJ, *et al.* Inhibition of mycobacterial arylamine N-acetyltransferase contributes to anti-mycobacterial activity of Warburgia salutaris. Bioorg Med Chem 2007; 15(10): 3579-86.
[http://dx.doi.org/10.1016/j.bmc.2007.02.011] [PMID: 17368035]

[17]   Munshi T, Gupta A, Evangelopoulos D, *et al.* Characterisation of ATP-dependent Mur ligases involved in the biogenesis of cell wall peptidoglycan in *Mycobacterium tuberculosis.* PLoS One 2013; 8(3): e60143.
[http://dx.doi.org/10.1371/journal.pone.0060143] [PMID: 23555903]

[18]   Bhakta S, Besra GS, Upton AM, *et al.* Arylamine N-acetyltransferase is required for synthesis of mycolic acids and complex lipids in *Mycobacterium tuberculosis* BCG and represents a novel drug target. J Exp Med 2004; 199(9): 1191-9.
[http://dx.doi.org/10.1084/jem.20031956] [PMID: 15117974]

[19]   Guzman JD, Pesnot T, Barrera DA, *et al.* Tetrahydroisoquinolines affect the whole-cell phenotype of *Mycobacterium tuberculosis* by inhibiting the ATP-dependent MurE ligase. J Antimicrob Chemother 2015; 70(6): 1691-703.
[http://dx.doi.org/10.1093/jac/dkv010] [PMID: 25656411]

[20]   Ghajavand H, Kargarpour Kamakoli M, Khanipour S, *et al.* Scrutinizing the drug resistance mechanism of multi- and extensively-drug resistant *Mycobacterium tuberculosis*: mutations *versus* efflux pumps. Antimicrob Resist Infect Control 2019; 8: 70.
[http://dx.doi.org/10.1186/s13756-019-0516-4] [PMID: 31073401]

[21]   Hassan STS, Šudomová M, Berchová-Bímová K, Gowrishankar S, Rengasamy KRR. Antimycobacterial, enzyme inhibition, and molecular interaction studies of psoromic acid in *Mycobacterium tuberculosis*: efficacy and safety investigations. J Clin Med 2018; 7(8): 226.
[http://dx.doi.org/10.3390/jcm7080226] [PMID: 30127304]

[22]   Dwivedi GR, Gupta S, Roy S, *et al.* Tricyclic sesquiterpenes from *Vetiveria zizanoides* (L.) Nash as antimycobacterial agents. Chem Biol Drug Des 2013; 82(5): 587-94.
[http://dx.doi.org/10.1111/cbdd.12188] [PMID: 23841574]

[23]   Patel K, Tyagi C, Goyal S, *et al.* Identification of chebulinic acid as potent natural inhibitor of *M. tuberculosis* DNA gyrase and molecular insights into its binding mode of action. Comput Biol Chem 2015; 59(Pt A): 37-47.
[http://dx.doi.org/10.1016/j.compbiolchem.2015.09.006]

[24]   Zheng P, Somersan-Karakaya S, Lu S, *et al.* Synthetic calanolides with bactericidal activity against replicating and nonreplicating *Mycobacterium tuberculosis.* J Med Chem 2014; 57(9): 3755-72.
[http://dx.doi.org/10.1021/jm4019228] [PMID: 24694175]

[25]   Eiznhamer DA, Creagh T, Ruckle JL, *et al.* Safety and pharmacokinetic profile of multiple escalating doses of (+)-calanolide A, a naturally occurring nonnucleoside reverse transcriptase inhibitor, in healthy HIV-negative volunteers. HIV Clin Trials 2002; 3(6): 435-50.
[http://dx.doi.org/10.1310/9GDE-F2R1-W2RL-E9FJ] [PMID: 12501127]

[26]   Xu ZQ, Barrow WW, Suling WJ, *et al.* Anti-HIV natural product (+)-calanolide A is active against both drug-susceptible and drug-resistant strains of *Mycobacterium tuberculosis.* Bioorg Med Chem 2004; 12(5): 1199-207.
[http://dx.doi.org/10.1016/j.bmc.2003.11.012] [PMID: 14980631]

[27]   Borovinskaya MA, Shoji S, Holton JM, Fredrick K, Cate JHD. A steric block in translation caused by the antibiotic spectinomycin. ACS Chem Biol 2007; 2(8): 545-52.
[http://dx.doi.org/10.1021/cb700100n] [PMID: 17696316]

[28]   Lee RE, Hurdle JG, Liu J, *et al.* Spectinamides: a new class of semisynthetic antituberculosis agents that overcome native drug efflux. Nat Med 2014; 20(2): 152-8.

[http://dx.doi.org/10.1038/nm.3458] [PMID: 24464186]

[29]   Liu J, Bruhn DF, Lee RB, *et al.* Structure-activity relationships of spectinamide antituberculosis agents: A dissection of ribosomal inhibition and native efflux avoidance contributions. ACS Infect Dis 2017; 3(1): 72-88.
[http://dx.doi.org/10.1021/acsinfecdis.6b00158] [PMID: 28081607]

[30]   Gavrish E, Sit CS, Cao S, *et al.* Lassomycin, a ribosomally synthesized cyclic peptide, kills *Mycobacterium tuberculosis* by targeting the ATP-dependent protease ClpC1P1P2. Chem Biol 2014; 21(4): 509-18.
[http://dx.doi.org/10.1016/j.chembiol.2014.01.014] [PMID: 24684906]

[31]   Akopian T, Kandror O, Raju RM, Unnikrishnan M, Rubin EJ, Goldberg AL. The active ClpP protease from M. tuberculosis is a complex composed of a heptameric ClpP1 and a ClpP2 ring. EMBO J 2012; 31(6): 1529-41.
[http://dx.doi.org/10.1038/emboj.2012.5] [PMID: 22286948]

[32]   Piacenza L, Trujillo M, Radi R. Reactive species and pathogen antioxidant networks during phagocytosis. J Exp Med 2019; 216(3): 501-16.
[http://dx.doi.org/10.1084/jem.20181886] [PMID: 30792185]

[33]   Freitas M, Lima JLFC, Fernandes E. Optical probes for detection and quantification of neutrophils' oxidative burst. A review. Anal Chim Acta 2009; 649(1): 8-23.
[http://dx.doi.org/10.1016/j.aca.2009.06.063] [PMID: 19664458]

[34]   Piccaro G, Pietraforte D, Giannoni F, Mustazzolu A, Fattorini L. Rifampin induces hydroxyl radical formation in *Mycobacterium tuberculosis*. Antimicrob Agents Chemother 2014; 58(12): 7527-33.
[http://dx.doi.org/10.1128/AAC.03169-14] [PMID: 25288092]

[35]   Galizia J, Acosta MP, Urdániz E, Martí MA, Piuri M. Evaluation of nitroxyl donors' effect on mycobacteria. Tuberculosis (Edinb) 2018; 109: 35-40.
[http://dx.doi.org/10.1016/j.tube.2018.01.006] [PMID: 29559119]

[36]   Vatansever F, de Melo WCMA, Avci P, *et al.* Antimicrobial strategies centered around reactive oxygen species--bactericidal antibiotics, photodynamic therapy, and beyond. FEMS Microbiol Rev 2013; 37(6): 955-89.
[http://dx.doi.org/10.1111/1574-6976.12026] [PMID: 23802986]

[37]   Podmore ID, Griffiths HR, Herbert KE, Mistry N, Mistry P, Lunec J. Vitamin C exhibits pro-oxidant properties. Nature 1998; 392(6676): 559.
[http://dx.doi.org/10.1038/33308] [PMID: 9560150]

[38]   Vilchèze C, Hartman T, Weinrick B, Jacobs WR Jr. *Mycobacterium tuberculosis* is extraordinarily sensitive to killing by a vitamin C-induced Fenton reaction. Nat Commun 2013; 4: 1881.
[http://dx.doi.org/10.1038/ncomms2898] [PMID: 23695675]

[39]   R. Hayman A. O. Gray D. Imidazole, a new natural product from the leguminosae. Phytochemistry 1987; 26: 3247-8.
[http://dx.doi.org/10.1016/S0031-9422(00)82479-6]

[40]   Howell Wescott HA, Roberts DM, Allebach CL, Kokoczka R, Parish T. Imidazoles Induce Reactive Oxygen Species in *Mycobacterium tuberculosis* Which Is Not Associated with Cell Death. ACS Omega 2017; 2(1): 41-51.
[http://dx.doi.org/10.1021/acsomega.6b00212] [PMID: 28180188]

[41]   Kolloli A, Subbian S. Host-directed therapeutic strategies for tuberculosis. Front Med (Lausanne) 2017; 4: 171.
[http://dx.doi.org/10.3389/fmed.2017.00171] [PMID: 29094039]

[42]   Guzmán-Beltrán S, Rubio-Badillo MÁ, Juárez E, Hernández-Sánchez F, Torres M. Nordihydroguaiaretic acid (NDGA) and α-mangostin inhibit the growth of *Mycobacterium tuberculosis* by inducing autophagy. Int Immunopharmacol 2016; 31: 149-57.

[http://dx.doi.org/10.1016/j.intimp.2015.12.027] [PMID: 26735610]

[43]   Dwivedi VP, Bhattacharya D, Singh M, *et al.* Allicin enhances antimicrobial activity of macrophages during *Mycobacterium tuberculosis* infection. J Ethnopharmacol 2019; 243: 111634.
[http://dx.doi.org/10.1016/j.jep.2018.12.008] [PMID: 30537531]

[44]   Lee H-J, Ko H-J, Kim SH, Jung YJ. Pasakbumin A controls the growth of *Mycobacterium tuberculosis* by enhancing the autophagy and production of antibacterial mediators in mouse macrophages. PLoS One 2019; 14(3): e0199799.
[http://dx.doi.org/10.1371/journal.pone.0199799] [PMID: 30865638]

[45]   Zhang Q, Sun J, Wang Y, *et al.* Antimycobacterial and anti-inflammatory mechanisms of baicalin *via* induced autophagy in macrophages infected with *Mycobacterium tuberculosis*. Front Microbiol 2017; 8: 2142.
[http://dx.doi.org/10.3389/fmicb.2017.02142] [PMID: 29163427]

[46]   Arteaga S, Andrade-Cetto A, Cárdenas R. *Larrea tridentata* (Creosote bush), an abundant plant of Mexican and US-American deserts and its metabolite nordihydroguaiaretic acid. J Ethnopharmacol 2005; 98(3): 231-9.
[http://dx.doi.org/10.1016/j.jep.2005.02.002] [PMID: 15814253]

[47]   Konno C, Lu ZZ, Xue HZ, *et al.* Furanoid lignans from *Larrea tridentata*. J Nat Prod 1990; 53(2): 396-406.
[http://dx.doi.org/10.1021/np50068a019] [PMID: 2166136]

[48]   Camacho-Corona MDR, Ramírez-Cabrera MA, González-Santiago O, Garza-González E, Palacios IDP, Luna-Herrera J. Activity against drug resistant-tuberculosis strains of plants used in Mexican traditional medicine to treat tuberculosis and other respiratory diseases. Phyther Res 2008.
[http://dx.doi.org/10.1002/ptr.2269]

[49]   Lü JM, Nurko J, Weakley SM, *et al.* Molecular mechanisms and clinical applications of nordihydroguaiaretic acid (NDGA) and its derivatives: an update. Med Sci Monit 2010; 16(5): RA93-RA100.
[http://dx.doi.org/10.1111/j.1600-6143.2008.02497.x.Plasma] [PMID: 20424564]

[50]   Kim SY, Kim TBJ, Moon KA, *et al.* Regulation of pro-inflammatory responses by lipoxygenases *via* intracellular reactive oxygen species *in vitro* and *in vivo*. Exp Mol Med 2008; 40(4): 461-76.
[http://dx.doi.org/10.3858/emm.2008.40.4.461] [PMID: 18779659]

[51]   Tsuchiya H, Sato M, Miyazaki T, *et al.* Comparative study on the antibacterial activity of phytochemical flavanones against methicillin-resistant *Staphylococcus aureus*. J Ethnopharmacol 1996; 50(1): 27-34.
[http://dx.doi.org/10.1016/0378-8741(96)85514-0] [PMID: 8778504]

[52]   Nakayama T, Hashimoto T, Kajiya K, Kumazawa S. Affinity of polyphenols for lipid bilayers. Biofactors 2000; 13(1-4): 147-51.
[http://dx.doi.org/10.1002/biof.5520130124] [PMID: 11237174]

[53]   Clemente-Soto AF, Balderas-Rentería I, Rivera G, Segura-Cabrera A, Garza-González E, del Rayo Camacho-Corona M. Potential mechanism of action of meso-dihydroguaiaretic acid on *Mycobacterium tuberculosis* H37Rv. Molecules 2014; 19(12): 20170-82.
[http://dx.doi.org/10.3390/molecules191220170] [PMID: 25474289]

[54]   Zhang Y, Xu S, Lin J, *et al.* mTORC1 is a target of nordihydroguaiaretic acid to prevent breast tumor growth *in vitro* and *in vivo*. Breast Cancer Res Treat 2012; 136(2): 379-88.
[http://dx.doi.org/10.1007/s10549-012-2270-7] [PMID: 23053656]

[55]   Guzmán-Beltrán S, Orozco-Ibarra M, González-Cuahutencos O, *et al.* Neuroprotective effect and reactive oxygen species scavenging capacity of mangosteen pericarp extract in cultured neurons. Curr Top Nutraceutical Res 2008; 6.

[56]   Zúñiga-Toalá A, Zatarain-Barrón ZL, Hernández-Pando R, *et al.* Nordihydroguaiaretic acid induces

Nrf2 nuclear translocation *in vivo* and attenuates renal damage and apoptosis in the ischemia and reperfusion model. Phytomedicine 2013; 20(10): 775-9.
[http://dx.doi.org/10.1016/j.phymed.2013.03.020] [PMID: 23643094]

[57]   Gonzalez Y, Aryal B, Chehab L, Rao VA. Atg7- and Keap1-dependent autophagy protects breast cancer cell lines against mitoquinone-induced oxidative stress. Oncotarget 2014; 5(6): 1526-37.
[http://dx.doi.org/10.18632/oncotarget.1715] [PMID: 24681637]

[58]   Friedlander TW, Weinberg VK, Huang Y, *et al.* A phase II study of insulin-like growth factor receptor inhibition with nordihydroguaiaretic acid in men with non-metastatic hormone-sensitive prostate cancer. Oncol Rep 2012; 27(1): 3-9.
[http://dx.doi.org/10.3892/or.2011.1487] [PMID: 21971890]

[59]   Masoprocol | C18H22O4 - PubChem n.d. https://pubchem.ncbi.nlm.nih.gov/ compound/ 71398#section=2D-Structure [(accessed April 26, 2020).];

[60]   Cyclandelate | C17H24O3 - PubChem n.d. https://pubchem.ncbi.nlm.nih.gov/compound/2893 [(accessed April 26, 2020).];

[61]   Agüero F, Al-Lazikani B, Aslett M, *et al.* Genomic-scale prioritization of drug targets: the TDR Targets database. Nat Rev Drug Discov 2008; 7(11): 900-7.
[http://dx.doi.org/10.1038/nrd2684] [PMID: 18927591]

[62]   Al-Massarani SM, El Gamal AA, Al-Musayeib NM, *et al.* Phytochemical, antimicrobial and antiprotozoal evaluation of *Garcinia mangostana* pericarp and α-mangostin, its major xanthone derivative. Molecules 2013; 18(9): 10599-608.
[http://dx.doi.org/10.3390/molecules180910599] [PMID: 24002136]

[63]   Chaivisuthangkura A, Malaikaew Y, Chaovanalikit A, *et al.* Prenylated xanthone composition of *Garcinia mangostana* (Mangosteen) fruit hull. Chromatographia 2009.
[http://dx.doi.org/10.1365/s10337-008-0890-1]

[64]   Ji X, Avula B, Khan IA. Quantitative and qualitative determination of six xanthones in *Garcinia mangostana* L. by LC-PDA and LC-ESI-MS. J Pharm Biomed Anal 2007; 43(4): 1270-6.
[http://dx.doi.org/10.1016/j.jpba.2006.10.018] [PMID: 17129697]

[65]   Peres V, Nagem TJ, de Oliveira FF. Tetraoxygenated naturally occurring xanthones. Phytochemistry 2000; 55(7): 683-710.
[http://dx.doi.org/10.1016/S0031-9422(00)00303-4] [PMID: 11190384]

[66]   Suksamrarn S, Suwannapoch N, Phakhodee W, *et al.* Antimycobacterial activity of prenylated xanthones from the fruits of *Garcinia mangostana*. Chem Pharm Bull (Tokyo) 2003; 51(7): 857-9.
[http://dx.doi.org/10.1248/cpb.51.857] [PMID: 12843596]

[67]   Ketsa S, Paull RE. Mangosteen (*Garcinia mangostana* L.). Postharvest Biol. Technol. Trop. Subtrop. Fruits. Elsevier 2011; pp. 1-32e.

[68]   Gutierrez-Orozco F, Chitchumroonchokchai C, Lesinski GB, Suksamrarn S, Failla ML. α-Mangostin: anti-inflammatory activity and metabolism by human cells. J Agric Food Chem 2013; 61(16): 3891-900.
[http://dx.doi.org/10.1021/jf4004434] [PMID: 23578285]

[69]   Mohan S, Syam S, Abdelwahab SI, Thangavel N. An anti-inflammatory molecular mechanism of action of α-mangostin, the major xanthone from the pericarp of *Garcinia mangostana*: an in silico, *in vitro* and *in vivo* approach. Food Funct 2018; 9(7): 3860-71.
[http://dx.doi.org/10.1039/C8FO00439K] [PMID: 29953154]

[70]   Fu T, Li H, Zhao Y, *et al.* Hepatoprotective effect of α-mangostin against lipopolysaccharide/d-galactosamine-induced acute liver failure in mice. Biomed Pharmacother 2018; 106: 896-901.
[http://dx.doi.org/10.1016/j.biopha.2018.07.034] [PMID: 30119260]

[71]   Sudta P, Jiarawapi P, Suksamrarn A, Hongmanee P, Suksamrarn S. Potent activity against multidrug-resistant *Mycobacterium tuberculosis* of α-mangostin analogs. Chem Pharm Bull (Tokyo) 2013; 61(2):

194-203.
[http://dx.doi.org/10.1248/cpb.c12-00874] [PMID: 23150066]

[72]   Koh J-J, Qiu S, Zou H, *et al.* Rapid bactericidal action of alpha-mangostin against MRSA as an outcome of membrane targeting. Biochim Biophys Acta 2013; 1828(2): 834-44.
[http://dx.doi.org/10.1016/j.bbamem.2012.09.004] [PMID: 22982495]

[73]   Nguyen PTM, Marquis RE. Antimicrobial actions of α-mangostin against oral streptococci. Can J Microbiol 2011; 57(3): 217-25.
[http://dx.doi.org/10.1139/W10-122] [PMID: 21358763]

[74]   Kim S-J, Hong E-H, Lee B-R, *et al.* α-mangostin reduced ER stress-mediated tumor growth through autophagy activation. Immune Netw 2012; 12(6): 253-60.
[http://dx.doi.org/10.4110/in.2012.12.6.253] [PMID: 23396851]

[75]   Chao AC, Hsu YL, Liu CK, Kuo PL. α-Mangostin, a dietary xanthone, induces autophagic cell death by activating the AMP-activated protein kinase pathway in glioblastoma cells. J Agric Food Chem 2011; 59(5): 2086-96.
[http://dx.doi.org/10.1021/jf1042757] [PMID: 21314123]

[76]   Chen JJ, Long ZJ, Xu DF, *et al.* Inhibition of autophagy augments the anticancer activity of α-mangostin in chronic myeloid leukemia cells. Leuk Lymphoma 2014; 55(3): 628-38.
[http://dx.doi.org/10.3109/10428194.2013.802312] [PMID: 23734655]

[77]   Ovalle-Magallanes B, Eugenio-Pérez D, Pedraza-Chaverri J. Medicinal properties of mangosteen (*Garcinia mangostana* L.): A comprehensive update. Food Chem Toxicol 2017; 109(Pt 1): 102-22.
[http://dx.doi.org/10.1016/j.fct.2017.08.021] [PMID: 28842267]

[78]   Kondo M, Zhang L, Ji H, Kou Y, Ou B. Bioavailability and antioxidant effects of a xanthone-rich Mangosteen (*Garcinia mangostana*) product in humans. J Agric Food Chem 2009; 57(19): 8788-92.
[http://dx.doi.org/10.1021/jf901012f] [PMID: 19807152]

[79]   Propantheline | C23H30NO3+ - PubChem n.d. https://pubchem.ncbi.nlm.nih.gov/compound/4934#section=Chemical-Vendors [(accessed April 26, 2020).];

[80]   Flupentixol | C23H25F3N2OS - PubChem n.d. https://pubchem.ncbi.nlm.nih.gov/compound/5281881 [(accessed April 26, 2020).];

[81]   Tiotixene | C23H29N3O2S2 - PubChem n.d. https://pubchem.ncbi.nlm.nih.gov/compound/941651 [(accessed April 26, 2020).];

[82]   DeJesus MA, Gerrick ER, Xu W, *et al.* Comprehensive essentiality analysis of the *Mycobacterium tuberculosis* genome *via* saturating transposon mutagenesis. MBio 2017; 8(1): e02133-16.
[http://dx.doi.org/10.1128/mBio.02133-16] [PMID: 28096490]

[83]   Shang A, Cao S-Y, Xu X-Y, *et al.* Bioactive compounds and biological functions of garlic (*Allium sativum* L.). Foods 2019; 8(7): 246.
[http://dx.doi.org/10.3390/foods8070246] [PMID: 31284512]

[84]   Keusgen M, Fritsch RM, Hisoriev H, Kurbonova PA, Khassanov FO. Wild Allium species (Alliaceae) used in folk medicine of Tajikistan and Uzbekistan. J Ethnobiol Ethnomed 2006; 2: 18.
[http://dx.doi.org/10.1186/1746-4269-2-18] [PMID: 16584547]

[85]   Viswanathan V, Phadatare AG, Mukne A. Antimycobacterial and antibacterial activity of *Allium sativum* bulbs. Indian J Pharm Sci 2014; 76(3): 256-61.
[PMID: 25035540]

[86]   Fernández-Bedmar Z, Demyda-Peyrás S, Merinas-Amo T, Del Río-Celestino M. Nutraceutic potential of two *Allium* species and their distinctive organosulfur compounds: A multi-assay evaluation. Foods 2019; 8(6): 222.
[http://dx.doi.org/10.3390/foods8060222] [PMID: 31234398]

[87]   Diretto G, Rubio-Moraga A, Argandoña J, Castillo P, Gómez-Gómez L, Ahrazem O. Tissue-specific

accumulation of sulfur compounds and saponins in different parts of garlic cloves from purple and white ecotypes. Molecules 2017; 22(8): 1359.
[http://dx.doi.org/10.3390/molecules22081359] [PMID: 28825644]

[88]   Szychowski K, Rybczyńska-Tkaczyk K, Gaweł-Bęben K, *et al.* Characterization of active compounds of different garlic (*Allium sativum* L.) Cultivars. Pol J Food Nutr Sci 2018; 68: 73-81.
[http://dx.doi.org/10.1515/pjfns-2017-0005]

[89]   Borlinghaus J, Albrecht F, Gruhlke MC, Nwachukwu ID, Slusarenko AJ. Allicin: Chemistry and biological properties. Molecules 2014; 19(8): 12591-618.
[http://dx.doi.org/10.3390/molecules190812591] [PMID: 25153873]

[90]   Miron T, Rabinkov A, Mirelman D, Wilchek M, Weiner L. The mode of action of allicin: Its ready permeability through phospholipid membranes may contribute to its biological activity. Biochim Biophys Acta 2000; 1463(1): 20-30.
[http://dx.doi.org/10.1016/S0005-2736(99)00174-1] [PMID: 10631291]

[91]   Reiter J, Levina N, van der Linden M, Gruhlke M, Martin C, Slusarenko AJ. Diallylthiosulfinate (Allicin), a volatile antimicrobial from garlic (*Allium sativum*), kills human lung pathogenic bacteria, including mdr strains, as a vapor. Molecules 2017; 22(10): 1711.
[http://dx.doi.org/10.3390/molecules22101711] [PMID: 29023413]

[92]   Curtis H, Noll U, Störmann J, Slusarenko AJ. Broad-spectrum activity of the volatile phytoanticipin allicin in extracts of garlic (*Allium sativum* L.) against plant pathogenic bacteria, fungi and Oomycetes. Physiol Mol Plant Pathol 2004; 65: 79-89.
[http://dx.doi.org/10.1016/j.pmpp.2004.11.006]

[93]   Yamada Y, Azuma K. Evaluation of the *in vitro* antifungal activity of allicin. Antimicrob Agents Chemother 1977; 11(4): 743-9.
[http://dx.doi.org/10.1128/AAC.11.4.743] [PMID: 856026]

[94]   Salama AA, AbouLaila M, Terkawi MA, *et al.* Inhibitory effect of allicin on the growth of babesia and theileria equi parasites. Parasitol Res 2014; 113(1): 275-83.
[http://dx.doi.org/10.1007/s00436-013-3654-2] [PMID: 24173810]

[95]   Son E-W, Mo S-J, Rhee D-K, Pyo S. Inhibition of ICAM-1 expression by garlic component, allicin, in gamma-irradiated human vascular endothelial cells *via* downregulation of the JNK signaling pathway. Int Immunopharmacol 2006; 6(12): 1788-95.
[http://dx.doi.org/10.1016/j.intimp.2006.07.021] [PMID: 17052669]

[96]   Chu YL, Ho CT, Chung JG, Rajasekaran R, Sheen LY. Allicin induces p53-mediated autophagy in Hep G2 human liver cancer cells. J Agric Food Chem 2012; 60(34): 8363-71.
[http://dx.doi.org/10.1021/jf301298y] [PMID: 22860996]

[97]   Lawson LD, Hunsaker SM. Allicin Bioavailability and Bioequivalence from Garlic Supplements and Garlic Foods. Nutrients 2018; 10(7): E812.
[http://dx.doi.org/10.3390/nu10070812] [PMID: 29937536]

[98]   Gruhlke MCH, Antelmann H, Bernhardt J, Kloubert V, Rink L, Slusarenko AJ. The human allicin-proteome: S-thioallylation of proteins by the garlic defence substance allicin and its biological effects. Free Radic Biol Med 2019; 131: 144-53.
[http://dx.doi.org/10.1016/j.freeradbiomed.2018.11.022] [PMID: 30500420]

[99]   Phosphonoacetohydroxamic acid | C2H6NO5P - PubChem n.d. https://pubchem.ncbi.nlm.nih.gov/compound/445375 [(accessed April 26, 2020).];

[100]   Zhao Q, Chen X-Y, Martin C. *Scutellaria baicalensis*, the golden herb from the garden of Chinese medicinal plants. Sci Bull (Beijing) 2016; 61(18): 1391-8.
[http://dx.doi.org/10.1007/s11434-016-1136-5] [PMID: 27730005]

[101]   Shan B, Cai Y-Z, Brooks JD, Corke H. The *in vitro* antibacterial activity of dietary spice and medicinal herb extracts. Int J Food Microbiol 2007; 117(1): 112-9.

[http://dx.doi.org/10.1016/j.ijfoodmicro.2007.03.003] [PMID: 17449125]

[102] Blaszczyk T, Krzyzanowska J, Lamer-Zarawska E. Screening for antimycotic properties of 56 traditional Chinese drugs. Phytother Res 2000; 14(3): 210-2.
[http://dx.doi.org/10.1002/(SICI)1099-1573(200005)14:3<210::AID-PTR591>3.0.CO;2-7] [PMID: 10815018]

[103] Tang Z, Peng M, Zhan C. Screening 20 Chinese herbs often used for clearing heat and dissipating toxin with nude mice model of hepatitis C viral infection. Zhongguo Zhong Xi Yi Jie He Za Zhi Zhongguo Zhongxiyi Jiehe Zazhi = Chinese J Integr Tradit West Med 2003; 23: 447-8.

[104] Zhao T, Tang H, Xie L, *et al.* Scutellaria baicalensis Georgi. (Lamiaceae): a review of its traditional uses, botany, phytochemistry, pharmacology and toxicology. J Pharm Pharmacol 2019; 71(9): 1353-69.
[http://dx.doi.org/10.1111/jphp.13129] [PMID: 31236960]

[105] Han J, Ye M, Xu M, Sun J, Wang B, Guo D. Characterization of flavonoids in the traditional Chinese herbal medicine-Huangqin by liquid chromatography coupled with electrospray ionization mass spectrometry. J Chromatogr B Analyt Technol Biomed Life Sci 2007; 848(2): 355-62.
[http://dx.doi.org/10.1016/j.jchromb.2006.10.061] [PMID: 17118721]

[106] Zhu W, Jin Z, Yu J, *et al.* Baicalin ameliorates experimental inflammatory bowel disease through polarization of macrophages to an M2 phenotype. Int Immunopharmacol 2016; 35: 119-26.
[http://dx.doi.org/10.1016/j.intimp.2016.03.030] [PMID: 27039210]

[107] Yu C, Zhang Z, Zhang H, *et al.* Pretreatment of baicalin and wogonoside with glycoside hydrolase: a promising approach to enhance anticancer potential. Oncol Rep 2013; 30(5): 2411-8.
[http://dx.doi.org/10.3892/or.2013.2726] [PMID: 24026776]

[108] Zhao QY, Yuan FW, Liang T, *et al.* Baicalin inhibits *Escherichia coli* isolates in bovine mastitic milk and reduces antimicrobial resistance. J Dairy Sci 2018; 101(3): 2415-22.
[http://dx.doi.org/10.3168/jds.2017-13349] [PMID: 29290430]

[109] Luo J, Dong B, Wang K, *et al.* Baicalin inhibits biofilm formation, attenuates the quorum sensing-controlled virulence and enhances Pseudomonas aeruginosa clearance in a mouse peritoneal implant infection model. PLoS One 2017; 12(4): e0176883.
[http://dx.doi.org/10.1371/journal.pone.0176883] [PMID: 28453568]

[110] Wu J, Hu D, Wang K-XX. Study of Scutellaria baicalensis and Baicalin against antimicrobial susceptibility of *Helicobacter pylori* strains *in vitro.* Zhong Yao Cai 2008; 31(5): 707-10.
[PMID: 18826148]

[111] Wang G, Gao Y, Wang H, Niu X, Wang J. Baicalin Weakens *Staphylococcus aureus* Pathogenicity by Targeting Sortase B. Front Cell Infect Microbiol 2018; 8: 418.
[http://dx.doi.org/10.3389/fcimb.2018.00418] [PMID: 30555803]

[112] Wan JY, Gong X, Zhang L, Li HZ, Zhou YF, Zhou QX. Protective effect of baicalin against lipopolysaccharide/D-galactosamine-induced liver injury in mice by up-regulation of heme oxygenase-1. Eur J Pharmacol 2008; 587(1-3): 302-8.
[http://dx.doi.org/10.1016/j.ejphar.2008.02.081] [PMID: 18420187]

[113] Zhang ZQ, Liua W, Zhuang L, Wang J, Zhang S. Comparative pharmacokinetics of baicalin, wogonoside, baicalein and wogonin in plasma after oral administration of pure baicalin, radix scutellariae and scutellariae-paeoniae couple extracts in normal and ulcerative colitis rats. Iran J Pharm Res 2013; 12(3): 399-409.
[http://dx.doi.org/10.22037/ijpr.2013.1331] [PMID: 24250647]

[114] Xing J, Chen X, Zhong D. Absorption and enterohepatic circulation of baicalin in rats. Life Sci 2005; 78(2): 140-6.
[http://dx.doi.org/10.1016/j.lfs.2005.04.072] [PMID: 16107266]

[115] Zhang J, Cai W, Zhou Y, *et al.* Profiling and identification of the metabolites of baicalin and study on

their tissue distribution in rats by ultra-high-performance liquid chromatography with linear ion trap-Orbitrap mass spectrometer. J Chromatogr B Analyt Technol Biomed Life Sci 2015; 985: 91-102.
[http://dx.doi.org/10.1016/j.jchromb.2015.01.018] [PMID: 25661005]

[116]   Huang T, Liu Y, Zhang C. Pharmacokinetics and bioavailability enhancement of baicalin: A review. Eur J Drug Metab Pharmacokinet 2019; 44(2): 159-68.
[http://dx.doi.org/10.1007/s13318-018-0509-3] [PMID: 30209794]

[117]   Hang Y, Qin X, Ren T, Cao J. Baicalin reduces blood lipids and inflammation in patients with coronary artery disease and rheumatoid arthritis: a randomized, double-blind, placebo-controlled trial. Lipids Health Dis 2018; 17(1): 146.
[http://dx.doi.org/10.1186/s12944-018-0797-2] [PMID: 29935544]

[118]   Apigenin | C15H10O5 - PubChem n.d. https://pubchem.ncbi.nlm.nih.gov/compound/5280443 [(accessed April 26, 2020).];

[119]   Diosmetin | C16H12O6 - PubChem n.d. https://pubchem.ncbi.nlm.nih.gov/compound/5281612 [(accessed April 26, 2020).];

[120]   Rengarajan J, Bloom BR, Rubin EJ. Genome-wide requirements for *Mycobacterium tuberculosis* adaptation and survival in macrophages. Proc Natl Acad Sci USA 2005; 102(23): 8327-32.
[http://dx.doi.org/10.1073/pnas.0503272102] [PMID: 15928073]

[121]   Evans Schultes R. Medicinal plants of East and Southeast Asia: Attributed properties. Econ Bot 1980; 34: 361-1.
[http://dx.doi.org/10.1007/BF02858311]

[122]   Kardono LBS, Angerhofer CK, Tsauri S, Padmawinata K, Pezzuto JM, Kinghorn AD. Cytotoxic and antimalarial constituents of the roots of *Eurycoma longifolia*. J Nat Prod 1991; 54(5): 1360-7.
[http://dx.doi.org/10.1021/np50077a020] [PMID: 1800638]

[123]   Farouk A-E, Benafri A. Antibacterial activity of *Eurycoma longifolia* Jack. A Malaysian medicinal plant. Saudi Med J 2007; 28(9): 1422-4.
[PMID: 17768473]

[124]   Bhat R, Karim AA. Tongkat Ali (*Eurycoma longifolia* Jack): a review on its ethnobotany and pharmacological importance. Fitoterapia 2010; 81(7): 669-79.
[http://dx.doi.org/10.1016/j.fitote.2010.04.006] [PMID: 20434529]

[125]   Rehman SU, Choe K, Yoo HH. Review on a traditional herbal medicine, *Eurycoma longifolia* jack (Tongkat Ali): Its traditional uses, chemistry, evidence-based pharmacology and toxicology. Molecules 2016; 21(3): 331.
[http://dx.doi.org/10.3390/molecules21030331] [PMID: 26978330]

[126]   Tung NH, Uto T, Hai NT, Li G, Shoyama Y. Quassinoids from the root of *Eurycoma longifolia* and their antiproliferative activity on human cancer cell lines. Pharmacogn Mag 2017; 13(51): 459-62.
[http://dx.doi.org/10.4103/pm.pm_353_16] [PMID: 28839372]

[127]   George A, Suzuki N, Abas AB, *et al.* Immunomodulation in middle-aged humans *via* the ingestion of Physta® standardized root water extract of *Eurycoma longifolia* Jack - A randomized, double-blind, placebo-controlled, parallel study. Phytother Res 2016; 30(4): 627-35.
[http://dx.doi.org/10.1002/ptr.5571] [PMID: 26816234]

[128]   Salman SAB, Amrah S, Wahab MSA, *et al.* Modification of propranolol's bioavailability by *Eurycoma longifolia* water-based extract. J Clin Pharm Ther 2010; 35(6): 691-6.
[http://dx.doi.org/10.1111/j.1365-2710.2009.01147.x] [PMID: 21054461]

[129]   Bevirimat | C36H56O6 - PubChem n.d. https://pubchem.ncbi.nlm.nih.gov/compound/457928 [(accessed April 27, 2020).];

[130]   Trioxsalen | C14H12O3 - PubChem n.d. https://pubchem.ncbi.nlm.nih.gov/compound/5585 [(accessed April 26, 2020).];

[131] Zumla A, Rao M, Wallis RS, *et al.* Host-directed therapies for infectious diseases: current status, recent progress, and future prospects. Lancet Infect Dis 2016; 16(4): e47-63.
[http://dx.doi.org/10.1016/S1473-3099(16)00078-5] [PMID: 27036359]

[132] Wallis RS, Hafner R. Advancing host-directed therapy for tuberculosis. Nat Rev Immunol 2015; 15(4): 255-63.
[http://dx.doi.org/10.1038/nri3813] [PMID: 25765201]

CHAPTER 3

Induction and Activation of Intracellular Antimicrobial Molecules for Mycobacterial Control

Laura E. Carreto-Binaghi and **Yolanda Gonzalez**[*]

Departamento de Investigación en Microbiología, Instituto Nacional de Enfermedades Respiratorias Ismael Cosío Villegas, CDMX, Mexico

Abstract: The primary function of antimicrobial molecules is the interaction with pathogens to clear infections. In this chapter, we discuss the role that antimicrobial peptides (AMPs), nitric oxide (NO), and reactive oxygen species (ROS) play in the elimination of intracellular bacteria and their induction by immunomodulators like vitamin D, focusing on the mycobacterial infection. AMPs are the major mechanisms to directly eliminate intracellular bacteria such as *Mycobacterium tuberculosis* or *Salmonella* sp. Cathelicidins (LL-37) and β-defensins (HBD-2) are the most studied AMPs, due to their relevance in the immunopathogenesis of several infectious diseases. Additionally, the production of ROS also kills intracellular bacteria directly, especially within the phagosome; patients with ROS deficiencies are susceptible to tuberculous mycobacterial infections. However, excessive production of ROS might induce cell death by apoptosis. The active form of vitamin D ($1\alpha,25(OH)_2D3$) is a key inducer of antimicrobial mechanisms. Vitamin D is involved in redox homeostasis, regulating the effect of ROS and NO to protect the cell integrity; and as an activator of anti-infective pathways for pathogen elimination through induction of AMPs and autophagy. The ability of induction of antimicrobial mechanisms confers these molecules a potential use as adjunct therapies in several infections.

Keywords: Antimicrobial peptides (AMPs), Autophagy, β-defensins, Cathelicidin, Hepcidin, IFN-γ, LL-37, *M. tuberculosis*, NADPH oxidase, Nitric oxide (NO), Reactive oxygen species (ROS), Vitamin D, Vitamin D receptor (VDR).

INTRODUCTION

The innate immunity is the first defense against microorganisms. The response to infections is a complex and dynamic process involving multiple cell types and

[*] **Corresponding author Yolanda Gonzalez:** Departamento de Investigación en Microbiología, Instituto Nacional de Enfermedades Respiratorias Ismael Cosío Villegas, CDMX, Mexico; Tel: 54871700, Ext. 5117; E-mail: ygonzalezh@iner.gob.mx

soluble factors such as cytokines, chemokines, and hormones coordinated through a series of cellular and molecular interactions. Antimicrobial peptides (AMPs) are a key part of these molecules. Their primary function is the elimination of pathogenic microorganisms. AMPs are mostly expressed on epithelial cells, which are the first barrier to invading or colonizing pathogens or stored in the intracellular granules of phagocytes [1]. Other functions of these peptides have been recently described, such as immunomodulation, wound repair, endotoxin neutralization, angiogenesis, and chemoattraction [1, 2]. AMPs are small molecules composed of cationic sequences of amino acids, conferring them hydrophobic properties [3, 4]; they induce phosphorylation of mitogen-activated protein kinases (MAPKs) to activate the pro-inflammatory cascade in the response against microbial pathogens [5]. In macrophages and epithelial cells, the antimicrobial mechanisms are inducible; they have potential use as adjunct therapies in several infections. Vitamin D is one of such inducers and will be discussed below.

The archetype of intracellular infections is *M. tuberculosis*, which is the causative agent of tuberculosis and a leading cause of morbidity and mortality worldwide [6]. *M. tuberculosis* is transmitted primarily by the respiratory route, and, in most cases, human tuberculosis is a pulmonary disease [7]. AMPs primarily control the infection with *M. tuberculosis*, and this chapter focuses on the role that AMPs and other antimicrobial effectors play in this infection.

ANTI-INFECTIVE MOLECULES AND THEIR NICHES OF ACTIVATION

Antimicrobial Peptides

The canonical AMPs comprise two families: cathelicidins and defensins, which are produced in immune cells, predominantly macrophages and neutrophils [3, 4], but also by non-immune cells. Both types of AMPs disrupt the integrity of the bacterial cell membrane, resulting in the death of microbes [2]. Cathelicidins are linear peptides that form α-helices. LL-37 is the only representative molecule of this family of AMPs described for both mice and humans. LL-37 has a broad spectrum of activity against both Gram-negative and Gram-positive bacteria, several viruses, and fungi [8]. Its precursor is called the human cationic antimicrobial peptide of 18 kDa (hCAP18) and is cleaved by cellular proteases to release the active form of LL-37 [5, 9]. Different cells express LL-37 including epithelial cells, neutrophils, NK cells, T and B cells, as well as urinary, respiratory, digestive, and epidermal cells [5, 10], with diverse effects that are tissue-dependent [11]. For chemoattraction, cathelicidin interacts with the formyl-peptide receptor-like 1, a G protein-coupled receptor that also promotes angiogenesis, and is present on monocytes, neutrophils, and CD4+ T lymphocytes; moreover, cathelicidin enhances the production of chemokines (IL-8 and monocyte-chemoattractant proteins 1 and 3) and histamine, thus increasing the migration of immune cells to tissues [1].

Cathelicidins offer innate unspecific responses to different kinds of pathogens [11, 12]. The immunomodulatory role of cathelicidin relies on its ability to bind lipopolysaccharide and lipoteichoic acid, preventing their receptor-ligand recognition. This lack of recognition eventually translates into the reduction of the transcription of pro-inflammatory molecules (*e.g.,* TNF-α, and NO), conferring LL-37 an anti-inflammatory role in Gram-negative infections [1]. In mycobacterial infections, cathelicidins also act as chemoattractants of CD4+ T cells, neutrophils, and monocytes, as well as immunomodulators of pro-inflammatory cytokines production, and inducers of apoptosis [12]. In mycobacterial pulmonary infections, pulmonary levels of LL-37 increase in a ROS-, nicotinamide adenine dinucleotide phosphatase (NADPH) oxidase-, and toll-like receptor 2 (TLR-2)-dependent manner [11], for mycobacterial phagocytosis and killing [13, 14].

Defensins are polypeptides folded mainly in β-sheets, classified as α-, β-, or θ-defensins according to the number of disulfide bridges and cysteine residues. Defensins play an important role in innate immunity, especially in the skin and lungs [15]. Human α- and β-defensins are mainly produced by immune (monocytes, macrophages, and dendritic cells) and mucosal epithelial cells (from the respiratory and urogenital tract, and skin) [10, 16]. Many human tissues express β-defensin 1 (HBD-1) constitutively. In contrast, other defensins (HBD-2, HBD-3, and HBD-4) are expressed in response to inflammatory stimuli, such as IL-1α, IL-1β, or TNF-α, mainly associated to microbial pathogens (bacteria, fungi, viruses, or parasites) [1, 10] (Fig. **1**).

The AMPs have three common ways to eliminate microorganisms: 1) the peptides bind to the bacterial cell membrane and arrange themselves forming a pore that consequently leads to bacterial lysis; 2) the peptides bind along the cell membrane as an external layer; 3) the peptides forming a pore bind the lipid head groups and disrupt the membrane [11, 12]. Bacterial membrane destruction leads to electrostatic alteration and modification of oxidative metabolism [11]. The AMPs also exert activities inside the bacteria, such as blocking DNA synthesis. The activities of AMPs extend to the host cell, by modulating gene transcription, apoptosis, or cytokine production, and the immune response against pathogens [12] (Fig. **2**).

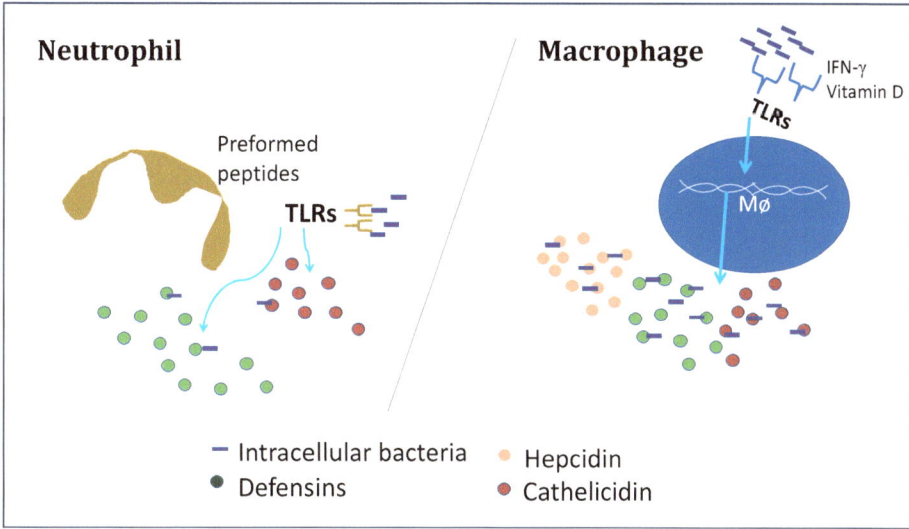

Fig. (1). Antimicrobial peptides in the immune response to an intracellular pathogen. Infection with intracellular pathogens induces immune cells like neutrophils and macrophages to produce pro-inflammatory cytokines and all the necessary mechanisms for bacterial elimination. For example, *M. tuberculosis* activates Toll-like receptors (TLRs) 2 and 4, which in turn, induce the release of preformed peptides by neutrophils or their synthesis in macrophages in the presence of IFN-γ and Vitamin D.

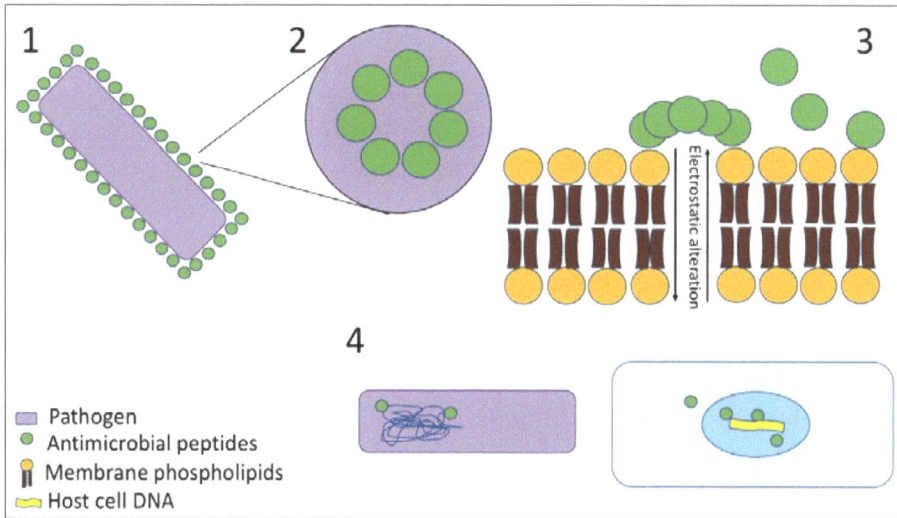

Fig. (2). Mechanisms of action of antimicrobial peptides (AMPs) to eliminate microorganisms. **1)** the peptides bind along the bacterial membrane to form an external layer; **2)** the peptides bind to the bacterial cell membrane and arrange themselves forming a pore; **3)** the peptides forming a pore attach to the lipid head groups and disrupt the membrane, leading to electrostatic alteration and modification of the oxidative metabolism. **4)** AMPs block bacterial DNA synthesis or interfere with the host cell processes (*e.g.,* gene transcription, apoptosis, or cytokine production), thus modulating the immune response against pathogens.

Antimicrobial Molecules (NO and ROS)

Nitric oxide (NO) and reactive oxygen intermediates are toxic molecules used by the immune system. NO is a significant mediator of cell-mediated antimycobacterial activities through the regulation of an array of genes that include reactive nitrogen intermediates produced in macrophages *via* NADPH oxidase (NOX2/gp91phox) and inducible nitric oxide synthase (iNOS) for bacterial degradation [17]. The importance of NO was demonstrated in an experimental model with iNOS-deficient mice, which lack inducible NO production, and are highly susceptible to *Mycobacterium tuberculosis* infection [18]. Previous results from our group showed that NO is released from *M. tuberculosis*-infected human blood monocytes and alveolar macrophages, conferring antimycobacterial activity. Moreover, NO was detectable in alveolar macrophages supernatants from household contacts of tuberculosis patients on days 4 and 7 post-infection [19]. Other reports also suggest that NO prevents *M. tuberculosis* growth and the subsequent inflammatory response, as well as the direct modulation of inflammation that impacts upon *M. tuberculosis* growth and function [20].

ROS (such as H_2O_2 and superoxide anion, O_2^-) are also produced *via* NADPH oxidase [17]. In mammals, O_2^- is generated by NADPH oxidase and xanthine oxidase systems; the superoxide radical is converted into several chemically distinct oxidants such as hydrogen peroxide H_2O_2, hypochlorite, hydroxyl radicals, and peroxynitrite. These ROS damage microbial DNA, lipids, proteins, as well as particularly susceptible cellular constituents such as iron-sulfur cluster proteins [21]. ROS are important to initiate inflammatory signaling cascades *via* protein kinase pathways, transcription factors, and genomic expression of pro-inflammatory regulators, leading to an overactivated immune system. ROS induction is essential for bacterial killing, as the infected macrophage initiates a respiratory burst and produces high ROS levels to counteract and kill mycobacteria [22]. ROS concentration is important for *M. tuberculosis* killing; concentrations of 0 - 5.0 mM of H_2O_2 have little effect on mycobacterial viability, whereas concentrations of 50 - 200 mM H_2O_2 are lethal to *M. tuberculosis* [17]. The importance of ROS and NADPH oxidase complex was observed in Chronic Granulomatous Disease, a life-threatening primary immunodeficiency affecting mainly phagocytes, this disease is caused by a mutation of any of the genes encoding one of the components of the NADPH oxidase complex, which is active in all phagocytes, including granulocytes, monocytes, and macrophages. In patients with tuberculosis, several mutations have been associated with the inability to produce NADPH-oxidase-dependent ROS, which are required for the phagocytic killing of microorganisms. The most important mutations are: CYBB (70% of cases), which is located on the X chromosome and encodes gp91phox;

CYBA (5% of cases), which encodes p22phox; NCF1 (20% of cases), which encodes p47phox; and NCF2 (5% of cases), which encodes p67phox. These mutations have been shown to confer a selective predisposition to tuberculous mycobacteria and a high susceptibility to pyogenic bacterial and fungal infections, particularly caused by *Staphylococcus aureus* and *Aspergillus fumigatus* [23].

The pathways of AMPs and ROS are interconnected in the activation of anti-infective mechanisms. AMPs promote the generation of ROS that may contribute to various apoptotic pathways as precursors of more potent ROS. The O_2^- is produced from oxygen and then converted to H_2O_2 by superoxide dismutase (SOD) in the mitochondria. H_2O_2 reacts with ferrous ion to produce highly reactive hydroxyl radicals through the Fenton and Haber-Weiss reactions. Due to this fact, it is straightforward for AMPs to induce plasma membrane disruption by direct damage or by indirect induction of apoptosis through intracellular ROS accumulation, especially hydroxyl radicals and the release of cytochrome C *via* complete depolarization of the mitochondrial membrane [24].

The anti-infective effect of NO and ROS occurs within the phagosome, where highly reactive intermediates are generated to induce oxidation and hence degradation of many proteins and lipids, leading to bacterial killing. In patients with tuberculosis, urinary levels of NO and nitrate increase during active disease as a defense mechanism against *M. tuberculosis*; then, these levels reduce with the anti-tuberculosis treatment [25]. Moreover, patients with active pulmonary tuberculosis present higher levels of NO in the lungs [26]. However, after long-time exposure, there is evidence that NO also damages lung tissue supporting the importance of an inflammatory control process. AMPs and the activation of the NADPH oxidase complex to produce ROS have multiple inducers; vitamin D is one of the best characterized in mycobacterial infections, either *in vivo* or *in vitro*.

INDUCTION AND ACTIVATION OF ANTIMICROBIAL PATHWAYS

Antimicrobial Molecules Induced by Vitamin D

Vitamin D (cholecalciferol, also vitamin D3) is a molecule with different functions in the organism that interacts with several types of cells. Neutrophils, monocytes, B and T lymphocytes, and NK cells bear a vitamin D receptor (VDR) that, upon vitamin D ligation, induces the production of cathelicidin [12] and the expression of other membrane receptors to enhance antimicrobial responses; apparently, this feature occurs mainly in humans [5] and non-human primates [10]. The active form of vitamin D, 1,25-dihydroxycholecalciferol ($1\alpha,25(OH)_2D3$) is produced from endogenous and dietary origins. In the skin, 7-dehydrocholesterol breaks by UV irradiation to form pre-vitamin D3; then, in the liver, it metabolizes into 25 hydroxyvitamin D (25(OH)D3), the principal circulating form of vitamin D. In immune cells, such as monocytes and macrophages, 25(OH)D3 metabolizes into 1α,25-dihydroxyvitamin D3 (1α,25(OH)$_2$D3), herein denominated vitamin D [27].

Vitamin D induces the production of AMPs, both cathelicidins, and defensins, which aid in the defense against viruses and bacteria, and modify cytokine profiles during infection activating the innate and adaptive immune system [28]. Hence, vitamin D deficiency predisposes to a wide variety of infections, including tuberculosis and viral respiratory tract ones [29]. In macrophages, vitamin D also induces the expression of toll-like receptors (TLRs) and enhances phagosome maturation, contributing to the antimicrobial activity related to LL-37 [10]. Vitamin D-induced TLR-2 enhances LL-37 production in mycobacterial infection, favoring phagolysosome fusion and, therefore, bacterial destruction [11]. Vitamin D also triggers LL-37-mediated autophagy to control mycobacterial infections [12] (Fig. **1**).

Additionally, vitamin D induces the HBD-2 gene through the activation of TLRs and other intracellular receptors, such as the nucleotide-binding oligomerization domain protein 2 (NOD-2), in monocytes and epithelial cells. Nevertheless, vitamin D is not a potent activator of inflammation; thus, other signaling pathways must be activated to generate an entire antimicrobial activity [10]; noteworthy, in stress conditions such as hypoxia, HBD-2 is upregulated through the vitamin D pathway [11]. The role of active vitamin D in controlling microbial infections has been well documented; a meta-analysis reported that people with low vitamin D levels in serum have a higher risk of developing active tuberculosis [30].

The relationship between reduced levels of vitamin D and the susceptibility to infections has been under scrutiny for many years. In children with rickets, vitamin D deficiency, the commonly experienced respiratory infections were called "rachitic lung" [31]. Liu *et al.* reported the ability of vitamin D to induce AMPs [13], demonstrating a relationship among pathogen-associated molecular patterns, TLRs activation, VDR, and vitamin D-1α-hydroxylase gene expression, leading to the production of cathelicidin and the killing of intracellular bacteria. They also reported that populations with high levels of skin melanin had an increased susceptibility to tuberculosis, which correlated with low serum levels of 25-hydroxyvitamin D3 (25(OH)D3) and low cathelicidin mRNA induction. These findings confirmed a link between TLRs and vitamin D-mediated innate immunity, suggesting that differences in the ability of human populations to produce vitamin D may contribute to susceptibility to microbial infections [32].

AMPs and autophagy are the main effectors triggered by vitamin D against *M.*

tuberculosis [32, 33]. Vitamin D-induced antimicrobial activity is completely inhibited in the presence of a siRNA for cathelicidin [33, 34]. Also, cathelicidin is essential for the induction of autophagy by vitamin D in bacterial infections [35]. *M. tuberculosis* antigens, such as the 19-kDa lipopeptide, are recognized by TLR-2/1, leading to the induction of cathelicidin and *M. tuberculosis* killing. In addition to the direct response to vitamin D, macrophages are capable of synthesizing vitamin D upon exposure to pathogens. Ligation of macrophage TLRs by *M. tuberculosis* antigens upregulates the expression of macrophage $25(OH)D3\text{-}1\alpha$-hydroxylase [32, 34].

Vitamin D exerts its immunomodulatory activities by binding to its receptor. Immune system cells display a VDR since the early stages of maturation, including B and T lymphocytes (both resting and activated), monocytes, and dendritic cells [36]. VDR belongs to the superfamily of nuclear transcription factors and is a direct inducer of innate antimicrobial immunity in humans. After induction by $1\alpha,25(OH)2D3$, VDR heterodimerizes with retinoid X receptors (RXRs) and translocate to the nucleus. Both elements bind to specific DNA motifs, known as VDR elements (VDRE), located in the promoters of *camp* (hCAP18) and *defb2* (HBD-2) genes [37, 38]. The expression of *camp* expression was strongly stimulated by $1\alpha,25(OH)_2D3$ in epithelial cells, macrophages/monocytes, and neutrophils [39], both at the mRNA and protein levels [32, 35, 37, 40] (Figs. **3** and **4**). In humans, cathelicidin contains activating vitamin D response elements in its promoter region, 507 bp upstream of its transcription initiation site [37]. People with serum vitamin D deficiency had lower induction LL-37 after TLR-2/1 stimulation that people without vitamin D deficiency [32]. Also, $1\alpha,25(OH)_2D3$ modulates other immune antimicrobial responses by binding the VDR, such as NOS (NOS2A) [41].

Because of the essential role of vitamin D for the innate and adaptive immune responses following viral and bacterial infections, vitamin D supplementation has been recommended [42]; however, the dose and regime of vitamin D supplementation required to optimize the outcome of infectious diseases are currently unknown. Its metabolism and functions are modulated by many factors, including physical activity and lifestyle, certain medications, environmental pollutants, and epigenetics, all of which also modify the balance between energy intake and expenditure through mitochondrial metabolic control [43]. However, for a reduction in the incidence of diseases and optimal health, a minimum level of 30-32 ng / mL 25(OH)D3 in serum is necessary [44]. Vitamin D is a suitable candidate for the treatment of mycobacterial infections because stimulation with *M. tuberculosis* and $1\alpha,25(OH)_2D3$ induces not only AMPs production but also upregulation of VDR expression [38, 45, 46].

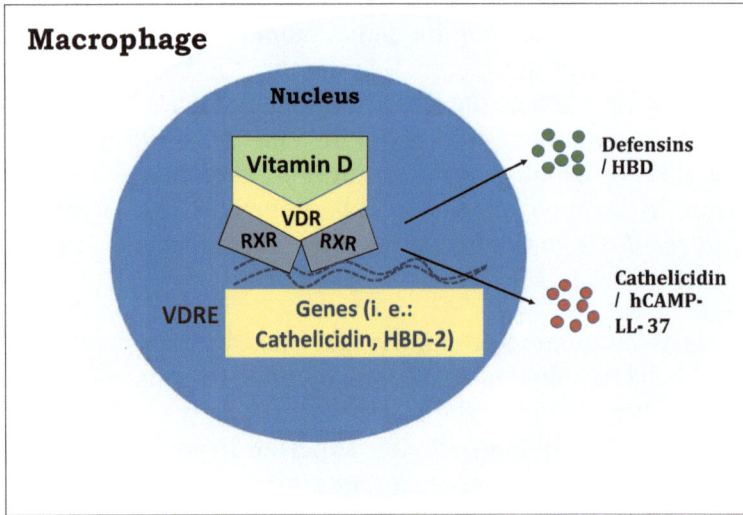

Fig. (3). Vitamin D-induced production of antimicrobial peptides (AMPs). The vitamin D receptor (VDR) is a nuclear receptor that forms a heterodimer with retinoid X receptors (RXRs) before binding to specific DNA motifs (VDR elements, VDRE), located in the promoters of AMP genes. Vitamin D, 1α,25(OH)$_2$D3. NF-κB, Nuclear Factor κB. HBD-2, human β-defensin-2 gene.

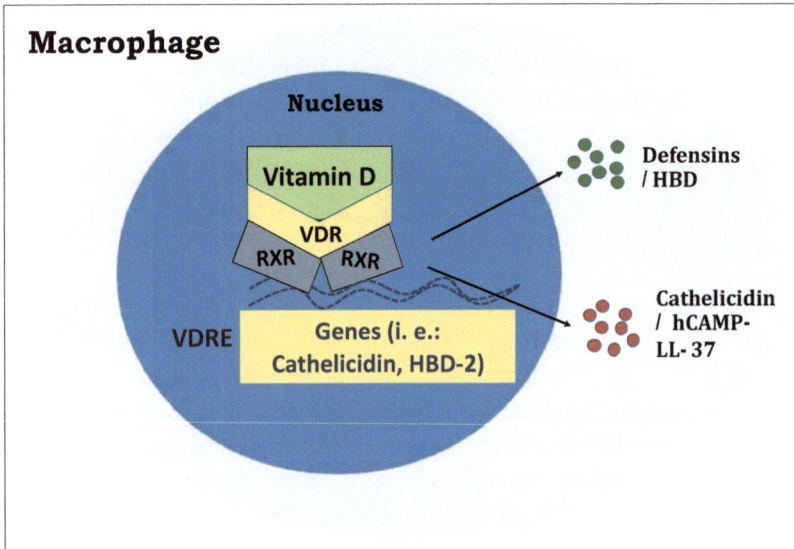

Fig. (4). Vitamin D induces inflammatory cytokines and antimicrobial peptides after intracellular bacterial infection. Antimicrobial activity is elicited after cathelicidin production in macrophages, mainly through the induction of inflammatory cytokines and chemokines. Vitamin D, 1α,25(OH)$_2$D3. NF-κB, Nuclear Factor κB. TLRs, Toll-like receptors. VDR, Vitamin D receptor. RXRs, retinoid X receptors.

Antimicrobial Molecules Induced by Vitamin D and IFN-γ

Vitamin D has no direct antimycobacterial activity, but its bactericidal activity against *M. tuberculosis* is enhanced by costimulation with IFN-γ [47]. IFN-γ is a cytokine produced by lymphocytes, with antiviral, immunoregulatory, and anti-tumoral properties. IFN-γ potentiates mycobacterial killing by upregulating the 1α-hydroxylase and inducing the 25(OH)D3-24-hydroxylase, a vital enzyme in the activation of 1α,25(OH)$_2$D3. Additionally, IFN-γ-induced antimicrobial activity enhances IL-15 production to upregulate CYP27B1, which results in intracellular conversion of 25(OH)D3 to its bioactive form; 1α,25(OH)$_2$D3 binds the VDR, which is required for downstream induction of AMPs, autophagy, and phagosome maturation, contributing to the antimicrobial response in monocytes and macrophages [47]. These processes facilitate the delivery of antimicrobial effector molecules, including AMPs and ubiquitinated peptides, to *M. tuberculosis*-containing vesicles, which otherwise block lysosomal fusion. Autophagy also can enclose pathogens that escape vacuoles and penetrate the cytoplasm, as has been reported to occur with *M. tuberculosis*. IFN-γ-induced autophagy is dependent on the expression of *Atg5* and *Beclin-1* [47]. IFN-γ directly induces autophagy and the recruitment of autophagy proteins to the mycobacterial phagosome in macrophages and also induces NO production, which in turn, promotes autophagy through an autocrine positive-feedback loop [35].

Autophagy is another mechanism to eradicate pathogens, amply described in chapter 5, that eliminates intracellular *M. tuberculosis* through lytic and antimicrobial properties unique to autolysosomes, which are more robust antimicrobial compartments than conventional phagosomes. The autophagosomal content is a mixture of neo-AMPs, known as cryptides, which have enhanced antimycobacterial properties and lysosomal enzymes that drive the autophagic proteolysis of *M. tuberculosis* together with other cytosolic proteins such as ribosomal proteins [48].

Antimicrobial Molecules Induced by Autophagy

Autophagy is induced by 1α,25(OH)$_2$D3 through the regulated expression of the autophagy-related genes *Beclin-1* and *Atg5*. The hCAP18/LL-37 is important for the autophagy maturation process because it is essential for autophagosome-lysosome fusion. Additionally, hCAP18/LL-37 acts as a secondary messenger to promote a variety of activities in innate and adaptive immunity; thus, cathelicidin is induced and modulated upstream of autophagy. Also, hCAP18/LL-37 plays a role in the activation of MAPKs and C/EBPβ, for transcriptional activation of *Beclin-1* or *Atg5* in monocytes, in response to 1α,25(OH)$_2$D3 [33]. In *Salmonella enterica* serovar *typhimurium* infection, active vitamin D may enhance VDR expression to maintain intestinal homeostasis, induce autophagic defense against *Salmonella* infection, and prevent secondary inflammatory bowel disease. $1\alpha,25(OH)_2D3$ enhances VDR mRNA and protein expression, which in turn increases Atg16L1 mRNA and protein expression in *Salmonella*-infected Caco-2 cells, subsequently resulting in Atg16L1-mediated autophagy [49]. Also, the induction of autophagy by IFN-γ was crucial in limiting the growth of *S. aureus*, *Streptococcus pyogenes*, and *Candida albicans* in infected Langerhans cells acting as antigen-presenting cells [50]. Thus, vitamin D-induced AMPs required the innate (TLR) and acquired (IFN-γ) mechanisms downstream the $1\alpha,25(OH)_2D3$-dependent pathways. Additional mechanisms may also contribute to IFN-γ induction of antimicrobial activity on T cells [47].

Antimicrobial Molecules Induced by Oxidative Stress and Vitamin D

Antimicrobial oxygen and nitrogen radicals are critical weapons of phagocytes. However, ROS attack both host cells and pathogens. Thus, the nuclear transcription factor Nrf2 plays a key role in protecting cells against oxidative stress; this transcription factor is modulated by vitamin D, which supports cellular redox control by maintaining normal mitochondrial functions [51]. Following $1\alpha,25(OH)_2D3$-VDR interaction, Nrf2 translocates from the cytoplasm to the nucleus and activates several genes with antioxidant activity [43]. The activation of the mitochondrial Nrf2/PGC-1α-SIRT3 pathway depends on the intracellular $1\alpha,25(OH)_2D3$ concentration and upregulates the expression of certain antioxidants and anti-inflammatory cytokines, thereby protecting tissues from toxins, micronutrient deficiency-related abnormalities, and parasitic and intracellular microbe-induced harm [51].

Vitamin D also upregulates the expression of glutathione (GSH) peroxidase, which converts H_2O_2 to water. This mechanism prevents the formation of GSH through the activation of the glucose-6-phosphate dehydrogenase that downregulates nitrogen oxide, a potent precursor of ROS, and upregulates SOD, which converts O_2^- to H_2O_2. These vitamin D-related actions collectively reduce the burden of intracellular ROS. Oxidative stress can be assessed in terms of the redox balance between GSH and cysteine. *In vitro*, $1\alpha,25(OH)_2D3$ directly upregulates key enzymes involved in GSH redox homeostasis, such as glutathione cysteine ligase and GSH reductase [43, 52].

The Vitamin D-VDR heterodimer, which interacts with the RXR, also binds to the VDRE located on the promoter of Nrf2, which has multiple roles in maintaining the integrity of cellular signaling systems. Nrf2, by increasing the cellular antioxidants, help to maintain the usually reducing environment within the cell

[53]. This phenomenon is important because the simultaneous presence of *M. tuberculosis* and $1\alpha,25(OH)_2D3$ induces an increased ROS generation. NOX2 and NOX-derived ROS may selectively control *M. tuberculosis* growth by inducing the expression of cathelicidin in $1\alpha,25(OH)_2D3$-treated macrophages [38]. Thus, the dual-role of vitamin D is to regulate the effect of ROS and NOS to protect cellular integrity and to induce the production of AMPs (LL-37) for pathogen elimination.

THE ROLE OF ANTIMICROBIAL PEPTIDES IN *M. TUBERCULOSIS* INFECTION

M. tuberculosis is the causative agent of tuberculosis and a leading cause of morbidity and mortality worldwide [6]. *M. tuberculosis* is transmitted primarily by the respiratory route and, in most cases, human tuberculosis is a pulmonary disease [7]. The principal AMPs related to tuberculosis are β-defensin and LL-37. Defensins play an important role in innate immunity especially in the skin and lungs [15].

Alveolar macrophages and alveolar epithelial cells are among the first host cells to encounter *M. tuberculosis*. HBD-2 is produced by epithelial cells in the respiratory tract, which may be relevant in the pathogenesis of several diseases, and plays a role in the early immune response to *M. tuberculosis* [54]. Previous results from our group have demonstrated that the earliest timing of the HBD-2 gene induction was 6 h following *M. tuberculosis* infection at a MOI of 10:1; HBD-2 gene induction was maintained until 48 h, with peaks at 18 and 24 h post-infection [54]. Late HBD-2 gene expression (at 48 h), raised the interrogation whether this expression was directly due to *M. tuberculosis* infection. *M. tuberculosis* induction of HBD-2 probably depends on the interaction of its mannose lipoarabinomannan with TLR-2. HBD-2 from lung epithelial cells may be a component of the innate immune response against *M. tuberculosis*, both in the primary infection and in the immunopathogenic human tuberculosis [54].

hCAP18 and the antimicrobial active fragment LL-37 have been detected in human lung macrophages [55] and are important to *M. tuberculosis* control. In a previous report, our group demonstrated that when lung epithelial cells were infected with *M. tuberculosis*, high levels of LL-37 were produced, primarily after 18 h, in a dose-dependent manner, suggesting HBD-2 and LL-37 AMPs may act synergistically against *M. tuberculosis* during a primary lung epithelial infection [14]. Also, LL-37 can be induced through TLR-9 ligands in lung epithelial cells after infection with *M. tuberculosis*, suggesting that cathelicidin from alveolar macrophages may be necessary during early infection in humans, probably after TLR-9 activation with *M. tuberculosis* DNA [14].

Another important non-canonical AMP is hepcidin, which is expressed in the liver after inflammatory stimuli. The hepcidin mRNA and protein can be induced by mycobacterial infection in mouse macrophages. Hepcidin and ferroportin are crucial molecules for intracellular iron sequestration; hepcidin activity and iron compartmentalization affect pathogens that require iron to survive, such as intracellular *M. tuberculosis* [56, 57]. In patients with active tuberculosis, high hepcidin concentrations correlate with low iron levels, suggesting the importance of iron limitations for *M. tuberculosis* control [58]. High levels of hepcidin and ferritin have been associated with increased risk of progression to tuberculosis disease in close household contacts of *M. tuberculosis*-infected individuals [59] (Fig. **1**).

Diabetes mellitus (DM) is frequently associated with tuberculosis, and the existence of both comorbidities modifies AMPs dynamics. DM has been associated with reduced T cell responses, neutrophil function, and disorders of humoral immunity and phagocytosis associated with the complement pathway [reviewed in 60]. Patients with DM have low levels of 25(OH)D3, which are associated with higher fasting glucose, insulin resistance, and metabolic syndrome [61]. The susceptibility to *M. tuberculosis* infection observed in DM patients suggests an impaired immune response, and vitamin D could be the link between these diseases [62]. In the Mexican population, we reported that 54% of the study participants with type two DM had inadequate serum levels of vitamin D, which were associated with decreased NO production in response to *M. tuberculosis* infection in monocytes, and a lower capacity to control the intracellular growth of *M. tuberculosis*. However, we did not find differences in the production of LL-37, HBD-2, or IL-10, suggesting that the altered immunological features observed could be associated with other mechanisms directly or indirectly regulated by vitamin D [63]. These observations could be partially explained in an ulterior report, where VDR glycosylation was induced by hyperglycemia, with glucose concentrations of 30mM; however, the expression of CYP24A1 and hCAP18 did not change with VDR O-GlcNAc glycosylation, and the bactericidal activity of a human monocytic cell line (THP-1) was not affected, suggesting that other mechanisms are involved. Possibly, other genes that depend partially on vitamin D might be affected by O-GlcNAc glycosylation [64].

CONCLUDING REMARKS

The anti-infective agents involve multiple pathways interconnected to pathogen control. The most relevant molecules are AMPs, represented by cathelicidins, defensins, hepcidin, and the antimicrobial metabolites (NOS and ROS), as well as those involved in particular processes, such as autophagy. The interaction of TLRs and pathogens usually triggers their induction. For intracellular microbes like *M. tuberculosis*, AMP production comprises a wide variety of pathways for activation, including induction of oxidative stress, IFN-γ, and other vitamin D-dependent mechanisms.

CONSENT FOR PUBLICATION

Not applicable.

CONFLICT OF INTEREST

The authors confirm that the content of this chapter has no conflict of interest.

ACKNOWLEDGEMENTS

We thank Gabriela Margarita Garcilazo Rojo for her assistance with the editing, which greatly improved the manuscript.

REFERENCES

[1]   Guaní-Guerra E, Santos-Mendoza T, Lugo-Reyes SO, Terán LM. Antimicrobial peptides: General overview and clinical implications in human health and disease. Clin Immunol 2010; 135(1): 1-11.
[http://dx.doi.org/10.1016/j.clim.2009.12.004] [PMID: 20116332]

[2]   Zhang LJ, Gallo RL. Antimicrobial peptides. Curr Biol 2016; 26(1): R14-9.
[http://dx.doi.org/10.1016/j.cub.2015.11.017] [PMID: 26766224]

[3]   Ageitos JM, Sánchez-Pérez A, Calo-Mata P, Villa TG. Antimicrobial peptides (AMPs): Ancient compounds that represent novel weapons in the fight against bacteria. Biochem Pharmacol 2017; 133: 117-38.
[http://dx.doi.org/10.1016/j.bcp.2016.09.018] [PMID: 27663838]

[4]   Lakshmaiah Narayana J, Chen JY. Antimicrobial peptides: Possible anti-infective agents. Peptides 2015; 72: 88-94.
[http://dx.doi.org/10.1016/j.peptides.2015.05.012] [PMID: 26048089]

[5]   Pinheiro da Silva F, Machado MC, Machado C. Antimicrobial peptides: Clinical relevance and therapeutic implications. Peptides 2012; 36(2): 308-14.
[http://dx.doi.org/10.1016/j.peptides.2012.05.014] [PMID: 22659161]

[6]   Centers For Disease Control and Prevention. World aids day 2010 mortality among patients with tuberculosis and associations with HIV. MMWR Morb Mortal Wkly Rep 2010; 59(46): 1510-38.

[7]   World Health Organization. Global Tuberculosis Report 2018 2018; 277.

[8]   Tjabringa GS, Ninaber DK, Drijfhout JW, Rabe KF, Hiemstra PS. Human cathelicidin LL-37 is a chemoattractant for eosinophils and neutrophils that acts *via* formyl-peptide receptors. Int Arch Allergy Immunol 2006; 140(2): 103-12.
[http://dx.doi.org/10.1159/000092305] [PMID: 16557028]

[9]   Dürr UHN, Sudheendra US, Ramamoorthy A. LL-37, the only human member of the cathelicidin family of antimicrobial peptides. Biochim Biophys Acta 2006; 1758(9): 1408-25.
[http://dx.doi.org/10.1016/j.bbamem.2006.03.030] [PMID: 16716248]

[10]   Campbell Y, Fantacone ML, Gombart AFA. Regulation of antimicrobial peptide gene expression by nutrients and by-products of microbial metabolism. Eur J Nutr 2012; 51(8): 899-907.
[http://dx.doi.org/10.1007/s00394-012-0415-4] [PMID: 22797470]

[11]   Padhi A, Sengupta M, Sengupta S, Roehm KH, Sonawane A. Antimicrobial peptides and proteins in mycobacterial therapy: Current status and future prospects. Tuberculosis (Edinb) 2014; 94(4): 363-73.
[http://dx.doi.org/10.1016/j.tube.2014.03.011] [PMID: 24813349]

[12]   AlMatar M, Makky EA, Yakıcı G, Var I, Kayar B, Köksal F. Antimicrobial peptides as an alternative to anti-tuberculosis drugs. Pharmacol Res 2018; 128: 288-305.
[http://dx.doi.org/10.1016/j.phrs.2017.10.011] [PMID: 29079429]

[13]   Liu PT. Toll-like receptor triggering of a vitamin d-mediated human antimicrobial response. Science (80-) 2006; 311(5768): 1770-3.

[14]   Rivas-Santiago B, Hernandez-Pando R, Carranza C, *et al.* Expression of cathelicidin LL-37 during *Mycobacterium tuberculosis* infection in human alveolar macrophages, monocytes, neutrophils, and epithelial cells. Infect Immun 2008; 76(3): 935-41.
[http://dx.doi.org/10.1128/IAI.01218-07] [PMID: 18160480]

[15]   Ganz T, Selsted ME, Szklarek D, *et al.* Defensins. Natural peptide antibiotics of human neutrophils. J Clin Invest 1985; 76(4): 1427-35.
[http://dx.doi.org/10.1172/JCI112120] [PMID: 2997278]

[16]   Mattar EH, Almehdar HA, Yacoub HA, Uversky VN, Redwan EM. Antimicrobial potentials and structural disorder of human and animal defensins. Cytokine Growth Factor Rev 2016; 28: 95-111.
[http://dx.doi.org/10.1016/j.cytogfr.2015.11.002] [PMID: 26598808]

[17]   Voskuil MI, Bartek IL, Visconti K, Schoolnik GK. The response of *Mycobacterium tuberculosis* to reactive oxygen and nitrogen species. Front Microbiol 2011; 2(MAY): 105.
[http://dx.doi.org/10.3389/fmicb.2011.00105] [PMID: 21734908]

[18]   Yang C-S, Yuk J-M, Jo E-K. The role of nitric oxide in mycobacterial infections. Immune Netw 2009; 9(2): 46-52.
[http://dx.doi.org/10.4110/in.2009.9.2.46] [PMID: 20107543]

[19]   Carranza C, Juárez E, Torres M, Ellner JJ, Sada E, Schwander SK. *Mycobacterium tuberculosis* growth control by lung macrophages and CD8 cells from patient contacts. Am J Respir Crit Care Med 2006; 173(2): 238-45.
[http://dx.doi.org/10.1164/rccm.200503-411OC] [PMID: 16210664]

[20]   Mishra BB, Lovewell RR, Olive AJ, *et al.* Nitric oxide prevents a pathogen-permissive granulocytic inflammation during tuberculosis. Nat Microbiol 2017; 2: 17072.
[http://dx.doi.org/10.1038/nmicrobiol.2017.72] [PMID: 28504669]

[21]   Nambi S, Long JE, Mishra BB, *et al.* The oxidative stress network of *Mycobacterium tuberculosis* reveals coordination between radical detoxification systems. Cell Host Microbe 2015; 17(6): 829-37.
[http://dx.doi.org/10.1016/j.chom.2015.05.008] [PMID: 26067605]

[22]   Goyal N, Kashyap B, Singh NP, Kaur IR. Neopterin and oxidative stress markers in the diagnosis of extrapulmonary tuberculosis. Biomarkers 2017; 22(7): 648-53.
[PMID: 27879161]

[23]   Boisson-Dupuis S, Bustamante J, El-Baghdadi J, *et al.* Inherited and acquired immunodeficiencies underlying tuberculosis in childhood. Immunol Rev 2015; 264(1): 103-20.
[http://dx.doi.org/10.1111/imr.12272] [PMID: 25703555]

[24]   Oyinloye BE, Adenowo AF, Kappo AP. Reactive oxygen species, apoptosis, antimicrobial peptides and human inflammatory diseases. Pharmaceuticals (Basel) 2015; 8(2): 151-75.
[http://dx.doi.org/10.3390/ph8020151] [PMID: 25850012]

[25]   Chan J, Tanaka K, Carroll D, Flynn J, Bloom BR. Effects of nitric oxide synthase inhibitors on murine infection with *Mycobacterium tuberculosis*. Infect Immun 1995; 63(2): 736-40.
[http://dx.doi.org/10.1128/IAI.63.2.736-740.1995] [PMID: 7529749]

[26]   Idh J, Andersson B, Lerm M, *et al.* Reduced susceptibility of clinical strains of *Mycobacterium*

tuberculosis to reactive nitrogen species promotes survival in activated macrophages. PLoS One 2017; 12(7): e0181221.
[http://dx.doi.org/10.1371/journal.pone.0181221] [PMID: 28704501]

[27]   Bikle D. Vitamin D: Production, metabolism, and mechanisms of action. In: Feingold KR, Anawalt B, Boyce A, Chrousos G, Dungan K, Grossman A, Eds. South Dartmouth, MA 2000.

[28]   Gunville CF, Mourani PM, Ginde AA. The role of vitamin D in prevention and treatment of infection. Inflamm Allergy Drug Targets 2013; 12(4): 239-45.
[http://dx.doi.org/10.2174/18715281113129990046] [PMID: 23782205]

[29]   Ginde AA, Mansbach JM, Camargo CAJ Jr. Vitamin D, respiratory infections, and asthma. Curr Allergy Asthma Rep 2009; 9(1): 81-7.
[http://dx.doi.org/10.1007/s11882-009-0012-7] [PMID: 19063829]

[30]   Nnoaham KE, Clarke A. Low serum vitamin D levels and tuberculosis: a systematic review and meta-analysis. Int J Epidemiol 2008; 37(1): 113-9.
[http://dx.doi.org/10.1093/ije/dym247] [PMID: 18245055]

[31]   Junaid K, Rehman A. Impact of vitamin D on infectious disease-tuberculosis-a review. Clin Nutr Exp 2019; 25: 1-10.
[http://dx.doi.org/10.1016/j.yclnex.2019.02.003]

[32]   Liu PT, Stenger S, Li H, *et al.* Toll-like receptor triggering of a vitamin D-mediated human antimicrobial response. Science 2006; 311(5768): 1770-3.
[http://dx.doi.org/10.1126/science.1123933] [PMID: 16497887]

[33]   Yuk JM, Shin DM, Lee HM, *et al.* Vitamin D3 induces autophagy in human monocytes/macrophages *via* cathelicidin. Cell Host Microbe 2009; 6(3): 231-43.
[http://dx.doi.org/10.1016/j.chom.2009.08.004] [PMID: 19748465]

[34]   Liu PT, Stenger S, Tang DH, Modlin RL. Cutting edge: vitamin D-mediated human antimicrobial activity against *Mycobacterium tuberculosis* is dependent on the induction of cathelicidin. J Immunol 2007; 179(4): 2060-3.
[http://dx.doi.org/10.4049/jimmunol.179.4.2060] [PMID: 17675463]

[35]   Wu S, Sun J. Vitamin D, vitamin D receptor, and macroautophagy in inflammation and infection. Discov Med 2011; 11(59): 325-35.
[PMID: 21524386]

[36]   Youssef DA, Miller CWT, El-Abbassi AM, *et al.* Antimicrobial implications of vitamin D. Dermatoendocrinol 2011; 3(4): 220-9.
[http://dx.doi.org/10.4161/derm.3.4.15027] [PMID: 22259647]

[37]   Wang T-T, Nestel FP, Bourdeau V, *et al.* Cutting edge: 1,25-dihydroxyvitamin D3 is a direct inducer of antimicrobial peptide gene expression. J Immunol 2004; 173(5): 2909-12.
[http://dx.doi.org/10.4049/jimmunol.173.5.2909] [PMID: 15322146]

[38]   Chun RF, Adams JS, Hewison M. Immunomodulation by vitamin D: implications for TB. Expert Rev Clin Pharmacol 2011; 4(5): 583-91.
[http://dx.doi.org/10.1586/ecp.11.41] [PMID: 22046197]

[39]   White JH. Vitamin D as an inducer of cathelicidin antimicrobial peptide expression: past, present and future. J Steroid Biochem Mol Biol 2010; 121(1-2): 234-8.
[http://dx.doi.org/10.1016/j.jsbmb.2010.03.034] [PMID: 20302931]

[40]   Peric M, Koglin S, Kim S-M, *et al.* IL-17A enhances vitamin D3-induced expression of cathelicidin antimicrobial peptide in human keratinocytes. J Immunol 2008; 181(12): 8504-12.
[http://dx.doi.org/10.4049/jimmunol.181.12.8504] [PMID: 19050268]

[41]   Rockett KA, Brookes R, Udalova I, Vidal V, Hill AVS, Kwiatkowski D. 1,25-Dihydroxyvitamin D 3 Induces Nitric Oxide Synthase and Suppresses Growth of. Society 1998; 66(11): 5314-21.

[42] Gois PHF, Ferreira D, Olenski S, Seguro AC. Vitamin D and infectious diseases: Simple bystander or contributing factor? Nutrients 2017; 9(7): 1-19.
[http://dx.doi.org/10.3390/nu9070651] [PMID: 28672783]

[43] Wimalawansa SJ, Vitamin D. Vitamin D deficiency: effects on oxidative stress, epigenetics, gene regulation, and aging. Biology (Basel) 2019; 8(2): 30.
[http://dx.doi.org/10.3390/biology8020030] [PMID: 31083546]

[44] Binkley N, Ramamurthy R, Krueger D. Low vitamin D status: definition, prevalence, consequences, and correction. Rheum Dis Clin North Am 2012; 38(1): 45-59.
[http://dx.doi.org/10.1016/j.rdc.2012.03.006] [PMID: 22525842]

[45] Liu PT, Modlin RL. Human macrophage host defense against *Mycobacterium tuberculosis*. Curr Opin Immunol 2008; 20(4): 371-6.
[http://dx.doi.org/10.1016/j.coi.2008.05.014] [PMID: 18602003]

[46] Hewison M. Vitamin D and the immune system: new perspectives on an old theme. Rheum Dis Clin North Am 2012; 38(1): 125-39.
[http://dx.doi.org/10.1016/j.rdc.2012.03.012] [PMID: 22525848]

[47] Fabri M, Stenger S, Shin D-M, *et al.* Vitamin D Is Required for IFN-γ–Mediated Antimicrobial Activity of Human Macrophages. Sci Transl Med 2011; 3(104): 104ra102 LP-.

[48] Ponpuak M, Davis AS, Roberts EA, *et al.* Delivery of cytosolic components by autophagic adaptor protein p62 endows autophagosomes with unique antimicrobial properties. Immunity 2010; 32(3): 329-41.
[http://dx.doi.org/10.1016/j.immuni.2010.02.009] [PMID: 20206555]

[49] Huang FC. Vitamin D differentially regulates *Salmonella*-induced intestine epithelial autophagy and interleukin-1β expression. World J Gastroenterol 2016; 22(47): 10353-63.
[http://dx.doi.org/10.3748/wjg.v22.i47.10353] [PMID: 28058015]

[50] Dang AT, Teles RMB, Liu PT, *et al.* Autophagy links antimicrobial activity with antigen presentation in Langerhans cells. JCI Insight 2019; 4(8): 126955.
[http://dx.doi.org/10.1172/jci.insight.126955] [PMID: 30996142]

[51] Alvarez JA, Grunwell JR, Gillespie SE, Tangpricha V, Hebbar KB. Vitamin D deficiency is associated with an oxidized plasma cysteine redox potential in critically Ill children. J Steroid Biochem Mol Biol 2018; 175(3): 164-9.
[http://dx.doi.org/10.1016/j.jsbmb.2016.09.013] [PMID: 27641738]

[52] Liu Y, Hyde AS, Simpson MA, Barycki JJ. Emerging regulatory paradigms in glutathione metabolism.Advances in Cancer Research. 2014; pp. 69-101.
[http://dx.doi.org/10.1016/B978-0-12-420117-0.00002-5]

[53] Berridge MJ. Vitamin D, reactive oxygen species and calcium signalling in ageing and disease. Philos Trans R Soc B Biol Sci 1700; 2016: 371.

[54] Rivas-Santiago B, Schwander SK, Sarabia C, *et al.* Human β-defensin 2 is expressed and associated with *Mycobacterium tuberculosis* during infection of human alveolar epithelial cells. Infect Immun 2005; 73(8): 4505-11.
[http://dx.doi.org/10.1128/IAI.73.8.4505-4511.2005] [PMID: 16040961]

[55] Agerberth B, Grunewald J, Castaños-Velez E, *et al.* Antibacterial components in bronchoalveolar lavage fluid from healthy individuals and sarcoidosis patients. Am J Respir Crit Care Med 1999; 160(1): 283-90.
[http://dx.doi.org/10.1164/ajrccm.160.1.9807041] [PMID: 10390413]

[56] Abreu R, Quinn F, Giri PK. Role of the hepcidin-ferroportin axis in pathogen-mediated intracellular iron sequestration in human phagocytic cells. Blood Adv 2018; 2(10): 1089-100.
[http://dx.doi.org/10.1182/bloodadvances.2017015255] [PMID: 29764842]

[57] Sow FB, Florence WC, Satoskar AR, Schlesinger LS, Zwilling BS, Lafuse WP. Expression and localization of hepcidin in macrophages: a role in host defense against tuberculosis. J Leukoc Biol 2007; 82(4): 934-45.
[http://dx.doi.org/10.1189/jlb.0407216] [PMID: 17609338]

[58] Javaheri-Kermani M, Farazmandfar T, Ajami A, Yazdani Y. Impact of hepcidin antimicrobial peptide on iron overload in tuberculosis patients. Scand J Infect Dis 2014; 46(10): 693-6.
[http://dx.doi.org/10.3109/00365548.2014.929736] [PMID: 25134646]

[59] Minchella PA, Donkor S, McDermid JM, Sutherland JS. Iron homeostasis and progression to pulmonary tuberculosis disease among household contacts. Tuberculosis (Edinb) 2015; 95(3): 288-93.
[http://dx.doi.org/10.1016/j.tube.2015.02.042] [PMID: 25764944]

[60] González-hernández Y, Sada Díaz E, Escobar-Gutiérrez A, Muños Torrico M, Torres Rojas M. Association of tuberculosis and diabetes mellitus: Immunological mechanisms involving susceptibility. Rev Inst Nac Enferm Respir 2009; 22(1)

[61] Nakashima A, Yokoyama K, Yokoo T, Urashima M. Role of vitamin D in diabetes mellitus and chronic kidney disease. World J Diabetes 2016; 7(5): 89-100.
[http://dx.doi.org/10.4239/wjd.v7.i5.89] [PMID: 26981182]

[62] Handel AE, Ramagopalan SV. Tuberculosis and diabetes mellitus: is vitamin D the missing link? Lancet Infect Dis 2010; 10(9): 596.
[http://dx.doi.org/10.1016/S1473-3099(10)70185-7] [PMID: 20797643]

[63] Herrera MT, Gonzalez Y, Hernández-Sánchez F, Fabián-San Miguel G, Torres M. Low serum vitamin D levels in type 2 diabetes patients are associated with decreased mycobacterial activity. BMC Infect Dis 2017; 17(1): 610.
[http://dx.doi.org/10.1186/s12879-017-2705-1] [PMID: 28882103]

[64] Hernández-Sánchez F, Guzmán-Beltrán S, Herrera MT, *et al.* High glucose induces O-GlcNAc glycosylation of the vitamin D receptor (VDR) in THP1 cells and in human macrophages derived from monocytes. Cell Biol Int 2017; 41(9): 1065-74.
[http://dx.doi.org/10.1002/cbin.10827] [PMID: 28710799]

CHAPTER 4

Immune Response Against *M. tuberculosis* in Human Pulmonary Tuberculosis

Angélica Moncada Morales and **María Teresa Herrera Barrios**[*]

Microbiology Department, National Institute of Respiratory Diseases Ismael Cosío Villegas, México City, México

Abstract: Tuberculosis (TB) is an infectious disease that represents a health problem in the world, with pulmonary tuberculosis (TBP) as the most frequent type of TB. This disease is caused by *Mycobacterium tuberculosis* (*M. tuberculosis*) that enters the host by inhalation. *M. tuberculosis* comes into contact with physiological barriers found in the upper respiratory tract (URT) and with innate immunity through airway epithelial cells (AECs). AECs are endowed with innate receptors (TLRs, NOD1, NOD2, NLRP3, TNFR, EGFR, and C-type lectins) that allow them to interact with microorganisms, or their components, and are a source of antimicrobial peptides (AMPs), such as α-defensins, β-defensins, cathelicidin (LL-37/hCAP-18), pro-inflammatory cytokines and chemokines. However, *M. tuberculosis* can resist and surpass innate defense mechanisms, descend to the lower respiratory tract (LRT) and arrives at the alveoli. At this site, *M. tuberculosis* comes into contact with alveolar macrophages (AMs), dendritic cells (DCs), type II epithelial cells, and neutrophils. *M. tuberculosis* interacts with AMs through TLRs (TLR2, TLR4, and TLR9) and triggers the production of pro-inflammatory (IL-1β, IL-6, TNF-α, IL-12) and anti-inflammatory cytokines (IL-4, IL-10). Innate immunity includes phagocytosis, killing, cytokines, and chemokines production with the participation of T cells, later, that orchestrate the elimination of mycobacteria. For *M. tuberculosis* clearance, it is fundamental that AMs or DCs present mycobacterial antigens to T cells and begin an acquired immune response for mycobacterial elimination. During the infection in the alveolar space, there are innate molecules such as AMPs, ROS, NO, pro-inflammatory cytokines (IL-1β, IL-6, IL-12, IL-18, TNF-α and IFN-γ), anti-inflammatory cytokines (IL-4, IL-10 and TGF-β), and immune specific T cells for *M. tuberculosis* clearance. Control of TB infection has been associated with IFN-γ production by T cells since it triggers and increases bactericidal AMs activity. However, the alveolar immune response against *M. tuberculosis* may not be effective due to the evasive mechanisms employed by the mycobacteria and the secretion of its virulent factors.

Keywords: Antimicrobial Peptides, Cytokines, Chemokines, *M. tuberculosis*, Macrophages, Neutrophils, Pulmonary Tuberculosis, Tuberculosis, T cells.

[*] **Corresponding author María Teresa Herrera Barrios:** Microbiology Department, National Instituto of Respiratory Diseases Ismael Cosío Villegas, Mexico City, Mexico; Tel: 54871700 (Extension 5117); E-mail: teresa_herrera@iner.gob.mx

INTRODUCTION

Mycobacterium tuberculosis (*M. tuberculosis*) is the main etiologic agent of human tuberculosis (TB). This infectious disease is one of the top 10 causes of death and the leading cause of a single infectious agent worldwide [1]. In 2018, 10 million people developed TB (5.7 million men, 3.2 million women, and 1.1 million children) and 1.5 million deaths resulted from this disease (including 251,000 HIV patients) [2].

About one-quarter of the world's population has been estimated to have latent TB. Consequently, people infected with *M. tuberculosis* without the active disease cannot transmit the disease, yet 5-15% of these people are at risk of developing TB [1, 2]. Pulmonary TB (TBP) is the most frequent form of TB because the respiratory tract is the main entrance of *M. tuberculosis* during inhalation and arrives at the alveoli after overcoming the pulmonary defense system [2]. Factors such as host genetic factors, smoking, HIV infection, diabetes and malnutrition contribute to developing TB [3 - 9].

IMMUNITY IN THE LUNG

The metabolism of the body's cells requires the exchange of very large quantities of oxygen and carbon dioxide across the alveolar-capillary interface in the peripheral lung [10, 11]. In humans, the dynamic process of ventilation moves millions of liters of air from the upper respiratory tract (URT) to the lower respiratory tract (LRT) and finally to the alveoli; the latter is lined by alveolar type I and type II epithelial cells [12].

In the process of oxygen delivery to the circulatory system, inert or toxic particles and microorganisms (virus, bacterial, fungi) from the environment are brought into the respiratory tract and come into contact with the human lung. This organ is exposed to a vast number of microorganisms capable of causing diseases that challenge the defense system in the lung.

The lung maintains its homeostasis with the participation of resident cells such as airway epithelial cells (AECs), dendritic cells (DCs), alveolar macrophages (AMs), and the innate and acquired immune response along the respiratory tract [13, 14].

Immunity involves both the innate and acquired systems of immunity. The innate immune response is characterized by nonspecific recognition with rapid response, detection of specific antigens, and recruitment of inflammatory cells against particular antigens, and inflammation is involved in this response. Conversely, the acquired immune response is antigen-specific, requires antigen presentation, takes a longer time to develop and memory cells are produced in the process. Both immune responses act together to fend off pathogens [15].

The Innate Immune Function Of Airway Epithelial Cells

Most of the research on the microorganism's infectious process has focused on AMs, DCs, and alveolar type II pneumocytes. However, AECs are the first to come into contact with microorganisms or particles and contribute to the body's early defense. AECs provide a physical and immunological barrier and stimulate the acquired immune response [16].

The mechanical clearance of mucus is considered the primary innate airway defense, and the role of AECs is to line the airway surface to provide the integral activity required for mucus transport, including ciliary activity and the regulation of salt and water *via* trans-epithelial ion transport [13, 17]. Mucus secreted by goblet cells and mucous glands entraps microorganisms or particles, propelled by ciliary movement, and provides the microenvironment necessary for the activity of antimicrobial substances [12, 18, 19].

AECs sense microorganisms or soluble molecules and respond by increasing their defense mechanisms and release different components into the airway surface fluid. The innate defense mechanism includes the secretion of components from different cells with antimicrobial activity such as lysozyme, lactoferrin (both work together and kill gram-negative pathogens by disrupting their membrane and exposing susceptible peptidoglycans) [20], secretory phospholipase A2, secretory leukocyte protease inhibitor (SLPI) and antimicrobial peptides. Other substances, such as complement, surfactant proteins A and D [14], Clara-cell protein (CC10, CCSP), and mucins (MUC 1, MUC 2, and MUC5AC), contribute to the defense mechanism [21].

In this scenario, human AECs from the respiratory tract are active cells. Their capability to participate in innate immunity has been reported through the production of reactive oxygen species (ROS) and the secretion of antimicrobial peptides (AMPs) such as α-defensins (HNP1-4), β-defensins (hBD-1, hBD-2), cathelicidin (LL-37/CAP18), and CCL20 into the airway surface fluid with action against different pathogens including *M. tuberculosis* (Table **1**) [16, 22].

Table 1. Production of innate components in the respiratory tract.

	Types	Mechanism of Expression	Source
α-defensins	HNP-1-4	Constitutive expression	Epithelial cells and neutrophil azurophil granules
β-defensins	hBD-1	Constitutive production	Epithelial respiratory tract, macrophages
	hBD-2	Induced by: TNF-α, IL-1α, IL-1β, flagellin, bacterial DNA, gram positives, gram negatives, dsRNA, *C. albicans*, LPS	
Cathelicidin	LL-37/hCAP18	Induced by microorganism	Epithelial respiratory tract Neutrophils that have arrived at the airways
CCL20		Induced by microorganism/ dust mite	Epithelial respiratory tract
Surfactant	A and D	Induced by microorganism	Type II epithelial respiratory tract
Lysozyme			
Lactoferrin			
ROS		Induced by microorganism	Neutrophils and macrophages
Mucin	MUC1, MUC2 and MUC5AC		Globet cells

HNP: Human neutrophils peptides, **hBD**: Human β-defensin, **ROS**: Reactive oxygen species, **LPS**: Lipopolysaccharide, **TNF**: Tumor necrosis factor, **IL**: Interleukin, **MUC**: Mucin.

Pattern Recognition Receptors (PRRs) Of Airway Epithelial Cells

Furthermore, AECs directly recognize pathogen-associated-molecular-patterns (PAMPs) of microorganisms or their soluble components through innate receptors called pattern-recognition receptors (PRRs). Innate receptors on AECs include the denominated toll-like receptor (TLR), surface receptors (TLR1, TLR2, TLR4, TLR5, TLR6), endosomal receptors (TLR3, TLR4, TLR7, TLR8, TLR9), cytosolic receptors such as the nucleotide oligomerization domain (NLR) (NOD 1, NOD 2), IL-1β-converting enzyme protease activation factor (IPAF), and NOD-like receptor pyrin domain-3 (NLRP3). Other surface receptors include the TNF receptor (TNFR) and the Epidermal Growth Factor Receptor (EGFR); both are an important source of CXCL8 (IL-8, which is chemotactic for neutrophils, basophils, and T cells). C-type lectin receptors are involved in recognition of β-glycans in fungi, yeast, mycobacteria, and type I IFNs. These innate receptors enable a rapid response for the production of pro-inflammatory cytokines, chemokines, antimicrobial peptides (AMPs), and other substances involved in the response against pathogens [10, 16, 23].

After the recognition of PAMPs by different AEC innate receptors, the inducible transcription nuclear factor NF-kB is activated through the canonical pathway and in turn activates genes involved in the production of inflammatory cytokines (IL-1β, IL-6, IL-8, TNF-α, IFN-γ), CXCR3 chemokines such as CXCL9 (MIG, Monokine Induced by Gamma interferon), CXCL10 (IP-10, Interferon gamma-induced Protein 10) and CXCL11 (I-TAC, Interferon–inducible T Cell Alpha Chemoattractant), type I IFNs and AMPs (α-defensins, LL-37, and CCL20) (Table **2**) [16, 23].

However, PAMPs, specifically LPS, can infiltrate the respiratory mucus layer, gain access to epithelial receptors, and stimulate inflammation with the production of pro-inflammatory cytokines (IL-1β, IL-6, IL-8), chemokines such as MIG, IP-10, and I-TAC. These chemokines stimulate the immune response with the recruitment of immune cells, for example, IP-10 that primarily attracts Th1/ T cells and is an antagonist for Th2 /T cells [24].

The inflammatory response characterized by pro-inflammatory cytokines and chemokines that follows the interaction of AECs, AMs, and DCs with microorganisms represents the innate immune response. It involves a rapid response and the recruitment and activation of neutrophils in response to IL-8 a pro-inflammatory chemokine associated with neutrophil chemotaxis as a defense mechanism to eliminate the pathogen [25]. However, this early response precedes an acquired immune response, which is specific and includes the participation of memory and T and B specific cells.

Table 2. Pattern Recognition Receptors (PRRs) in airway epithelial cells and its ligands.

Receptor	Types	PAMPs	Localized
TLRs	1	Tri-acyl lipopeptides	Surface
	2	Lipoteichoic acid, peptidoglycan, zymosan, microbial lipoproteins and lipopeptides, HSP70 (host),	Surface
	6	Di-acyl lipopeptides	Surface
	4	LPS	Surface
	5	Flagellin	Surface
	3	Double-stranded RNA	Endosomal
	4	LPS, HSP60 and 70, hyaluronic acid fragments (host)	Endosomal
	7	ssRNA	Endosomal
	8 and 9	CpG DNA	Endosomal
RIG-1		RNA viruses	Cytosolic

(Table 2) cont.....

MDA5		RNA viruses	Cytosolic
IPAF		Flagellin	Cytosolic
NLRP3		ATP	Cytosolic
NOD1		Peptidoglycan (iE-DAP)	Cytosolic
NOD2		Peptidoglycan (*N-acetyl* MDP)	Cytosolic
TNFR		Protein A from *S. aureus*-mediates IgG binding and IL-8 release	Surface
EGFR		Protein A from *S. aureus*-mediates IgG binding and IL-8 release	Surface
C-type lectins	Dectin-1 Dectin-2 Mincle	β-glycans on fungi, yeast, and *Mycobacterium* cell walls.	Surface

PAMPs: Pathogen-Associated Molecular Patterns, **TLR:** Toll-like receptor, **RIG-1**: Retinoic Acid Inducible Gene-1, **MDA5**: Melanoma Differentiation -Associated protein 5, **IPAF**: IL-1β-converting enzyme Protease Activation Factor, **NLRP3**: NOD-like Receptor Pyrin Domain-3; **NOD1**: Nucleotide Oligomerization Domain-1; **NOD2**: Nucleotide Oligomerization Domain-2, **TNFR**: TNF receptor, **EGFR**: Epidermal Growth Factor Receptor; C-Type lectins, **HSP**: Heat shock protein, **MDP**: Muramyl-dipeptide, **LPS**: Lipopolysaccharide.

The Immune Response Of Airway Epithelial Cells

The initial interaction of the pathogenic microorganism with the host usually takes place on the inside or outside of body surfaces. AECs are the primary site of contact with the microorganism. Some of the consequences of contact with the host tissue are: **a)** the local innate immune response (mucus, lysozyme, lactoferrin, phospholipase A2, SPLI, SPA, SPD, mucins, ROS, and calprotectin) (Table **1**) accompanied by cough and mucociliary clearance, which if efficient, eliminates the microorganisms without an inflammatory response or the activation of acquired immunity. This event normally occurs in the LRT and in a short period; **b-c)** the microorganisms surpass this level of innate immune response and as a consequence, the immune response is upregulated with direct antimicrobial activity and the production of AMPs (α- and β-defensins, LL-37). Also, the innate receptors (Table **2**) on AECs and AMs, recognize the microorganism, or its soluble components, and begin the production of pro-inflammatory cytokines and chemokines. These, in turn, initiate the recruitment of inflammatory cells (neutrophils, macrophages) at the site of infection, which results in the elimination of the microorganism. In this context, the innate immune response controls the growth of the microorganism and maintains local homeostasis. AMs and DCs carry out antigen presentation to T or B cells and begin the development of the acquired immune response. However, when the microorganism surpasses the innate and acquired immunities, together with a strong inflammatory response, the host's health may be compromised. Additionally, the microorganism may colonize the airways for a long time if the immune response is deficient (Fig. **1**).

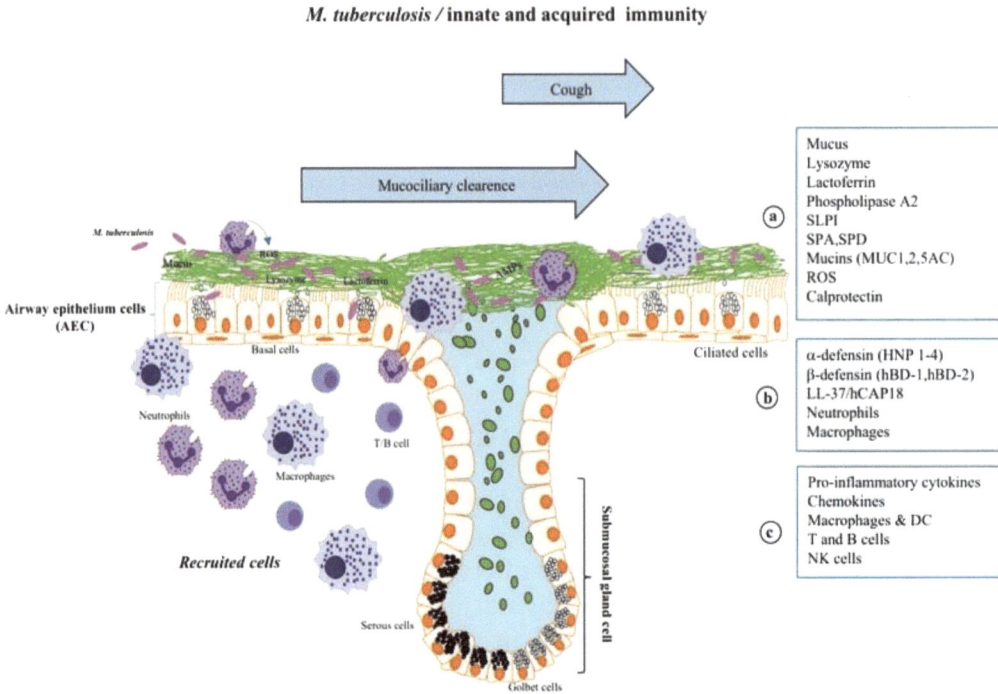

Fig. (1). The immune response levels of airway epithelial cells in the respiratory tract in *M. tuberculosis* infection. The microorganism in the lung induces an innate immune response associated with inflammation. The initial immune response can eliminate the microorganism without inflammation a). However, the microorganism can outgrow the immune response that results in the recognition of PAMPs by AECs and AMs, the production of pro-inflammatory cytokines and chemokines with the recruitment of neutrophils and T and B cells at the site where DCs and AMs present antigens, and begin the acquired immune response (b, c).

Characteristics of *M. tuberculosis*

M. tuberculosis is the etiologic agent of TB and displays slow growth that doubles in a period of 12-24 h under optimal conditions. Its major characteristic is its cell wall structure that provides a strong impermeable barrier to drugs and noxious components, thus playing a fundamental role in its virulence. The mycobacteria possess an outer membrane with an asymmetric lipid bilayer made of long fatty acids in the inner leaflet (mycolic acids), and glycolipids and waxy components on the outer layer. Between the outer and inner membranes, a periplasmic space is formed, with a thin layer of peptidoglycan in the innermost side covalently linked to arabinogalactan and lipoarabinomannan, which in turn are bound to mycolic acids. Synthesis of mycolic acids and arabinogalactan is the target of isoniazid and ethambutol, thus making evident the importance of the mycobacterial cell wall in the biology of this microorganism [26, 27].

Effects of Mycobacterial Virulent Factors on the Immune Response

M. tuberculosis is an extremely successful intracellular pathogen armed with multiple tactics to subvert host immunity, in part due to its complex structure conformed of nearly 60% lipids with virulent factors that reduce the host's immune response for survival. The culture filtrate protein 10 kDa (CFP-10) and early secretory antigen target- 6 kDa (ESAT-6) from *M. tuberculosis*, reduce bacteriostatic components as nitric oxide (NO) and reactive oxygen species (ROS) production on macrophages by direct action on inducible nitric oxide synthase (iNOS) enzyme activity [28].

Alternatively, the cell wall Rv1808 (PPE32) surface protein is a virulent component of mycobacteria that prolongs its survival within the macrophage and accelerates the macrophage's death. Additionally, the interaction of Rv1808-TLR2 with macrophages increases the production of anti-inflammatory IL-10, and pro-inflammatory TNF-α and IL-6 cytokines *via* co-activation of NF-kB and MAPK, and NF-kB signaling pathways [29].

Also glycolipids of the cell envelope of *M. tuberculosis* act as antagonists of TLR2, and are a strategy of *M. tuberculosis* to undermine the innate immune response, avoid NF-kB activation, and the production of pro-inflammatory cytokines and chemokines [30].

M. tuberculosis in Lung Infection

In TBP, *M. tuberculosis* enters the host through inhalation and comes into contact with physical barriers and innate immunity characterized by AECs susceptible to infection by *M. tuberculosis*, despite their capacity to respond by producing AMPs, cytokines, and chemokines [31].

When AECs become infected with *M. tuberculosis*, the uptake of *M. tuberculosis* H37Rv is five times less effective compared to DCs. In DCs, the percentage of infection is greater (94.1%) than in the bronchial epithelial cell line and in large airway epithelial cells (24.8% and 26.3% respectively). Nevertheless, AECs play an important role in the transition from the innate to the acquired immune response. They possess the capability to present mycobacterial antigens to non-classical Mtb reactive CD8$^+$ T cells (MAIT) mediated by HLA-I, and they induce a strong IFN-γ production, an important cytokine in the control of the mycobacterial infection [32]. Also, activated AECs produce pro-inflammatory cytokines and chemokines with the recruitment of neutrophils.

Alveolar Macrophages and Their Response Against *M. tuberculosis*

After *M. tuberculosis* overcomes the innate immunity mediated by AECs, it finally arrives at the alveoli, and AMs are the first defense against *M. tuberculosis*, after which an inflammatory response is induced. This response is mediated by the recognition of different mycobacterial components by TLRs on surface (TLR1, TLR2 and TLR4) or endosomal (TRL3, TRL8, and TLR9) localization, affecting the innate and acquired immune response which can contribute to the clearance of mycobacteria and prevent the development of TBP [33, 34]. In human AMs, NOD1 and NOD2 receptors are involved in recognition, pro-inflammatory cytokine production (IL-1β, IL-6, and TNF-α), and autophagy, with potential implications in the clearance of *M. tuberculosis* [35, 36]. AMs involve other innate receptors such as the mannose receptor (MR), CD14, MARCO, DC-SIGN, and scavenger receptors (CD36) (Table **3**) [37].

Table 3. Pattern Recognition Receptors (PRRs) in alveolar macrophages and their mycobacterial ligands.

Receptor	Ligand	Effect
TLR2	Rv1808 (PPE32)	Manipulation of MyD88, MAPK; NF-kB signaling pathways
	MPT83	Th1 activation, MMP-9 induction
	Rv0577, Rv3628	DCs activation, Th1 response, Ag-specific memory T cell expansion
	Acylated lipoprotein	Regulatory protection
	LprG, LpqH	T CD4+ activation
	Peptidoglycan	NK activation, IFN-γ production
	Mycolic acid	Macrophage activation
	ESAT-6	Macrophage apoptosis
	Rv2660	Macrophage stimulation, cytokine secretion, maintenance of Mtb in latent phase

TLR4	Acylated LM, HSP60, 65, 50S ribosomal protein	Immune cells activation
	Rv0652, Chaperonin 60	Macrophage stimulation
	E5531	Blocking of TNF-α production in alveolar macrophages
	Phosphatidylinositol mannoside	Inhibition of TLR4, nitric oxide, and inflammatory cytokines
	HBHA, Rv0652	DC maturation, Th1 response
	RpfB	DC incitation, Th1, 17 response, pro-inflammatory cytokines secretion
TLR1, 2	Tri-acylated lipoproteins	T cell co-stimulation
TLR2, 4	38kDa Ag	TNF-α and IL-6 induction
TLR4, 9	CpG	Th1 response enhancement, protection against aerosolized Mtb
TLR3, 4, 9	CAF09, MLP/TDM, CpG	IFN-γ CD4+ T cells induction
TLR 9 & 8	Unmethylated CpG, small oligonucleotide	Macrophage and DC activation Pro-inflammatory induction including IL-12
NOD2	*N-acetyl* MDP	Inflammatory response
cGAS	Mycobacterial DNA	Type I IFN production and autophagy
CLRs (Glycolipids):		
Mincle	TDM, GMM and GroMM	Pro-inflammatory cytokines, granuloma formation
MCL	TDM	
DCAR	Tri- and Tetra-acylated PIMs (AcPIM2 and Ac2PIM2	Production of MCP-1, IFN-γ by T cells
Dectin-2	Man LAM	IL-2 and IL-10 cytokines
Dectin-1		Pro-inflammatory cytokines
Mannose receptor	Man LAM, LM	Pro-inflammatory cytokines
DC-SIGN	Man LAM	Pro-inflammatory cytokines

LM: Lipomannan, **HSP**: Heat shock protein, **HBHA**: Heparin-binding hemagglutinin, **Rpf**: Resuscitation-promoting factor, **CAF**: Cationic adjuvant formulation, **MLP**: Monophosphoryl lipid-A, **TDM**: Threhalose - 6,6′-dimycolate, **ESAT**: Early secreted antigen, **NK cell**: Natural killer cell, **Th**: T helper, **MMP**: Matrix metalloprotease, **MAPK**: Mitogen-activated protein kinase, **NF-kB**: Nuclear factor kappa-light-chan-enhancer of activated B cells, **TNF**: Tumor necrosis factor, **Mincle:** Macrophage-inducible C-type lectin, **MCL:** Macrophage C-type lectin, **DCAR:** Dendritic Cell Immunoactivating Receptor, **TDM:** trehalose-6,6--dimycolate, **GMM:** Glucose monomycolate, **GroMM:** Glycerol monomycolate, **PIM:** Phosphatydilinositol mannoside, **LAM:** Lipoarabinomannan, **Man LAM:** mannose-capped-LAM, **IL:** Interleukin, **DC:** Dendritic cell, **MCP-1:** monocyte chemoattractant protein-1.

Interaction Between Alveolar Cells and *M. tuberculosis*

It is commonly assumed that *M. tuberculosis* primarily infects human AMs, but it also infects neutrophils, monocytes, and type II alveolar epithelial cells [38]. The infection of these cells triggers the production of cathelicidin LL-37, involved in the clearance of *M. tuberculosis*. This peptide has been localized on the cell surface and in the cytoplasm of phagocytosed mycobacteria and co-localized with a main component of the mycobacteria lipoarabinomannan (LAM). The production of LL-37 is mediated by TLR2, TLR4, and TLR9, but is most efficiently produced in AMs by TLR9 [39].

AMs production as LL-37 and hBD-2 in active human TBP in children has been evidenced in bronchoalveolar lavage (BAL) [40]. Furthermore, recognition of mycobacterial components by TLRs induce cytokine production involved in the control of the infection. Studies in human AMs have demonstrated the contribution of TLR2, TLR4, and TLR9 in pro-inflammatory cytokine production such as IL-1β, IL-6, and TNF-α under specific-ligand interaction (Pam3Cys, LPS, and Mtb DNA), important in the control of mycobacterial infections [41].

Because *M. tuberculosis* also infects type II alveolar epithelial cells, studies with the A549 human cell line (type II alveolar epithelial) demonstrated that invasion by *M. tuberculosis* H37Rv is more efficient than H37Ra, *M. avium*, and *E. coli*. This process is mediated by the vitronectin receptor (CD51) and the β1 integrin (CD29). Intracellular replication is also more efficient in *M. tuberculosis* H37Rv and H37Ra. The bacterial invasion probably employs a mycobacterial evasion mechanism that avoids the actions of bactericidal soluble proteins and the immune response [42].

AMs have the innate capability to recognize PAMPs, as well as to directly recognize the pathogen which is fundamental to innate immunity; opsonization allows the diversification of pathogen recognition [43, 44]. Phagocytosis of *M. tuberculosis* by AMs involves ligand-receptor interactions, including the mannose receptor (MR) that recognizes mycobacterial components such as lipoarabinomannan (LAM) and Man-LAM. Phagocytosis is also promoted by Fc receptors (FcR) after opsonization with specific immunoglobulins, or by complement receptors (CR1, CR3, and CR4) after non-specific opsonization with complement [34, 43]. Phagocytosis is an important event because antigen presentation by AMs or DCs to T cells constitutes the beginning of the development of acquired immunity specific against *M. tuberculosis*.

T CELLS PLAY AN IMPORTANT ROLE IN ACQUIRED IMMUNITY

The control of *M. tuberculosis* infection depends on the development of the cellular immune response development after mycobacterial antigen presentation by DCs or AMs to T cells, characterized by the recruitment of different cellular populations at the site of infection such as macrophages, monocytes, DC, neutrophils, CD4$^+$, CD8$^+$, γδ T cells and natural killer (NK) cells and the production of pro-inflammatory cytokines (IL-1β, IL-6, IL-12, IL-18, TNF-α and IFN-γ) and chemokines CCL5, MIG and IP-10 which promote the recruitment of Th1 cells characterized by production of pro-inflammatory cytokines (IL-2, IFN-γ, and TNF-α) and antagonize Th2 recruitment source of anti-inflammatory cytokines (IL-4, IL-10 and TGF-β) [24].

After mycobacterial antigen presentation to specific-antigens CD4+ and CD8+ T cells subpopulations are activated and produce pro-inflammatory cytokines such as IL-2, IFN-γ, and TNF-α, that promote cellular immunity and confer protection in TB, but anti-inflammatory cytokines IL-4, IL-10 and TGF-β are also produced.

Inflammation against *M. tuberculosis* infection is characterized by pro-inflammatory cytokines (IL-1β, IL-6, IL-12, IL-18, TNF-α and IFN-γ) production related with infection control [45]. However, *M. tuberculosis*-induced host immune evasion by suppressive mechanism associated with pro-inflammatory cytokines production (IL-4, IL-0 and TGF-β) that promote humoral immunity that is less important in anti-mycobacterial defense [46].

BAL from TBP patients has been characterized by the production of cytokines and chemokines characteristic of Th2 such as IL-4 and CCL4, with highly specific mycobacterial IgG antibodies and SOCS3, in moderate to severe disease [47].

The growth control of *M. tuberculosis* depends in part on AMs and CD8+ T cells [48], through CCL5 production and the release of granulysin and perforin. Taken together, this report provides evidence that a subset of CD8+ T cells is thereby providing a host mechanism to attract *M. tuberculosis*-infected macrophages to kill the intracellular pathogen [49].

A main role of T cells is to be source of IFN-γ because induce macrophages activation and promote the mycobacterial elimination [50].

Neutrophils

Alveolar neutrophils considered "professional phagocytes", are an important cell population in the control of *M. tuberculosis* because they arrive early at the site of infection by chemotaxis in response to IL-8 and begin phagocytosis of mycobacteria to eliminate and control the initial infection. Simultaneously, activated neutrophils release different antibacterial components through three types of granules: i) azurophilic/primary granules, which mainly myeloperoxidase (MPO), elastase, cathepsin G and proteinase 3 and produce large amounts of ROS in a MPO-dependent and NADPH oxidase-dependent manner into the phagosome where the microorganism is eliminated. ii) Gelatinase/secondary granules with lactoferrin and the large source of lysozyme. iii) Gelatinase/tertiary granules that may represent partly emptied secondary granules without lactoferrin [51]. However, *M. tuberculosis* can survive inside neutrophils by escaping the oxidative killing [52]. Activated neutrophils produce soluble factors such as IL-1β, IL-8, IL-12 and LL-37 and are the first defense and recruit cells from the immune system. Also, infected neutrophils produce neutrophil extracellular traps from DNA (NETs) with MPO and elastase enzymes with bactericidal function which trap mycobacteria, but are unable to kill them [53].

Cytokines and Chemokine Release By Alveolar Macrophages and T Cells

This secction, include the cytokines and chemokines produced in TB and its interaction with different cells populations involved in the defense against *M. tuberculosis*.

Interleukin-12 (IL-12)

IL-12 is an early cytokine produced in macrophages, DCs, monocytes, neutrophils and, to a lesser extent, in other cells [54]. Phagocytosis of *M. tuberculosis* by macrophages triggers IL-12 production is detected at 3 h, peaks at 6-12 h, and decays to basal levels at 18-24 h [55]. Its production is regulated by cytokines, such as IFN-γ, that increase its production and by contrast, a reduction is observed in IL-4, IL-10, IL-11, IL-13, TGF-β and type I IFNs [54, 56, 57].

This cytokine is important in regulating the balance between Th1 and Th2 cells; Th1 cells secrete pro-inflammatory cytokines IL-2, TNF-α and IFN-γ promoting cell-mediated immunity importante in TB infection control, while Th2 cells produce anti-inflammatory cytokines IL-4, IL-5, IL-10, and IL-13, facilitating the humoral response.

IL-12 favors: **a)** the differentiation of naïve T cells during the initial encounter with antigen into Th1-cells capable of producing large amounts of IFN-γ, **b)** serves as a co-stimulus required for maximum secretion of IFN-γ by differentiated CD4+ Th1 cells that respond to a specific antigen, **c)** stimulates resting memory T cells to produce IFN-γ and, **d)** induces proliferation and increases cytotoxic activity in T and NK cells. Indirectly, IL-12 participates in acquired immunity because IFN-γ induces activation of phagocytic cells and increases their capability of killing, processing, and antigen presentation to CD4+ and CD8+ T cells for a specific immune response [54, 57]. IL-12 also enhances the expression of the IL-18 receptor. IL-18 is a cytokine produced by macrophages after infection with *M. tuberculosis* and indirectly contributes to the control of the mycobacterial infection by inducing IFN-γ production [58].

As previously mentioned, IL-12 is important for immunity against infection from *M. tuberculosis* because it is a potent inductor of IFN-γ. The interaction of IFN-γ with the IFN-γ receptor (IFN-γ R) on the surface of macrophages induces its activation followed by the expression of over 200 genes related with the efficient processing of MHC-mediated antigen presentation, synthesis of NO, the induction of components of cascade, apoptosis, and increased bactericidal activity of phagocytic cells. Thus it is important in infection by intracellular pathogens such as *M. tuberculosis* [50].

The importance of IFN-γ in the control of mycobacterial infections is demonstrated in mice model [59] and in patients with primary immunodeficiencies, like Mendelian Susceptibility to Mycobacterial Diseases (MSMD) with genetic alterations that affect the IL-12/IL-23/IFN-γ axis, and as a consequence, the production or response to IFN-γ is impaired. These patients have recurrent infections caused by mycobacteria and other intracellular pathogens like Salmonella [9, 60 - 63].

BAL from TBP patients revealed an increase of T cells and neutrophils in alveolar cells after infection by *M. tuberculosis* or PPD, which stimulated the production of high levels of IFN-γ, mainly from CD4+(CD45RO+) followed by CD8+, γδTCR cells, CD56+ T cell subpopulations and NK cells (CD3-CD56+) in association with IL-12 and IL-4 cytokine production [64, 65]. Furthermore, chemokines such as IP-10, MIG, Regulated upon activation, normal T cell expressed and secreted (RANTES), macrophage chemotactic protein-1 (MCP-1), macrophage inflammatory protein-1α (MIP-1α), IL-8, and TNF-α are released by infected human AMs to recruit different cell populations for granuloma formations, as a protection strategy [66, 67].

Tumoral Necrosis Factor-α (TNF-α)

TNF-α is a pro-inflammatory cytokine produced by activated macrophages, DCs, and T cells. In human AMs treated with MDP, the NOD2-specific ligand revealed that significant levels of IL-1β, IL-6, and TNF-α improved control of intracellular growth, an activity associated with IL-6 and TNF-α. This cytokine is important to recruit immune cells at the site of infection for the formation and maintenance of granuloma, and when neutralized, the granuloma is disrupted and the infection is exacerbated [68]. In human AMs, infection with *M. tuberculosis*, from H37Ra or H37Rv strains, caused cytolysis through a TNF-α-dependent mechanism of apoptosis [69].

However, the pathogen can exploit this mechanism to escape the intracellular bactericidal mechanism of the macrophage. This cytokine acts in synergy with IFN-γ, inducing iNOS enzyme expression in human AMs after *M. tuberculosis* infection. It is associated with NO production and has demonstrated growth inhibition of mycobacteria, suggesting the role of NO in the elimination of the microorganism [65, 70] Exacerbed TNF-α production causes necrosis with damage in host tissue and can be exploited by *M. tuberculosis*.

M. tuberculosis express surface antigens that can induce IL-10 and IL-4 (Th2 response), which typically have anti-inflammatory effects with the apparent capability to promote tissue damage in association with TNF-α. Some studies suggest that IL-4 (alone or with TNF-α) may destroy the cell and/or cause cell death during infection by *M. tuberculosis*. There is evidence of IL-4 production by AMs in TB patients [64, 65].

Interleukin-10 (IL-10)

IL-10 is an anti-inflammatory cytokine produced by AMs and T cells that can inhibit the production of pro-inflammatoty cytokines (IFN-γ, TNF-α and IL-12) and the action of antigen-presenting cells, blocking CD4+T cell activation by inhibiting MHC class II molecule expression. Because successful phagosomal maturation is important for the innate immune response, *M. tuberculosis* can manipulate and inhibit this response and survive within macrophages. However, this process can be modulated by cytokines. Human macrophages treated with IFN-γ may accelerate *M. tuberculosis* antigen processing and presentation, whereas IL-10 favors the trafficking of vesicles without lysosomal-associated membrane protein-1 (LAMP-1). Thus, this cytokine can promote the persistence of *M. tuberculosis* by contributing to *M. tuberculosis*-phagosome maturation arrest, in human macrophages [71, 72].

In TBP, the immune response involves participation of different cell populations, production of cytokines, chemokines and other bactericidal molecules, in a complex interaction, which is integrated in the Fig. (**2**).

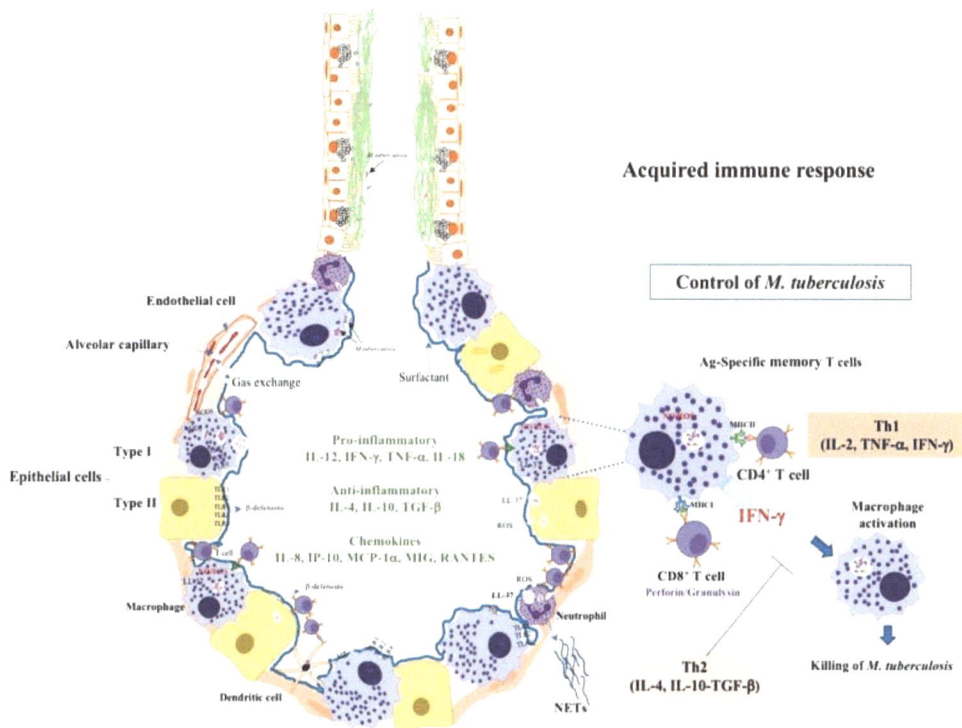

Fig. (2). Immunity development in the alveoli against *M. tuberculosis* infection. In human TBP, defense against *M. tuberculosis* in the alveoli is a complex and dynamic network with the participation of innate (macrophages, neutrophils) and acquired immune cells (T cells -Th1/ Th2), and epithelial cells (Type I and II). The immune response is characterized by the production of pro- and anti-inflammatory cytokines, chemokines, antimicrobial peptides (β-defensins, LL-37), surfactant, NET´s, NO, and ROS.

Effect of Host Genetic Factors, TB Treatment, Smoking, HIV And Diabetes on The Immune Response During Tuberculosis

Protection in TB is related to an acquired cellular immune response characterized by specific-antigen CD4+ T cells which are the main source of IFN-γ production, followed by CD8+T cells and NK cells [59]. This cytokine has been associated with the control of intracellular pathogens, such as *M. tuberculosis* because after IFN-γ interacts with the IFN-γ receptor (IFN-γR) on the surface of macrophages, macrophage activation is induced [50]. Evidence of the role of IFN-γ in mycobacterial clearance has been demonstrated in human macrophages the induction of autophagy, phagosomal maturation, AMPs production (cathelicidin and DEFB4) and the elimination of *M. tuberculosis* in a vitamin D-dependent pathway [73]. The importance of host genetic factors in the susceptibility to TBP had been demonstrated in patients with primary immunodeficiencies, such as

MSMD, with a deficient production of, or response to, IFN-γ, caused by mutations in the IL-12/IL-23/IFN-γ axis. Mutations on seven autosomal genes (*IFNR1, IFNR2, STAT1, IL12B, IL-12RB1, ISG15* and *IRF8)* and two x-linked (*NEMO and CYBB*) have been reported and result in impaired macrophage or T cells function, and cytokine production including IFN-γ, IL-23 or TNF-α, involved in the control of intracellular pathogens such as *M. bovis* BCG, environmental mycobacteria (EM) and *M. tuberculosis* [9, 60, 74].

Recently, mutations on the *SPPL2a, IL12Rβ2,* and *IL23R,* and *TYK2* P1104A genes have been discovered, resulting in selective impairment of response to IL-12 and IL-23, required for the optimal IFN-γ function [75].

These patients also have recurrent mycobacterial infections which give evidence to the important role of IFN-γ production in mycobacterial infection control [60, 61]. However, in bronchoalveolar cells (BAC) in active TBP, IFN-γ production by CD4+ and CD8+ T cells is increased when compared to healthy individuals. Therefore, failure to control *M. tuberculosis* growth may be due to immunosuppressive mechanisms that subvert the antimycobacterial activity of IFN-γ [64].

Additionally, natural killer (NK) cells play an important role in the early control of mycobacterial infections since they are a source of IFN-γ and participate in the intracellular control of *M. tuberculosis* infection. In the Manitoba population, a study that analyzed the frequency of killer cells immunoglobulin-like receptors (KIRs) found that TB patients had a centromeric AA-haplotype compared with the controls. This can result in differential cytokine expression and genetic susceptibility to TB [76].

In Indian population, the susceptibility to TB is due to single nucleotide polymorphism (SNPs-) on TLR1 (*TLR1-N248S*) innate receptor which prevents recognition of *M. tuberculosis*, and is characterized by reduction of TNF-α production, an important cytokine for the macrophage activation and granuloma formation during the TB infection [77].

Meanwhile, susceptibility to TBP is associated with allele A of the SNPs on rs352139 (in Mexican Amerindians), rs352143 (Vietnam population), and rs352142 with meningeal TB on TLR9 gene [78, 79].

Anti-TB treatment in patients with HIV-TB and TB has repercussions on the cytokine production and CD4+T phenotype cells involved in the immune response. The reduction of the mycobacterial burden is associated with an increased frequency of CD4+T cells that produce IFNγ+IL-2+TNF-α+, and with a decline in MIP-1β, IL-2 and TNF-α production. There is an increase in central memory T cells (CM), a reduction of effector memory cells (EM), and the inhibitory activation of T cell pathways (CTLA-4 and PD-1) as well [80]. Conversely, peripheral blood mononuclear cells (PBMC) from active TBP patients, produce lower levels of IFN-γ and higher levels of IL-10 in response to a 30 kDa mycobacterial antigen. After anti-TB treatment, IFN-γ expression and production increase and are probably associated with the reduction of the mycobacterial load [81]. Similarly, a significant increase of IFN-γ production was observed during isoniazid treatment in individuals with latent TB [82].

Smoking is other risk factor for TB, an observation supported by active TBP patients with reduced IFN-γ production. Thus, smoking reduces the cellular immune response important in the control and elimination of *M. tuberculosis* [83].

HIV-1 infection is the strongest risk factor for extrapulmonary TB with an effect on CD4+ T cells resulting in their reduction, and consequently, the source of IFN-γ thereby increasing the risk for TB in HIV patients [2, 84, 85].

HIV-1 infection alters the immune response by preventing the development of the cellular immune response against *M. tuberculosis*. Some studies show that HIV-1 increases *M. tuberculosis* growth in human macrophages, and HIV-TB co-infection reduces macrophage viability associated with high levels of TNF-α and IL-10 production [35, 86 - 88]. Apoptosis is an innate response to control *M. tuberculosis* infection and limit the disease. HIV-1 reduced apoptosis and significant TNF-α production [89]. Autophagy is another macrophage mechanism to eliminate *M. tuberculosis,* however, some HIV-1 viral proteins (Env, Tat, Vif) interfere with the early steps of autophagy in CD4+ T cells and macrophages [90].

Anti-retroviral therapy (ART) and anti-TB treatment, in HIV-TB and TB patients, have a similar effect on the CD4+ T cell count and cytokine production, EM, CM, and the inhibitory pathways previously mentioned. This evidence leads to conclude that these changes are related to anti-TB treatment rather than ART [80].

ART reduces HIV-1 replication with an increase of CD4+ T cells and early reconstitution of CM and naïve T cells but fewer in T cells is completely differentiated [86].

When HIV-infected patients on TB treatment start ART, approximately 15.9% acquire TB-associated immune reconstitution inflammatory syndrome (TB-IRIS), an early complication of ART, which reflects the immunopathological reaction to mycobacterial antigens by the recovering immune system. It is characterized by excessive inflammatory reactions against *M. tuberculosis* antigens with the recurrence of TB symptoms and commonly requires hospitalization [84, 86]. TB-IRIS is associated with polyfunctional expansions of PPD-specific IFN-γ-producing CD4+T cells that co-express pro-inflammatory cytokines IFN-γ+TNF-α+ and IL-2+ with the EM phenotype, and are highly active [91].

Diabetes patients have a high risk for developing TB [6, 7] and it is thought that chronic hyperglycemia affects the immune response [92]. Studies on peripheral monocytes from type 2 diabetes (T2D) patients, with low serum levels of vitamin D, show impaired control of intracellular *M. tuberculosis* with reduced NO production, but no effect on phagocytosis and IL-10, β-defensin, and LL-37 expression [93]. LL-37 is an AMP in innate immunity involved in the control of TB [39, 94]. The hyperglycemic conditions in T2D cause the vitamin D receptor (VDR) to be O-GlcNAcylated, without affecting LL-37 production [95].

However, some studies found that phagocytosis is reduced *via* the Fc-gamma receptor and complement in T2D patients [96].

CONCLUDING REMARKS

The immune response in human pulmonary tuberculosis requires the participation and the complex interaction of different cell types and is mediated by cytokines and chemokines. The cellular immune response, characterized by pro-inflammatory cytokines, plays an important role in the control of the infection. However, *M. tuberculosis* has different mechanisms to evade the immune response that give it an advantage and allow its survival in the host.

CONSENT FOR PUBLICATION

Not applicable.

CONFLICT OF INTEREST

The authors confirm that this chapter contents have no conflict of interest.

ACKNOWLEDGEMENTS

None declared.

REFERENCES

[1]   WHO | Global tuberculosis report 2019 World Health Organization (2020)
        [http://dx.doi.org/1037//0033-2909.I26.1.78]

[2]   WHO. https://www.who.int/news-room/fact-sheets/detail/tuberculosis

[3]   Khan AH, Israr M, Khan A, Aftab RA, Khan TM. Smoking on treatment outcomes among tuberculosis patients. Am J Med Sci 2015; 349(6): 505-9.
        [http://dx.doi.org/10.1097/MAJ.0000000000000473] [PMID: 26030612]

[4]   Reed GW, Choi H, Lee SY, *et al.* Impact of diabetes and smoking on mortality in tuberculosis. PLoS One 2013; 8(2): e58044.

[http://dx.doi.org/10.1371/journal.pone.0058044] [PMID: 23469139]

[5]   Stevenson CR, Forouhi NG, Roglic G, *et al.* Diabetes and tuberculosis: The impact of the diabetes epidemic on tuberculosis incidence. BMC Public Health 2007; 7: 234.
      [http://dx.doi.org/10.1186/1471-2458-7-234] [PMID: 17822539]

[6]   Jeon CY, Murray MB. Diabetes mellitus increases the risk of active tuberculosis: A systematic review of 13 observational studies. PLoS Med 2008; 5(7): e152.
      [http://dx.doi.org/10.1371/journal.pmed.0050152] [PMID: 18630984]

[7]   Baker MA, Harries AD, Jeon CY, *et al.* The impact of diabetes on tuberculosis treatment outcomes: A systematic review. BMC Med 2011; 9: 81.
      [http://dx.doi.org/10.1186/1741-7015-9-81] [PMID: 21722362]

[8]   Feleke BE, Feleke TE, Biadglegne F. Nutritional status of tuberculosis patients, a comparative cross-sectional study. BMC Pulm Med 2019; 19(1): 182.
      [http://dx.doi.org/10.1186/s12890-019-0953-0] [PMID: 31638950]

[9]   Bustamante J, Boisson-Dupuis S, Abel L, Casanova JL. Mendelian susceptibility to mycobacterial disease: genetic, immunological, and clinical features of inborn errors of IFN-γ immunity. Semin Immunol 2014; 26(6): 454-70.
      [http://dx.doi.org/10.1016/j.smim.2014.09.008] [PMID: 25453225]

[10] Hartl D, Tirouvanziam R, Laval J, *et al.* Innate immunity of the lung: From basic mechanisms to translational medicine. J Innate Immun 2018; 10(5-6): 487-501.
      [http://dx.doi.org/10.1159/000487057] [PMID: 29439264]

[11] Schoene RB. Limits of human lung function at high altitude. J Exp Biol 2001; 204(Pt 18): 3121-7.
      [PMID: 11581325]

[12] Whitsett JA, Alenghat T. Respiratory epithelial cells orchestrate pulmonary innate immunity. Nat Immunol 2015; 16(1): 27-35.
      [http://dx.doi.org/10.1038/ni.3045] [PMID: 25521682]

[13] Lloyd CM, Marsland BJ. Lung homeostasis: Influence of age, microbes, and the immune system. Immunity 2017; 46(4): 549-61.
      [http://dx.doi.org/10.1016/j.immuni.2017.04.005] [PMID: 28423336]

[14] Whitsett JA, Wert SE, Weaver TE. Alveolar surfactant homeostasis and the pathogenesis of pulmonary disease. Annu Rev Med 2010; 61: 105-19.
      [http://dx.doi.org/10.1146/annurev.med.60.041807.123500] [PMID: 19824815]

[15] B. Moldoveanu, P. Otmishi, P. Jani, *et al.* Inflammatory mechanisms in the lung. J Inflamm Res 2009; 1-12.

[16] Parker D, Prince A. Innate immunity in the respiratory epithelium. Am J Respir Cell Mol Biol 2011; 45(2): 189-201.
      [http://dx.doi.org/10.1165/rcmb.2011-0011RT] [PMID: 21330463]

[17] Knowles MR, Boucher RC. Innate defenses in the lung. J Clin Invest 2002; 109: 571-7.
      [http://dx.doi.org/10.1172/JCI0215217] [PMID: 11877463]

[18] Bals R. Epithelial antimicrobial peptides in host defense against infection. Respir Res 2000; 1(3): 141-50.
      [http://dx.doi.org/10.1186/rr25] [PMID: 11667978]

[19] Middleton AM, Chadwick MV, Nicholson AG, *et al.* Interaction between mycobacteria and mucus on a human respiratory tissue organ culture model with an air interface. Exp Lung Res 2004; 30(1): 17-29.
      [http://dx.doi.org/10.1080/01902140490252876] [PMID: 14967601]

[20] Ellison Iii R T, Giehl T J, Laforcet F M. Damage of the outer membrane of enteric gram-negative bacteria by lactoferrin and transferrin. Infect Immun 1988; 56(11): 2774-81.

[21]   Ridley C, Thornton DJ. Mucins: the frontline defence of the lung. Biochem Soc Trans 2018; 46(5): 1099-106.
[http://dx.doi.org/10.1042/BST20170402] [PMID: 30154090]

[22]   Tecle T, Tripathi S, Hartshorn KL. Review: Defensins and cathelicidins in lung immunity. Innate Immun 2010; 16(3): 151-9.
[http://dx.doi.org/10.1177/1753425910365734] [PMID: 20418263]

[23]   Liu T, Zhang L, Joo D, Sun SC. NF-κB signaling in inflammation. Signal Transduct Target Ther 2017; 2: 17023.
[http://dx.doi.org/10.1038/sigtrans.2017.23] [PMID: 29158945]

[24]   Bals R, Hiemstra PS. Innate immunity in the lung: How epithelial cells fight against respiratory pathogens. Eur Respir J 2004; 23(2): 327-33.
[http://dx.doi.org/10.1183/09031936.03.00098803] [PMID: 14979512]

[25]   Harada A, Sekido N, Akahoshi T, *et al.* Essential involvement of interleukin-8 (IL-8) in acute inflammation. J Leukocyte Bio 1994; 56(5): 559-64.
[http://dx.doi.org/doi:10.1002/jlb.56.5.559]

[26]   Delogu G, Sali M, Fadda G. The biology of *Mycobacterium tuberculosis* infection. Mediterr J Hematol Infect Dis 2013; 5(1): e2013070.
[http://dx.doi.org/10.4084/mjhid.2013.070] [PMID: 24363885]

[27]   Forrellad MA, Klepp LI, Gioffré A, *et al.* Virulence factors of the *Mycobacterium tuberculosis* complex. Virulence 2013; 4(1): 3-66.
[http://dx.doi.org/10.4161/viru.22329] [PMID: 23076359]

[28]   Seghatoleslam A, Hemmati M, Ebadat S, Movahedi B, Mostafavi-Pour Z. Macrophage Immune Response Suppression by Recombinant *Mycobacterium tuberculosis* Antigens, the ESAT-6, CFP-10, and ESAT-6/CFP-10 Fusion Proteins. Iran J Med Sci 2016; 41(4): 296-304.

[29]   Deng W, Li W, Zeng J, *et al. Mycobacterium tuberculosis* PPE family protein Rv1808 manipulates cytokines profile *via* co-activation of MAPK and NF-κB signaling pathways. Cell Physiol Biochem 2014; 33(2): 273-88.
[http://dx.doi.org/10.1159/000356668] [PMID: 24525621]

[30]   Blanc L, Gilleron M, Prandi J, *et al. Mycobacterium tuberculosis* inhibits human innate immune responses *via* the production of TLR2 antagonist glycolipids. Proc Natl Acad Sci USA 2017; 114(42): 11205-10.
[http://dx.doi.org/10.1073/pnas.1707840114] [PMID: 28973928]

[31]   Hernández-Pando R, Jeyanathan M, Mengistu G, *et al.* Persistence of DNA from *Mycobacterium tuberculosis* in superficially normal lung tissue during latent infection. Lancet 2000; 356(9248): 2133-8.
[http://dx.doi.org/10.1016/S0140-6736(00)03493-0] [PMID: 11191539]

[32]   Harriff MJ, Cansler ME, Toren KG, *et al.* Human lung epithelial cells contain *Mycobacterium tuberculosis* in a late endosomal vacuole and are efficiently recognized by CD8⁺ T cells. PLoS One 2014; 9(5): e97515.
[http://dx.doi.org/10.1371/journal.pone.0097515] [PMID: 24828674]

[33]   Faridgohar M, Nikoueinejad H. New findings of Toll-like receptors involved in *Mycobacterium tuberculosis* infection. Pathog Glob Health 2017; 111(5): 256-64.
[http://dx.doi.org/10.1080/20477724.2017.1351080] [PMID: 28715935]

[34]   Ishikawa E, Mori D, Yamasaki S. Recognition of Mycobacterial Lipids by Immune Receptors. Trends Immunol 2017; 38(1): 66-76.
[http://dx.doi.org/10.1016/j.it.2016.10.009] [PMID: 27889398]

[35]   Juárez E, Carranza C, Hernández-Sánchez F, *et al.* Nucleotide-oligomerizing domain-1 (NOD1) receptor activation induces pro-inflammatory responses and autophagy in human alveolar

macrophages. BMC Pulm Med 2014; 14: 152.
[http://dx.doi.org/10.1186/1471-2466-14-152] [PMID: 25253572]

[36] Juárez E, Carranza C, Hernández-Sánchez F, *et al.* NOD2 enhances the innate response of alveolar macrophages to *Mycobacterium tuberculosis* in humans. Eur J Immunol 2012; 42(4): 880-9.
[http://dx.doi.org/10.1002/eji.201142105] [PMID: 22531915]

[37] Danelishvili L, Cirillo SLG, Cirillo JD, Bermudez LE. Virulent mycobacteria and the many aspects of macrophage uptake. Future Microbiol 2007; 2(5): 461-4.
[http://dx.doi.org/10.2217/17460913.2.5.461] [PMID: 17927465]

[38] Ganbat D, Seehase S, Richter E, *et al.* Mycobacteria infect different cell types in the human lung and cause species dependent cellular changes in infected cells. BMC Pulm Med 2016; 16: 19.
[http://dx.doi.org/10.1186/s12890-016-0185-5] [PMID: 26803467]

[39] Rivas-Santiago B, Hernandez-Pando R, Carranza C, *et al.* Expression of cathelicidin LL-37 during *Mycobacterium tuberculosis* infection in human alveolar macrophages, monocytes, neutrophils, and epithelial cells. Infect Immun 2008; 76(3): 935-41.
[http://dx.doi.org/10.1128/IAI.01218-07] [PMID: 18160480]

[40] Cakir E, Torun E, Gedik AH, *et al.* Cathelicidin and human β-defensin 2 in bronchoalveolar lavage fluid of children with pulmonary tuberculosis. Int J Tuberc Lung Dis 2014; 18(6): 671-5.
[http://dx.doi.org/10.5588/ijtld.13.0831] [PMID: 24903937]

[41] Juarez E, Nuñez C, Sada E, Ellner JJ, Schwander SK, Torres M. Differential expression of Toll-like receptors on human alveolar macrophages and autologous peripheral monocytes. Respir Res 2010; 11: 2.
[http://dx.doi.org/10.1186/1465-9921-11-2] [PMID: 20051129]

[42] Bermudez LE, Goodman J. *Mycobacterium tuberculosis* invades and replicates within type II alveolar cells. Infect Immun 1996; 64(4): 1400-6.
[http://dx.doi.org/10.1128/IAI.64.4.1400-1406.1996] [PMID: 8606107]

[43] Aderem A, Underhill DM. Mechanisms of phagocytosis in macrophages. Annu Rev Immunol 1999; 17: 593-623.
[http://dx.doi.org/10.1146/annurev.immunol.17.1.593] [PMID: 10358769]

[44] Ernst JD. Macrophage receptors for *Mycobacterium tuberculosis*. Infect Immun 1998; 66(4): 1277-81.
[http://dx.doi.org/10.1128/IAI.66.4.1277-1281.1998] [PMID: 9529042]

[45] Schwander S, Dheda K. Human lung immunity against *Mycobacterium tuberculosis*: insights into pathogenesis and protection. Am J Respir Crit Care Med 2011; 183(6): 696-707.
[http://dx.doi.org/10.1164/rccm.201006-0963PP] [PMID: 21075901]

[46] Achkar JM, Chan J, Casadevall A. B cells and antibodies in the defense against *Mycobacterium tuberculosis* infection. Immunol Rev 2015; 264(1): 167-81.
[http://dx.doi.org/10.1111/imr.12276] [PMID: 25703559]

[47] Ashenafi S, Aderaye G, Bekele A, *et al.* Progression of clinical tuberculosis is associated with a Th2 immune response signature in combination with elevated levels of SOCS3. Clin Immunol 2014; 151(2): 84-99.
[http://dx.doi.org/10.1016/j.clim.2014.01.010] [PMID: 24584041]

[48] Carranza C, Juárez E, Torres M, Ellner JJ, Sada E, Schwander SK. *Mycobacterium tuberculosis* growth control by lung macrophages and CD8 cells from patient contacts. Am J Respir Crit Care Med 2006; 173(2): 238-45.
[http://dx.doi.org/10.1164/rccm.200503-411OC] [PMID: 16210664]

[49] Stegelmann F, *et al.* Defense Mechanism against *Mycobacterium tuberculosis* 1. J Immunol 2005.
[PMID: 16301655]

[50] Boehm U, Klamp T, Groot M, Howard JC. Cellular responses to interferon-γ. Annu Rev Immunol 1997; 15: 749-95.

[http://dx.doi.org/10.1146/annurev.immunol.15.1.749] [PMID: 9143706]

[51]   Gunzer M. Traps and hyper inflammation - new ways that neutrophils promote or hinder survival. Br J Haematol 2014; 164(2): 189-99.
[http://dx.doi.org/10.1111/bjh.12608] [PMID: 24138538]

[52]   Corleis B, Korbel D, Wilson R, Bylund J, Chee R, Schaible UE. Escape of *Mycobacterium tuberculosis* from oxidative killing by neutrophils. Cell Microbiol 2012; 14(7): 1109-21.
[http://dx.doi.org/10.1111/j.1462-5822.2012.01783.x] [PMID: 22405091]

[53]   Ramos-Kichik V, Mondragón-Flores R, Mondragón-Castelán M, *et al.* Neutrophil extracellular traps are induced by *Mycobacterium tuberculosis*. Tuberculosis (Edinb) 2009; 89(1): 29-37.
[http://dx.doi.org/10.1016/j.tube.2008.09.009] [PMID: 19056316]

[54]   Watford WT, Moriguchi M, Morinobu A, O'Shea JJ. The biology of IL-12: coordinating innate and adaptive immune responses. Cytokine Growth Factor Rev 2003; 14(5): 361-8.
[http://dx.doi.org/10.1016/S1359-6101(03)00043-1] [PMID: 12948519]

[55]   Fulton SA, Johnsen JM, Wolf SF, Sieburth DS, Boom WH. Interleukin-12 production by human monocytes infected with *Mycobacterium tuberculosis*: role of phagocytosis. Infect Immun 1996; 64(7): 2523-31.
[http://dx.doi.org/10.1128/IAI.64.7.2523-2531.1996] [PMID: 8698475]

[56]   Fulton SA, Cross JV, Toossi ZT, Boom WH. Regulation of interleukin-12 by interleukin-10, transforming growth factor-β, tumor necrosis factor-α, and interferon-γ in human monocytes infected with *Mycobacterium tuberculosis* H37Ra. J Infect Dis 1998; 178(4): 1105-14.
[http://dx.doi.org/10.1086/515698] [PMID: 9806041]

[57]   Gately MK, Renzetti LM, Magram J, *et al.* The interleukin-12/interleukin-12-receptor system: role in normal and pathologic immune responses. Annu Rev Immunol 1998; 16: 495-521.
[http://dx.doi.org/10.1146/annurev.immunol.16.1.495] [PMID: 9597139]

[58]   Robinson CM, O'Dee D, Hamilton T, Nau GJ. Cytokines involved in interferon-γ production by human macrophages. J Innate Immun 2010; 2(1): 56-65.
[http://dx.doi.org/10.1159/000247156] [PMID: 20375623]

[59]   Flynn JL, Chan J, Triebold KJ, Dalton DK, Stewart TA, Bloom BR. An essential role for interferon γ in resistance to *Mycobacterium tuberculosis* infection. J Exp Med 1993; 178(6): 2249-54.
[http://dx.doi.org/10.1084/jem.178.6.2249] [PMID: 7504064]

[60]   Rosain J, Oleaga-Quintas C, Deswarte C. A variety of Alu-mediated copy number variations can underlie IL-12Rβ1 deficiency. J Clin Immunol 2018; 38(5): 617–27.
[http://dx.doi.org/10.1007/s10875-018-0527-6]

[61]   Pedraza-Sánchez S, Herrera-Barrios MT, Aldana-Vergara R, *et al.* Bacille Calmette-Guérin infection and disease with fatal outcome associated with a point mutation in the interleukin-12/interleukin-23 receptor beta-1 chain in two Mexican families. Int J Infect Dis 2010; 14 (Suppl. 3): e256-60.
[http://dx.doi.org/10.1016/j.ijid.2009.11.005] [PMID: 20171917]

[62]   Dorman SE, Holland SM. Mutation in the signal-transducing chain of the interferon-γ receptor and susceptibility to mycobacterial infection. J Clin Invest 1998; 101(11): 2364-9.
[http://dx.doi.org/10.1172/JCI2901] [PMID: 9616207]

[63]   Pedraza S, Lezana JL, Samarina A, *et al.* Clinical disease caused by Klebsiella in 2 unrelated patients with interleukin 12 receptor β1 deficiency. Pediatrics 2010; 126(4): e971-6.
[http://dx.doi.org/10.1542/peds.2009-2504] [PMID: 20855390]

[64]   Herrera MT, Torres M, Nevels D, *et al.* Compartmentalized bronchoalveolar IFN-γ and IL-12 response in human pulmonary tuberculosis. Tuberculosis (Edinb) 2009; 89(1): 38-47.
[http://dx.doi.org/10.1016/j.tube.2008.08.002] [PMID: 18848499]

[65]   Cavalcanti YVN, Brelaz MCA, Neves JKDAL, Ferraz JC, Pereira VRA. Role of TNF-alpha, IFN-gamma, and IL-10 in the development of pulmonary tuberculosis. Pulm Med 2012; 2012: 745483.

[http://dx.doi.org/10.1155/2012/745483] [PMID: 23251798]

[66]   Sadek MI, Sada E, Toossi Z, Schwander SK, Rich EA. Chemokines induced by infection of mononuclear phagocytes with mycobacteria and present in lung alveoli during active pulmonary tuberculosis. Am J Respir Cell Mol Biol 1998; 19(3): 513-21.
[http://dx.doi.org/10.1165/ajrcmb.19.3.2815] [PMID: 9730880]

[67]   Fenton MJ, Vermeulen MW, Kim S, Burdick M, Strieter RM, Kornfeld H. Induction of gamma interferon production in human alveolar macrophages by *Mycobacterium tuberculosis*. Infect Immun 1997; 65(12): 5149-56.
[http://dx.doi.org/10.1128/IAI.65.12.5149-5156.1997] [PMID: 9393809]

[68]   Jacobs M, Samarina A, Grivennikov S, *et al*. Reactivation of tuberculosis by tumor necrosis factor neutralization. Eur Cytokine Netw 2007; 18(1): 5-13.
[http://dx.doi.org/10.1684/ecn.2007.0083] [PMID: 17400533]

[69]   Keane J, Balcewicz-Sablinska MK, Remold HG, *et al*. Infection by *Mycobacterium tuberculosis* promotes human alveolar macrophage apoptosis. Infect Immun 1997; 65(1): 298-304.
[http://dx.doi.org/10.1128/IAI.65.1.298-304.1997] [PMID: 8975927]

[70]   Rich EA, Torres M, Sada E, Finegan CK, Hamilton BD, Toossi Z. *Mycobacterium tuberculosis* (MTB)-stimulated production of nitric oxide by human alveolar macrophages and relationship of nitric oxide production to growth inhibition of MTB. Tuber Lung Dis 1997; 78(5-6): 247-55.
[http://dx.doi.org/10.1016/S0962-8479(97)90005-8] [PMID: 10209679]

[71]   Bobadilla K, Sada E, Jaime ME, *et al*. Human phagosome processing of *Mycobacterium tuberculosis* antigens is modulated by interferon-γ and interleukin-10. Immunology 2013; 138(1): 34-46.
[http://dx.doi.org/10.1111/imm.12010] [PMID: 22924705]

[72]   O'Leary S, O'Sullivan MP, Keane J. IL-10 blocks phagosome maturation in *Mycobacterium tuberculosis*-infected human macrophages. Am J Respir Cell Mol Biol 2011; 45(1): 172-80.
[http://dx.doi.org/10.1165/rcmb.2010-0319OC] [PMID: 20889800]

[73]   Fabri M, Stenger S, Shin DM, *et al*. Vitamin D is required for IFN-γ-mediated antimicrobial activity of human macrophages. Sci Transl Med 2011; 3(104): 104ra102.
[http://dx.doi.org/10.1126/scitranslmed.3003045] [PMID: 21998409]

[74]   de Beaucoudrey L, Samarina A, Bustamante J, *et al*. Revisiting human IL-12Rβ1 deficiency: a survey of 141 patients from 30 countries. Medicine (Baltimore) 2010; 89(6): 381-402.
[http://dx.doi.org/10.1097/MD.0b013e3181fdd832] [PMID: 21057261]

[75]   Bustamante J. Mendelian susceptibility to mycobacterial disease: recent discoveries. Hum Genet 2020; 139(6-7): 993-1000.
[http://dx.doi.org/10.1007/s00439-020-02120-y] [PMID: 32025907]

[76]   Braun K, Wolfe J, Kiazyk S, Kaushal Sharma M. Evaluation of host genetics on outcome of tuberculosis infection due to differences in killer immunoglobulin-like receptor gene frequencies and haplotypes. BMC Genet 2015; 16: 63.
[http://dx.doi.org/10.1186/s12863-015-0224-x] [PMID: 26077983]

[77]   Dittrich N, Berrocal-Almanza LC, Thada S, *et al*. Toll-like receptor 1 variations influence susceptibility and immune response to *Mycobacterium tuberculosis*. Tuberculosis (Edinb) 2015; 95(3): 328-35.
[http://dx.doi.org/10.1016/j.tube.2015.02.045] [PMID: 25857934]

[78]   Torres-García D, Cruz-Lagunas A, García-Sancho Figueroa MC, *et al*. Variants in toll-like receptor 9 gene influence susceptibility to tuberculosis in a Mexican population. J Transl Med 2013; 11: 220.
[http://dx.doi.org/10.1186/1479-5876-11-220] [PMID: 24053111]

[79]   Graustein AD, Horne DJ, Arentz M, *et al*. TLR9 gene region polymorphisms and susceptibility to tuberculosis in Vietnam. Tuberculosis (Edinb) 2015; 95(2): 190-6.
[http://dx.doi.org/10.1016/j.tube.2014.12.009] [PMID: 25616954]

[80]   Saharia KK, Petrovas C, Ferrando-Martinez S, *et al*. Tuberculosis therapy modifies the cytokine profile, maturation state, and expression of inhibitory molecules on *Mycobacterium tuberculosis*-specific CD4+ T-Cells. PLoS One 2016; 11(7): e0158262.
[http://dx.doi.org/10.1371/journal.pone.0158262] [PMID: 27367521]

[81]   Torres M, Herrera T, Villareal H, Rich EA, Sada E. Cytokine profiles for peripheral blood lymphocytes from patients with active pulmonary tuberculosis and healthy household contacts in response to the 30-kilodalton antigen of *Mycobacterium tuberculosis*. Infect Immun 1998; 66(1): 176-80.
[http://dx.doi.org/10.1128/IAI.66.1.176-180.1998] [PMID: 9423855]

[82]   Torres M, García-García L, Cruz-Hervert P, *et al*. Effect of isoniazid on antigen-specific interferon-γ secretion in latent tuberculosis. Eur Respir J 2015; 45(2): 473-82.
[http://dx.doi.org/10.1183/09031936.00123314] [PMID: 25359354]

[83]   Altet N, Latorre I, Jiménez-Fuentes MÁ, *et al*. Assessment of the influence of direct tobacco smoke on infection and active TB management. PLoS One 2017; 12(8): e0182998.
[http://dx.doi.org/10.1371/journal.pone.0182998] [PMID: 28837570]

[84]   Sterling TR, Pham PA, Chaisson RE. HIV infection-related tuberculosis: clinical manifestations and treatment. Clin Infect Dis 2010; 50 (Suppl. 3): S223-30.
[http://dx.doi.org/10.1086/651495] [PMID: 20397952]

[85]   Kedzierska K, Crowe SM. Cytokines and HIV-1: interactions and clinical implications. Antivir Chem Chemother 2001; 12(3): 133-50.
[http://dx.doi.org/10.1177/095632020101200301] [PMID: 12959322]

[86]   Walker NF, Meintjes G, Wilkinson RJ. HIV-1 and the immune response to TB. Future Virol 2013; 8(1): 57-80.
[http://dx.doi.org/10.2217/fvl.12.123] [PMID: 23653664]

[87]   Pathak S, Wentzel-Larsen T, Asjö B. Effects of *in vitro* HIV-1 infection on mycobacterial growth in peripheral blood monocyte-derived macrophages. Infect Immun 2010; 78(9): 4022-32.
[http://dx.doi.org/10.1128/IAI.00106-10] [PMID: 20624908]

[88]   Imperiali FG, Zaninoni A, La Maestra L, Tarsia P, Blasi F, Barcellini W. Increased *Mycobacterium tuberculosis* growth in HIV-1-infected human macrophages: role of tumour necrosis factor-α. Clin Exp Immunol 2001; 123(3): 435-42.
[http://dx.doi.org/10.1046/j.1365-2249.2001.01481.x] [PMID: 11298131]

[89]   Patel NR, Zhu J, Tachado SD, *et al*. HIV impairs TNF-α mediated macrophage apoptotic response to *Mycobacterium tuberculosis*. J Immunol 2007; 179(10): 6973-80.
[http://dx.doi.org/10.4049/jimmunol.179.10.6973] [PMID: 17982088]

[90]   Espert L, Beaumelle B, Vergne I. Autophagy in *Mycobacterium tuberculosis* and HIV infections. Front Cell Infect Microbiol 2015; 5: 49.
[http://dx.doi.org/10.3389/fcimb.2015.00049] [PMID: 26082897]

[91]   Bourgarit A, Carcelain G, Samri A, *et al*. Tuberculosis-associated immune restoration syndrome in HIV-1-infected patients involves tuberculin-specific CD4 Th1 cells and KIR-negative gammadelta T cells. J Immunol 2009; 183(6): 3915-23.
[http://dx.doi.org/10.4049/jimmunol.0804020] [PMID: 19726768]

[92]   Torres M, Herrera MT, Fabián-San-Miguel G, Gonzalez Y. The intracellular growth of *M. tuberculosis* is more associated with high glucose levels than with impaired responses of monocytes from T2D patients. J Immunol Res 2019; 2019: 1462098.
[http://dx.doi.org/10.1155/2019/1462098] [PMID: 31815150]

[93]   Herrera MT, Gonzalez Y, Hernández-Sánchez F, Fabián-San Miguel G, Torres M. Low serum vitamin D levels in type 2 diabetes patients are associated with decreased mycobacterial activity. BMC Infect Dis 2017; 17(1): 610.

[http://dx.doi.org/10.1186/s12879-017-2705-1] [PMID: 28882103]

[94]   Martineau AR, Wilkinson KA, Newton SM, *et al.* IFN-γ- and TNF-independent vitamin D-inducible human suppression of mycobacteria: the role of cathelicidin LL-37. J Immunol 2007; 178(11): 7190-8.
[http://dx.doi.org/10.4049/jimmunol.178.11.7190] [PMID: 17513768]

[95]   Hernández-Sánchez F, Guzmán-Beltrán S, Herrera MT, *et al.* High glucose induces O-GlcNAc glycosylation of the vitamin D receptor (VDR) in THP1 cells and in human macrophages derived from monocytes. Cell Biol Int 2017; 41(9): 1065-74.
[http://dx.doi.org/10.1002/cbin.10827] [PMID: 28710799]

[96]   Gomez DI, Twahirwa M. S., S. L. & I., R. B. Reduced association of mycobacterium with monocytes from diabetes patients with poor glucose control. Tuberc 2013; 93: 192-7.
[http://dx.doi.org/10.1016/j.tube.2012.10.003] [PMID: 23131496]

CHAPTER 5

Inducing Autophagy to Eliminate Intracellular Bacteria

Andy Ruiz[1,3] and **Esmeralda Juárez**[2,*]

¹ Departamento de Inmunología Integrativa, Instituto Nacional de Enfermedades Respiratorias Ismael Cosío Villegas, Ciudad de México, México

² Departamento de Investigación en Microbiología, Instituto Nacional de Enfermedades Respiratorias Ismael Cosío Villegas, Ciudad de México, México

³ Posgrado en Ciencias Biológicas, UNAM, México

Abstract: Autophagy is a lysosome-based degradation pathway of cytosolic cargos activated to prolong survival during starvation and diverse stress conditions by recycling of cellular content. In selective macroautophagy, specific cargos that could be misfolded proteins, damaged organelles, or intracellular pathogens selectively undergo degradation within autolysosomal compartments. However, some pathogens exhibit highly evolved tactics for evading autophagic recognition and are capable of surviving and replicating within the cytoplasm. Because autophagy is inducible in cells infected with pathogens that block autophagy, this mechanism has been proposed to be useful for therapy. In this chapter, we focus on *Mycobacterium tuberculosis*, one of the top causes of death worldwide and an archetype of intracellular pathogens, and its interaction with the autophagy machinery. First, we describe the generalities of the autophagic process and give examples of the bacterial strategies to evade or exploit autophagy. Also, we discuss the induction of autophagy as a therapeutic approach to circumvent the escape of bacteria from autophagy by using three types of autophagy inducers, the natural compounds, the microbial compound, and drugs. Also, we argue the main concerns that should be taken into account when using autophagy inducers as therapeutic agents.

Keywords: Autophagy, LC3, Tuberculosis, Macrophage, Immunomodulator, Rapamycin, Loperamide, MDP, Tri-DAD, NDGA.

INTRODUCTION

Autophagy is the name generally used for lysosome-based degradation pathways of cytosolic cargos (extensively reviewed in [1]). Autophagy was initially characterized by its ability to prolong survival during starvation and diverse stress

* **Corresponding author Esmeralda Juárez:** Instituto Nacional de Enfermedades Respiratorias Ismael Cosío Villegas. Departamento de Investigación en Microbiología. Ciudad de México, México; Tel: 54871700, Ext 5117; E-mail: ejuarez@iner.gob.mx

Gloria G. Guerrero Manriquez (Ed.)

conditions by recycling of cellular content, including organelles, to generate energy and nutrients by sacrificing parts of the cytosol. Currently, multiple studies have demonstrated that this catabolic pathway is a central element of immunological functions, such as innate and adaptive immune activation and antimicrobial host defense against viral, parasitic, and bacterial infections [2, 3]. Taking into consideration that multiple players involved in the autophagy machinery comprise elements with complex names, there is an alphabetically ordered list at the end of this chapter of all the acronyms and protein names used here (Box **1**).

There are three types of autophagy. 1) Microautophagy, which involves the direct acquisition of substrates by invaginating endosomal or lysosomal membranes. 2) Chaperone-mediated autophagy, which mediates selective degradation of proteins containing a KFERQ-like motif, whose recognition is mediated by heat shock cognate 71 kDa (Hsc70) chaperones, and they are further translocated across the lysosomal membrane in a lysosomal-associated membrane protein 2A (LAMP2A)-dependent fashion. 3) Macroautophagy, which requires the formation of autophagosomes, double-membrane vesicles that enclose a portion of the cytosol and fuse with late endosomes and lysosomes [4, 5]. Because of its involvement in eliminating intracellular pathogens, we are focusing on macroautophagy in this chapter.

For autophagosome origination and delivery to lysosomes, autophagy-related gene (atg) products are critical (Fig. **1**). These Atgs are organized in complexes that integrate metabolic signs to regulate macroautophagy and modify membranes by lipid phosphorylation and ubiquitin-like protein conjugation to lipids. The result is the autophagosome biogenesis (at the beginning it is called phagophore) and the expansion of the lipid membrane to complete the autophagosome. The Atg1/ ULK1 complex, regulated through phosphorylation by mammalian target of rapamycin (mTOR) inhibition and AMP-activated protein kinase (AMPK) activation, sense nutrient or growth factor exhaustion *via* decreased mTOR activity and low-energy levels. Atg1/ULK1 phosphorylates Atg6/ Beclin-1, resulting in a phosphoinositide mark on membranes. Atg16L1 is then recruited to the phagophore and establishes a complex to conjugate Atg8/LC3/GABARAP to phosphatidylethanolamine (PE), which participates in the recruitment of cargo into the autophagosome. The cysteine protease Atg4 cleaves Atg8/LC3 to generate microtubule-associated protein 1A/1B-light chain 3 (LC3 dissociated form, also known as LC3-I), which is subsequently conjugated to PE on the autophagosomal membranes *via* Atg3 and Atg7, forming the lipidated, membrane-associated LC3-II form. LC3-II is involved in the final sealing steps that allow the completion of an autophagosome and is considered a gold standard marker of autophagic compartments. The newly formed autophagosome then fuses with the lysosome to form an acidified autophagolysosome fully equipped to degrade the cargo [1, 6 - 9].

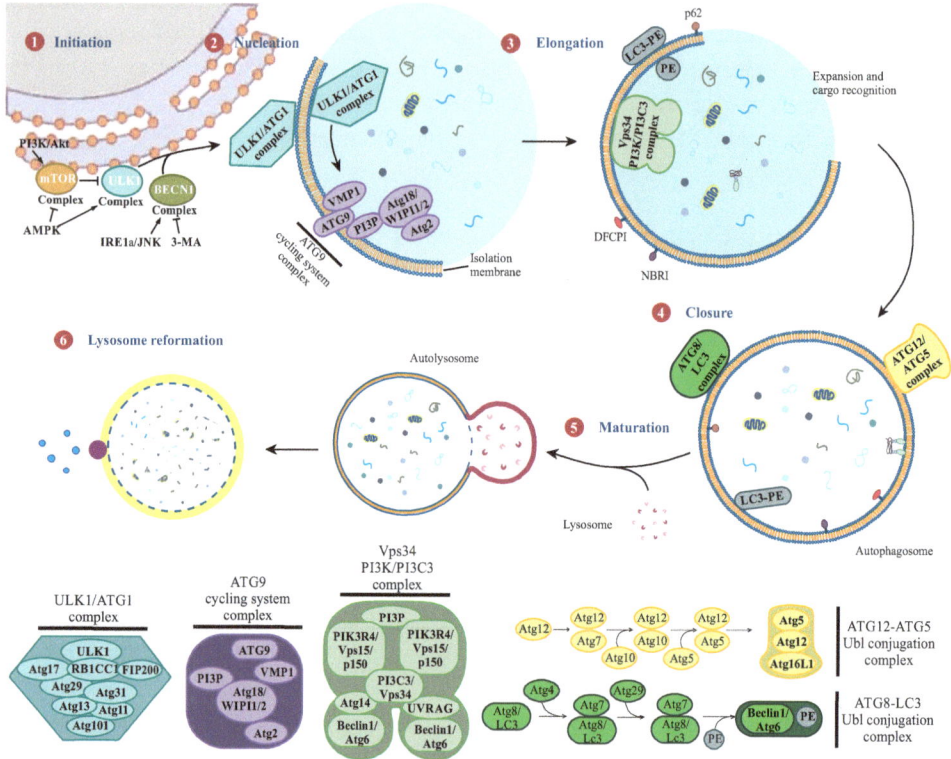

Fig. (1). Autophagosome biogenesis. Autophagy is controlled primarily by ATG proteins. The ATG family and other proteins operate in a complex conjugation cascade. A simplified scheme for autophagy includes four sub-groups of core proteins involved in three steps of autophagosome formation: initiation (1), nucleation (2), and elongation (3). The ATG1/ULK1 complex initiates autophagy under negative and positive regulation by mTOR and AMP kinase (AMPK), respectively, as well as mTOR-independent pathways. The ATG9 cycling system coordinates the nucleation and the Vps34 complex the elongation. The closure (4) of the autophagosome depends on ATG12/ATG5 and ATG8/LC3 ubiquitin-dependent conjugation. Maturation (5) requires lysosomal fusion with the autophagosome to form the autolysosome and lysosome reformation (6). Complexes are described in the inset.

Under starvation environments, macroautophagy operates nonselectively by recycling components of the cytosol for nutritional purposes. However, macroautophagy can also be selective, with specific substrates ranging from protein aggregates to damaged organelles for specific degradation of excessive or toxic structures. In this instance, selective macroautophagy operates under nutrient-rich conditions. In selective macroautophagy, specific cargos such as misfolded proteins, damaged organelles, or intracellular pathogens are first ubiquitinated. After that, the ubiquitinated products are recognized by the cargo receptors or adaptors such as the yeast Atg19, and two related mammalian proteins p62 (also known as SQSTM1, sequestosome-1) and neighbor of BRCA1 gene 1 protein (NBR1) to link the cargo to the autophagic machinery and elicit directed autophagosome formation and further degradation of the cargo [10 - 14].

Because selective macroautophagy clears several subcellular structures, various terms have been devised to reflect the specificity of the process. Selective autophagy classification includes mitophagy (degradation of damaged mitochondria), pexophagy (peroxisomes), lipophagy (lipid droplets), glycophagy (glycogen), ribophagy (ribosomes), ER-phagy (endoplasmic reticulum, ER), and xenophagy (intracellular pathogens such as bacteria, viruses, and parasites) [3, 11]. The diversity of potential targets for autophagic degradation suggests their implication in regulating diverse physiological processes, including cellular homeostasis, inflammation, and the fate of intracellular infection. Xenophagy is the central point in this chapter, and we will give special attention to *Mycobacterium tuberculosis*, the archetype of intracellular pathogens.

Importance of Xenophagy

The expected outcome of host-pathogen interaction in intracellular infections is the elimination of the intracellular microbial niche, exposing the intracellular pathogen to immune degradation and activating the adaptive immune system. Xenophagy is an essential arm of cell immunity to intracellular bacteria. This process targets a broad range of gram-positive and gram-negative bacteria such as *Listeria monocytogenes*, *Salmonella enterica* serovar *typhimurium*, *Shigella flexneri*, *Francisella tularensis*, *Staphylococcus aureus*, group A Streptococcus, *Yersinia enterocolitica*, *Burkholderia pseudomallei*, and *Mycobacterium tuberculosis*. Xenophagy begins with the permeation of the bacterium-containing vacuole, followed by ubiquitination and recruitment of autophagy adaptor proteins, including p62, nuclear dot protein 52 kDa (NDP52), ring finger protein 166 (RNF166), and optineurin, leading to the recruitment of LC3 and the formation of an autophagosome. The autophagosome then fuses with lysosomal-associated membrane protein 1 (LAMP1)-positive lysosomes, and the targeted microbe degrades [15 - 21]. Thus, xenophagy (hereafter referred to as autophagy) is necessary to limit bacterial replication.

Autophagy is a crucial mechanism through which macrophages reduce intracellular *M. tuberculosis* burden [22]. *M. tuberculosis*, the causative agent of tuberculosis, is a highly infectious and successful human pathogen that, despite being treatable, takes more adult lives than any other single infectious disease [23]. *M. tuberculosis* reaches the human lungs, where it first encounters alveolar macrophages. In response to *M. tuberculosis* infection, the host macrophages defend by targeting the pathogen either by induction of apoptosis, phagosome-lysosome fusion, production of reactive oxygen and nitrogen species (ROS and RNS), and induction of autophagy. Upon phagosome damage mediated by the 6-kDa early secretory antigenic target (ESAT-6) secretion system 1 (ESX-1) secretory system, *M. tuberculosis* is tagged for autophagy by ubiquitination. Ubiquilin 1 (UBQLN1), a member of a protein family that contains a ubiquitin-like domain, a ubiquitin-associated domain, and stress inducible protein 1 (STI1) motifs, recruits ubiquitin. Ubiquitination is an essential step required for the recruitment of the autophagic adaptors p62 and NDP52 and LC3 to *M. tuberculosis*-containing vacuoles ensuring delivery of both the bacteria and self-proteins to lysosomal degradation [24 - 26].

An exciting aspect of autophagic bacterial clearance has been described in *M. tuberculosis*- associated autophagy. Autophagosomes collect cytosolic components together with the pathogen, and the autophagic machinery generates antimicrobial peptides *de novo*. Mycobactericidal peptides are generated from cargo delivered to mycobacteria containing phagosomes such as the ubiquitin itself [27]. Also, p62 has recently been discovered not to be required to pull mycobacteria into autophagosomes but to generate mycobactericidal activity by producing antimicrobial peptides from ribosomal proteins [28].

Intracellular Bacteria Subvert Autophagy

Intracellular bacteria have evolved numerous mechanisms to evade or exploit autophagy to grant survival. Intracellular bacteria subvert autophagy at different levels by preventing autophagy initiation, recruitment into autophagosomes, or autophagosome-lysosome fusion. For example, some pathogens, such as *Francisella tularensis* and *Shigella flexneri* avoid tagging, and thus recognition, by autophagy receptors impairing the recruitment of the autophagic machinery to the bacterial site [29, 30]. Other microbes evade from autophagy at different points *Legionella pneumophila* extracts lipidated LC3 from autophagosome membranes to disassemble de the autophagic machinery [31]. Autophagy can be exploited by bacterial pathogens to source nutrients for their survival, taking advantage of the nutrient recycling part of the process. Moreover, *Brucella abortus* has evolved mechanisms to sabotage the autophagy pathway and establish a replicative compartment within autophagosomes [32]. For additional examples, see Table **1**.

M. tuberculosis successfully manipulates host membrane trafficking, remodels mycobacteria-containing phagolysosomes, and modulates cell death signaling for colonization, persistence, and replication. The ability of the pathogen to inhibit phagosome-lysosome fusion is central to the initiation of the infection, which is, in turn, linked to many virulent mechanisms. Furthermore, despite the crucial role of autophagy as an antimycobacterial mechanism, *M. tuberculosis* has developed a means to escape from it.

M. tuberculosis uses sophisticated mechanisms to escape autophagy and replicate inside host cells. *M. tuberculosis* antigens inhibit autophagy at different stages. For example, enhanced intracellular survival (EIS) protein-induced histone acetylation mediates the suppression of the autophagic control of *M. tuberculosis* by modulation of cytokine production, proline-glutamic acid_polymorphic GC-rich repetitive sequence 47 (PE_PGRS47) protein prevents the formation of the autophagosome, and ESAT6 inhibits autophagy by blocking autophagosome-lysosome fusion in an mTOR-dependent fashion [33 - 35]. Also, the induction of several microRNAs (miRNAs) by *M. tuberculosis* has been recently discovered to inhibit autophagy by interfering with different aspects of cellular physiology.

Infection of macrophages with *M. tuberculosis* resulted in the upregulation of miR-125a, which through targeting with the Atg UV radiation resistance-associated gene (UVRAG) protein, a binding partner of the Beclin 1–class III PI3K complex, inhibits the initiation of autophagosome formation [36]. Also, at the initiation of autophagosome formation, the induction of miR33 and miR33* expression manipulates cellular metabolism and energy levels, and the induction of miR30A decreases Beclin 1 expression levels [37, 38]. *M. tuberculosis* also induces the expression of miR144*, which downregulates the expression of DNA damage-regulated autophagy modulator 2 (DRAM2), and of miR-23a-5p, which inhibits the formation of LC3-II, downregulates toll-like receptor 2 (TLR2), and reduces the nuclear translocation of nuclear factor kappa-light-chain-enhancer of activated B cells (NFκB), thereby facilitating bacterial survival. The dynamics of those miRNA expressions may be a part of a complex mechanism that regulates many autophagy-related molecules converging on immune escape and promoting intracellular growth of *M. tuberculosis*. Although bacteria have evolved several mechanisms to evade detection and killing by the host, the host cell elicits multiple pathways to countermeasure bacterial evasion. Noteworthy, induction can rescue autophagy blockade.

Table 1. Mechanisms of evasion of autophagy by intracellular bacteria.

Bacteria	Host Cell	Autophagy-related Evasion Mechanism	References
Bacillus Calmette-Guérin expressing ESAT6	Murine macrophages Raw264.7/ACM.	ESAT6 activates mTOR through phosphorylation of S2481.	[34]

(Table 1) cont.....

Bacteria	Host Cell	Autophagy-related Evasion Mechanism	References
MRSA	Human macrophage-like THP1 cells, and a wide range of cells.	Elevated expression of virulence factor IsaB.	[39]
Francisella spp.	Murine macrophages, murine bone marrow☐derived macrophages (BMMs), and Human monocyte-derived macrophages (MDMs).	Prevention of autophagy by O-antigen polysaccharide, and activation of noncanonical autophagy for nutrient scavenging.	[40]
Brucella spp.	Murine bone marrow☐derived macrophages and HeLa cells	The hijacking of autophagy components like ATG9 and WIPI.	[40]
Salmonella typhimurium	Mouse embryonic fibroblasts, Mouse macrophages (PEMS, BMDMs)	Use of virulence factors T3SS-1, TS3SS-2 for survival within *Salmonella*- containing vacuoles. Activation of the Akt/mTOR pathway by recruitment of FAK kinase to the surface of *Salmonella*-containing vacuoles.	[41, 42]
Listeria monocytogenes	Mouse macrophages (BMDMs)	Expression of phospholipases PlcA and PlcB and ActA surface protein promotes escape from phagosomes. Expression of ActA promotes actin polymerization avoiding autophagy by escaping of LC3 phagosomes.	[43, 44]
Borrelia pseudomallei	RAW 264.7 cells	The type III secretion system cluster 3 (TTSS3) facilitates bacterial escape from phagosomes.	[45]
Legionella pneumophila	MCF-7 cells THP-1 cells, HEK-293T cells	The effector protein RavZ deconjugates Atg8/LC3 proteins coupled to PE on autophagosomal membranes. Secretion of a protein homologous of LpSPL whose lyase activity changes the host's sphingolipid metabolism.	[31] [46]
Group A *Streptococcus*	Macrophages	SLO-dependent autophagy evasion, the co-toxin NADase inhibits granule fusion with the phagosomes of neutrophils.	[47]
Streptococcus pyogenes	HMEC-1 and A549 cells	Prevention of ubiquitination of GAS.	[48]
Mycobacterium tuberculosis	BMDMs, THP-1 macrophages	Induction of miR-33 and miR-33* expression to repress AMPKα and downstream transcription factors and inhibit autophagy. ESAT6 inhibits autophagic flux. EIS inhibits autophagy and induces IL10.	[38] [34] [33]

(Table 1) cont.....

Bacteria	Host Cell	Autophagy-related Evasion Mechanism	References
Helicobacter pylori	Cell line HFE-145	Downregulation of acid phosphatase, β-NAG, and cathepsin D. VacA disrupts the autolysosomal system.	[49]

Abbreviations: MRSA, Methicillin-resistant *Staphylococcus aureus*; IsaB, Immunodominant surface antigen B; PEMs, mouse peritoneal macrophages; BMDMs, bone marrow-derived macrophages; PLCs A and B, phospholipase C, A, and B; ActA, A surface protein; T3SS-1 and T3SS-2, Type III secretion systems 1 and 2; PE, phosphatidylethanolamine; GAS, group A Streptococcus; NADase, NAD-glycohydrolase; HMEC-1, Human microvascular endothelial cell line-1; A549, Lung epithelial A549 cells; LpSPL, Protein highly similar to eukaryotic SGPL1of *L. pneumophila*; HFE-145, human gastric epithelial cell line; SLO, streptolysin O; AMPKα, adenosine 5' monophosphate-activated protein kinase; ESAT6, early secretory antigen 6; EIS, enhanced intracellular survival protein; β-NAG, N-acetyl-β-D-glucosaminidase; VacA, vacuolating cytotoxin A.

INDUCTION OF AUTOPHAGY AS A THERAPEUTIC APPROACH

Autophagy can eliminate intracellular microbes, including those that are naturally resistant to this mechanism, such as *Mycobacterium tuberculosis*. Therefore, the induction of autophagy in infected cells may be relevant for bacterial clearance. Because physiological, pharmacological, and immunological stimuli induce autophagy *via* elements, such as mTOR (a negative regulator of autophagy), AMPK (a positive regulator of autophagy), Atg1 (the most upstream autophagy-specific kinase), and Beclin 1 (mammalian Atg6), several therapeutic options can be procured [1].

A great diversity of natural compounds represents a powerful tool for drug discovery, and many of them induce autophagy. Immunological stimulation activates autophagy in infected cells by using microbial compounds as stimulants. Besides, several drugs approved for human consumption induce autophagy. In the following sections, we will discuss these autophagy inducers and give special attention to *M. tuberculosis* infection because the search for an adjunctive therapeutic strategy for tuberculosis has gained the interest of many researchers and clinicians.

Tuberculosis is the leading global cause of death from the bacterial infectious disease [23]. The main concern in this pressing issue is the rapid spread of drug-resistant strains of *M. tuberculosis*, with mortality rates from extensively drug-resistant strains reaching up to 98% [50]. The treatment of tuberculosis is complex and requires the extensive use of expensive, toxic anti-tuberculosis drugs that are not highly effective. The slow progression in the development and evaluation of new drugs for tuberculosis emphasizes the need for adjunctive therapy.

The Natural Compounds Approach

Physiological, pharmacological, and immunological stimuli induce autophagy.

Natural compounds could be applied as new drugs with potential antimicrobial activity themselves or by modulating the immune response to enhance the removal of the infective agent [51]. Several examples are described below.

1.- Sesquiterpenoids. Various sesquiterpenoids such as drimane from *Drimys winteri*, germacrene from *Podanthus mitiqui,* and dihydro agarofuran from *Maytenus boaria* have shown a broad range of trypanocidal activities. The biological effects of sesquiterpenoids involve mitochondrial dysfunction, ROS production, and autophagic response in *Trypanosoma cruzi* [52].

2.- Resveratrol (3,5,40-trans-trihydroxy stilbene) is a polyphenolic stilbene found in grapes and red wine and is considered as a novel food ingredient. Its role as a global autophagy inducer is well-recognized. Resveratrol stimulates xenophagy *in vivo* (in intestinal epithelial cells and macrophages) and *in vitro* (infection in a transgenic GFP-LC3 zebrafish model) against *Salmonella Typhimurium* and Crohn's disease-associated Adherent-Invasive *Escherichia coli* [53].

3.- Alkaloids. Oxindole, an alkaloid from *Uncaria rhynchophylla,* is routinely used in traditional Chinese medicine formulas for the treatment of symptoms relevant to Parkinson's disease. Several neuronal autophagy inducers come from oxindole alkaloids such as corynoxine (Cory) and corynoxine B (Cory B) that induce autophagy in neuronal cells in an mTOR-independent but Beclin--dependent manner [54]. Conophylline, a vinca alkaloid isolated from the tropical plants *Tavertaemontana divaricate* and *Ervatamia microphylla*, induce autophagy in non-neuronal and neuronal cell lines in an mTOR independent manner, promoted the degradation of α-synuclein aggregates, and reduced cell death induced by the neurotoxin 1-methyl-4-phenylpyridinium (MPP^+) [54].

4.-Polyphenols. Curcumin (16-hydroxycleroda-3,13-dien-15,16-olid, polyphenol) is an active component of turmeric (*Curcuma longa*). Curcumin is neuroprotective in experimental models of Parkinson's disease through multiple mechanisms, such as preventing oxidative stress and inflammation and inhibiting α-synuclein aggregation and fibrillation. Curcumin and the polyphenol prodigiosin are autophagy inducers that trigger cell death and could be used as an alternative medicine for cancer therapy [54, 55].

5.-Vitamins. The active metabolite of vitamin A, all trans-retinoic acid (ATRA) solution, induces bactericidal responses both in murine and in human macrophages infected with *M. tuberculosis* and *Bordetella pertussis*. ATRA reduces bacterial burden by inducing autophagy [56, 57]. The contribution of vitamin D in immunomodulation and induction of autophagy is amply described in chapter 3 of this book.

We investigated the effect of two plant-derived bioactive and immunostimulatory compounds in macrophages infected with *M. tuberculosis* [58]. We evaluated the ability of nordihydroguaiaretic acid (NDGA) and α-mangostin to affect the survival of *M. tuberculosis* both *in vitro* and inside infected THP-1, and human monocyte-derived macrophages (MDMs). NDGA is the most abundant lignan of *Larrea tridentate,* and α-mangostin is the most abundant xanthone of *Garcinia mangostana* [59, 60] Extracts from *L. tridentata* and *G. mangostana* show bactericidal activity against strains of *M. tuberculosis* [60, 61]. Moreover, several anti-infective properties have been attributed to NDGA and α-mangostin against viruses and bacteria [62 - 64].

We found that NDGA caused a dose-dependent decrease in bacterial growth at doses from 8 to 250 µg/mL when the bacteria were cultured in a liquid medium, and this bactericidal effect of NDGA was comparable with the previously reported antimycobacterial activity of α-mangostin [65]. The obtained MICs were 250 µg/mL and 62.5 µg/mL for NDGA and α-mangostin, respectively. Neither NDGA nor α-mangostin were capable of completely inhibit the growth of bacteria in a manner comparable to rifampicin. When we evaluated the effect of this treatment on infected macrophages, we found that lower doses of NDGA (7 µg/mL) or α-mangostin (6 µg/mL) significantly reduced the intracellular bacterial growth. We observed bacterial load reductions of up to 75% after five days of incubation. Treatment with rifampicin resulted in a significant bactericidal effect of more than 98%. NDGA and α-mangostin induced autophagy in uninfected and infected macrophages, which explains the antibacterial outcome.

Moreover, in infected macrophages, the intracellular bacteria were recruited into autophagosome vesicles. These findings allow us to suggest that these compounds or designed analogs could be used in combination with conventional therapy and may contribute to the treatment of drug-sensitive or drug-resistant tuberculosis. NDGA exerts bactericidal activity over other pathogens, such as *Staphylococcus aureus*, S. epidermidis, and *Helicobacter pylori*, but whether autophagy has a role in this process remains uncertain [66, 67].

The Microbial Compounds Approach

Recent advances in immunomodulators indicate the usefulness of microbial components to address microbial control issues. For example, stimulation with ultrapure LPS through CD40 and TLR-4 induces autophagy and might be a valid Host Directed Therapy against *M. tuberculosis* [68]. Also, CpG oligodeoxynucleotides (CpG-ODN) promote phagocytosis and autophagy through JNK/p38 signal pathway in *Staphylococcus aureus*-stimulated macrophages [69]. In our work, we demonstrated that DNA isolated from *M. tuberculosis* also induces autophagy in M1 macrophages, enhancing their antimicrobial activity against mycobacteria [70].

We also conducted a study to investigate the ability of two bacterial-derived compounds to stimulate macrophages infected with the virulent strain of *M. tuberculosis* for antimicrobial responses [71, 72]. Tri-diaminopimelic acid (tri-DAP) and muramyldipeptide (MDP) are major components of the bacterial cell walls that are recognized by innate immune sensors NOD1 and NOD2, respectively [73, 74]. The NOD proteins, members of the NLR family, are cytoplasmic receptors implicated in the recognition of bacterial molecules produced during the synthesis or degradation of peptidoglycan [75]. Activation of NOD1 and NOD2 by bacterial products can stimulate two major signaling pathways to activate pro-inflammatory responses, including the NF-κB pathway and the inflammasome pathway [74, 76]. Experimental models suggested the advantage of using MDP to induce control of *M. tuberculosis* replication. However, the mechanism responsible for this result was uncertain [77, 78], but at the time we performed our investigation, there was no data to support the use of Tri-DAP to enhance antimycobacterial responses.

We found that stimulation with MDP (10 µg/ml) and Tri-DAP (5 µg/ml) for 24 h induced autophagy in human alveolar macrophages infected with virulent *M. tuberculosis*. Autophagy was determined by either measuring the induction of autophagy-related proteins LC3, IRGM, ATG9, and ATG16L1, or their recruitment to the mycobacteria-containing vacuole. Also, stimulation with MDP induced the expression of the antimicrobial peptide LL-37. Both Tri-DAP and MDP significantly induced the production of proinflammatory cytokines, but such production was moderate compared to the highly proinflammatory stimulus of LPS. In addition, both Tri-DAP and MDP prevented the intracellular growth of *M. tuberculosis*. This immune response may be beneficial for the host because all the anti-infective responses were activated with only 24 h of treatment. Our findings suggest that autophagy is a key mechanism by which human alveolar macrophages eliminate *M. tuberculosis* and that it may be involved in the early innate control of *M. tuberculosis* primary infections, the modulation of proinflammatory cytokines, or the induction of antimicrobial peptides. Interestingly, alveolar macrophages were higher responders to Tri-DAP and MDP stimulation than MDMs, or in some cases than monocytes. The latter may be essential for the development of immunological therapies that could activate good local responses in pulmonary tuberculosis.

The Drug Approach

Several drugs approved for human consumption induce autophagy. The archetype of autophagy inducing drugs is rapamycin. Rapamycin, which was isolated from a microorganism in the soil of Easter Island (Rapa Nui), was initially developed as an antibiotic; currently, rapamycin is used as an immunosuppressant, of very high activity to inhibit the activation of mTOR, to prevent rejection in organ transplants. It also has a high antiproliferative activity, which makes it an anticancer agent, and rapamycin also induces antibacterial activity against *B. cepacia* through autophagy [79, 80]. Other drugs recognized as autophagy inducers appear in Table **2**.

Table 2. Autophagy-inducing drugs in experimental assays.

Drug	Experimental Setting	Experimental Outcome	References
AR-12/MPs	RAW 264.7 cells and human MDMs infected with *Salmonella typhi* were treated with AR-12/MPs for 5, 7, and 22 h.	AR-12/MPs induced autophagosome formation and enhanced clearance of *S. typhi*.	[81]
Artesunate	Artesunate was used as a treatment in a rat model of rheumatoid arthritis (RA) *in vivo* for a total of 12 days.	Artesunate inhibits chondrocyte proliferation and accelerates cell apoptosis and autophagy *via* suppression of the PI3K/Akt/mTOR signaling pathway.	[82]
3-Arylidene azetidin-2-ones	Several 3-arylidene azetidin-2-ones were used as an antifungal agent against *Alternaria solani* after administration during 12, 24, and 48 h.	One of these compounds leads to intracellular accumulation of reactive oxygen species, dissipation of mitochondrial transmembrane potential, and an autophagy-like cell death process in *A. solani*.	[83]
Carbamazepine (CBZ)	Zebrafish infected with *Mycobacterium marinum* were treated with CBZ and chloroquine for 24 h. Autophagosome formation was confirmed in RAW 264.7 macrophages and primary human macrophages.	CBZ stimulates autophagy *in vivo* and enhances the clearance of *M. marinum* in mice infected with a highly virulent multidrug-resistant *M. tuberculosis* strain. CBZ reduced bacterial burden, improved lung pathology, and stimulated adaptive immunity.	[84]
Clarithromycin	PMNs from healthy humans treated with clarithromycin at 500 mg b.i.d. for ten days *in vivo* were studied after *Acinetobacter baumannii* infection *ex vivo*.	Clarithromycin induces NETs formation and autophagy in PMNs.	[85]
AR-12	RAW264.7 infected with *Salmonella* serovar *Typhimurium* with AR-12.	AR-12 can effectively kill *Salmonella* serovar *typhimurium* in infected macrophages at submicromolar concentrations by inducing autophagy- and Akt-dependent mechanisms; it also decreases bacterial loads in infected mice and increases their survival.	[86]

(Table 2) cont.....

Drug	Experimental Setting	Experimental Outcome	References
OMS-A and OMS-B	BMDMs were infected with *M. tuberculosis* for 4 h and then treated with OMS-A or OMS-B or co-treated with OMS-A and OMS-B for three days.	OMS-A and OMS-B promote antimicrobial responses through autophagy activation *via* the AMP-activated protein kinase pathway.	[87]
Rapamycin	Mouse macrophages and ΔF508 macrophages were infected with *Burkholderia cenocepacia* and treated with rapamycin for 2 h post-infection.	Rapamycin markedly decreases *B. cepacia* infection *via* autophagy both *in vitro* and *in vivo* in the lungs of CF mice and drastically reduces signs of lung inflammation.	[80]
Cysteamine	BMDMs (*in vitro*) and CF model mice (*in vivo*) were infected with *Pseudomonas aeruginosa* PAO1 and treated with 250 μM cysteamine for 10 min or 3 h.	Cysteamine re-establishes the ability to clear *P. aeruginosa* in cystic fibrosis.	[88]
Tamoxifen	MCF7 cells and MEFs were transiently transfected with an LC3-GFP expression and were infected with *toxoplasma gondii*, and 2 h later treated with tamoxifen 10 μM.	Tamoxifen is a potent inducer of autophagy and restricts *T. gondii* growth by inducing xenophagy.	[89]
Small-molecule BRD5631	Atg5+/+ and Atg5−/− MEFs were transfected with *eGFP-HDQ74* construct followed by treatment with BRD5631 (10 μM for 48 h).	BRD5631 suppresses NPC1-Induced Cell Death in a hiPSC-Derived Neuronal Model of Niemann–Pick Type C1 disease, enhances bacterial clearance, and decreases IL-1β secretion.	[90]
Statins (Simvastatin)	PBMCs and MDMs from patients with familial hypercholesterolemia under statin therapy were infected with *M. tuberculosis*, and the bacterial burden was determined.	Statins mediated reduction in cholesterol levels within phagosomal membranes counteract *M. tuberculosis* and promote host-induced autophagy.	[91]
Vitexin	Human colorectal carcinoma HCT-116 cells were exposed to vitexin, and the induction of HSF-1 downstream target proteins was assessed.	Vitexin suppressed tumor growth through activation of an autophagic cascade in the HCT-116 xenograft model.	[92]
VitD3-PMQ	Murine model of *Pneumocystis* pneumonia.	VitD3-PMQ therapy upregulates the expression of autophagy genes (ATG5 and beclin-1).	[93]

Additional Abbreviations: MDMs, monocyte-derived macrophages; RA, rheumatoid arthritis; BMDMs, bone marrow-derived macrophages; HSF-1, heat shock factor 1; VitD3-PMQ, Vitamin D3 plus primaquine.

Regarding tuberculosis, several attempts to identify more effective treatments are currently under study, with particular attention set on drugs that modulate immune responses [94, 95]. Thus, the use of drugs that enhance the immunological mechanisms involved in the intracellular killing of *M. tuberculosis* would be ideal. Because the macrophage-mediated killing of *M. tuberculosis* involves autophagy, we carried out a study that focused on U.S. Food and Drug Administration–approved drugs that already had been described as autophagy inducers, regardless of their primary therapeutic use, to address the need to boost immune responses to *M. tuberculosis* [96]. We included rapamycin, carbamazepine, valproic acid, verapamil, and loperamide. Rapamycin is an immunosuppressant used in solid organ transplants that inhibits mTOR and induce autophagy [97]. Carbamazepine and valproic acid are anticonvulsants that trigger autophagy independently of mTOR [84]. Verapamil and loperamide are calcium channel blockers commonly used to treat hypertension and diarrhea, respectively [98]. We found that loperamide, an antidiarrheal drug, was the best drug to induce autophagy in alveolar macrophages infected with the virulent strain of *M. tuberculosis*.

Our study revealed that human and murine alveolar macrophages exhibited increased autophagy after treatment with carbamazepine, loperamide, verapamil, and valproic acid *in vitro*. However, *M. tuberculosis* localization to autophagosomes concomitant with a decreased intracellular bacterial burden only occurred after treatment with loperamide. Because none of the drugs under study had been reported to reach the lungs at the moment, we intraperitoneally administered loperamide, verapamil, and valproic acid to uninfected mice daily for three days. We obtained the alveolar macrophages 24 h after the last drug administration and found activation of autophagy in lung macrophages of loperamide- and valproic acid-treated mice. Furthermore, these alveolar macrophages were infected *ex vivo,* and without additional treatment or stimulation, loperamide treated-mouse macrophages were able to control the intracellular growth of virulent *M. tuberculosis*. The lack of bactericidal effect observed for the valproic acid-treated mouse macrophages was due to its induction of unproductive autophagy. Later, we found that the ability of loperamide to enhance macrophage's anti-infective mechanisms depended on its ability to activate the μ opioid receptors and that this response extended to other mycobacteria [99].

With those studies, we concluded that loperamide enhances the natural antimicrobial capacity of lung macrophages to control tuberculosis infection. However, two aspects of autophagy induction as therapeutic strategy came to attention. First, autophagy inducers must reach the specific organ that is the intended target, so the studies searching for this approach should demonstrate the organ-specific effects of their compounds. Second, inducing autophagy is not enough. It has to be productive autophagy; that is, the process should progress to autophagolysosomal degradation of the cargo. Some compounds can induce unproductive autophagy with no anti-infective results, which suggests caution when using them as therapeutic agents.

The Drawbacks of Inducing Autophagy

A large number of natural products, microbial compounds, and drugs are involved in autophagy modulation through multiple signaling pathways and transcriptional regulators. Most of the studies focus on the ability of the compound to induce autophagy, but only a few consider the fact that induction alone is not enough. Thus, autophagy may be either protective or toxic. We observed such for valproic acid [96], but there are other cases. For instance, the natural product climacostol induces autophagosome formation; there is an increase of LC3 puncta and lipidated LC3-II levels in melanoma cells from climacostol-treated mice [100]. Those characteristics would be enough to claim that the compound is an autophagy inducer; however, the actual outcome of climacostol treatment was induction of autophagy, but suppression of autolysosomal maturation. This phenomenon is termed disruption of the autophagic flux, which is detrimental for the host and has been reported for several autophagy inducers such as conessine, a steroidal alkaloid isolated from the bark of *Holarrhena floribunda* [101], and azithromycin, a potent macrolide antibiotic [102].

Another example involves the differential outcomes that occur depending on the experimental settings. Rapamycin is the typical autophagy inducer; however, in macrophages coinfected with HIV and *M. tuberculosis*, stimulation of autophagy with rapamycin led to increased *M. tuberculosis* survival by inducing a dysfunctional autophagic flux [103]. Also, intranasal rapamycin treatment reduces *P. aeruginosa* bacterial burdens in murine lungs, but it does not improve survival disputing the actual benefit of the treatment [104]. In addition, it is necessary to consider the immunosuppressive effects of rapamycin, which could also cause reactivation and progression of some infections, outweighing any benefit of activating autophagy.

Tumor cells, in some cases, regulate autophagy to survive and increase their growth and aggressiveness. Autophagy, in this case, benefits the tumor because of the inherent deficiencies of the microenvironment and the increase in the metabolism and biosynthetic demands imposed by dysregulated proliferation. The mechanisms by which autophagy promotes cancer include the suppression of the p53 tumor suppressor protein induction, the maintenance of the metabolic function of the mitochondria, and the delivery of a variety of substrates to fuel cellular metabolism [100, 105, 106]. Thus, inducing autophagy needs to be reconsidered when the patient has susceptibility to tumor development.

Box 1. List of acronyms and detailed names of the proteins used in this chapter.

A549, Lung epithelial A549 cells	**MEF**, mouse embryonic fibroblasts
ActA, A surface protein	**MIC**, minimum inhibitory concentration
Akt, also known as protein kinase B or PKB	**MRSA**, Methicillin-resistant *Staphylococcus aureus*
AMP, adenosine monophosphate	**miRNAs** or **miR**, microRNAs
AMPK, AMP-activated protein kinase	**MPP⁺**, 1-methyl-4-phenylpyridinium
AR-12/MPs, AR-12 microparticles	**NADase**, NAD-glycohydrolase
Atg, autophagy-related gene	**β-NAG**, N-acetyl-β-D-glucosaminidase
ATRA, all trans-retinoic acid	**NBR1,** Neighbor of BRCA1 gene 1
BMDMs, bone marrow-derived macrophages	**NETs**, neutrophil extracellular traps
CBZ, carbamazepine	**NFκB**, nuclear factor kappa-light-chain-enhancer of
CD40, cluster of differentiation 40	activated B cells
CF, cystic fibrosis	**NOD1** and **2**, Nucleotide oligomerization domain 1 and 2
CpG-ODN, CpG oligodeoxynucleotides	**NLR**, NOD-like receptor
DRAM2, DNA damage-regulated autophagy	**NDP52**, nuclear dot protein 52 kDa
modulator 2	**NDGA**, nordihydroguaiaretic acid
ER, endoplasmic reticulum	**NPC1**, Niemann-Pick disease, type C1 protein
EIS, enhanced intracellular survival	**PE_PGRS47**, proline-glutamic acid_ polymorphic GC-
ESAT6, early secretory antigenic target 6	rich repetitive sequence 47
ESX-1, 6-kDa early secretory antigenic target	**PEMs**, mouse peritoneal macrophages
(ESAT-6) secretion system 1	**PI3K**, phosphatidil inositol 3 kinase
FAK, focal adhesion kinase	**PLCs A and B**, phospholipase C, A, and B
GABARAP, gamma-aminobutyric acid	**PE**, phosphatidylethanolamine
receptor-associated protein	**SGPL1**, sphingosine-1-phosphate lyase 1
GAS, group A Streptococcus	**SLO**, streptolysin O
GFP, green fluorescence protein	**RA**, rheumatoid arthritis
HFE-145, human gastric epithelial cell line	**OMS-A and OMS-B**, ohmyungsamycins A and B
HMEC-1, Human microvascular endothelial cell	**PMNs**, polymorphonuclear leukocytes
line-1	**ROS**, reactive oxygen species
Hsc70, heat shock cognate 71 kDa protein	**RNS**, reactive nitrogen species
HSF-1, heat shock factor 1	**RNF166**, ring finger protein 166
IRGM, interferon related GTP-ase M	**SQSTM1**, sequestosome-1, also known as p62
IsaB, Immunodominant surface antigen B JNK	**STI1**, stress inducible protein 1
JNK, Jun N-Terminal Kinase	**TLR**, toll-like receptor
KFERQ, lysine, phenylalanine, glutamic acid,	**T3SS-1** and **T3SS-2**, Type III secretion systems 1 and 2
arginine, glutamine	**Tri-DAP**, tri-diaminopimelic acid
LAMP1, lysosomal-associated membrane	**UBQLN1**, ubiquilin 1
protein 1	**ULK1**, Unc-51 like autophagy activating kinase
LAMP2A, lysosomal-associated membrane	**UVRAG**, UV radiation resistance-associated gene
protein 2A	**VacA**, vacuolating cytotoxin A
LC3 or LC3-I, microtubule-associated protein	**VitD3-PMQ**, Vitamin D3 plus primaquine.
1A/1B-light chain 3	**Vps34**, class III PI 3-kinase vacuolar protein sorting 34
LC3-II, lipidated, membrane-associated LC3	**WIPI**, WD repeat protein interacting with
LL-37, human cathelicidin LL-37 peptide LPS	phosphoinositides
LPS, lipopolysaccharide	**WT**, wild-type
LpSPL, *Legionella peumophila* SGPL1	
mTOR, mammalian target of rapamycin NBR1	
MDMs, human monocyte-derived macrophages	
MDP, muramyldipeptide	

CONCLUDING REMARKS

Autophagy provides a means for infected macrophages to overcome the infection of intracellular pathogens. Several strategies are under study to find a suitable autophagy inducer but given the ability of intracellular bacterial pathogens to evade and exploit xenophagy and the impact of autophagy-associated proteins on diverse immune responses, pursuing autophagy as a therapeutic target requires the consideration of some issues. For example, manipulating the activity of autophagy proteins may affect both autophagy-dependent and -independent processes that have incalculable effects on disease outcomes. Moreover, any attempts to stimulate xenophagy may be futile if the downstream steps of autophagy are blocked– such as autophagolysosome formation– then induction of autophagy may not be effective and may be detrimental to the cell.

Besides, as more autophagy-promoting drugs are evaluated against *M. tuberculosis*, it will be essential to ascertain if particular pathways offer better efficacy advantages as host-directed therapies. At the same time, it will be necessary and informative to test whether candidate drugs adversely influence the balance of protective versus damaging immunity through mechanisms like mTOR inhibition. The likely complications resulting from the pleiotropic effects of these pharmacologic agents need to be considered. Also, it remains elusive how the results obtained using single cell type processes will translate into animal models where multiple cell types are exposed to a drug.

CONSENT FOR PUBLICATION

Not applicable.

CONFLICT OF INTEREST

The authors confirm that this chapter contents have no conflict of interest.

ACKNOWLEDGEMENT

Declared none.

REFERENCES

[1]   Mizushima N, Yoshimori T, Ohsumi Y. The role of Atg proteins in autophagosome formation. Annu Rev Cell Dev Biol 2011; 27(1): 107-32.
      [http://dx.doi.org/10.1146/annurev-cellbio-092910-154005] [PMID: 21801009]

[2]   Münz C. Autophagy proteins in phagocyte endocytosis and exocytosis. Front Immunol 2017; 8: 1183.
      [http://dx.doi.org/10.3389/fimmu.2017.01183] [PMID: 29018446]

[3]   Selleck EM, Orchard RC, Lassen KG, *et al.* A noncanonical autophagy pathway restricts *toxoplasma gondii* growth in a strain-specific manner in ifn-γ-activated human cells. MBio. Boyle J, Boothroyd JC, *et al.* 2015; 6: pp. (5)1-2.

[4]   Hatakeyama R, Péli-Gulli M-P, Hu Z, *et al.* Spatially distinct pools of torc1 balance protein homeostasis. Mol Cell 2019; 73(2): 325-338.e8.
[http://dx.doi.org/10.1016/j.molcel.2018.10.040] [PMID: 30527664]

[5]   Iwama R, Ohsumi Y. Analysis of autophagy activated during changes in carbon source availability in yeast cells. J Biol Chem 2019; jbc.RA118.005698..

[6]   Colecchia D, Strambi A, Sanzone S, *et al.* MAPK15/ERK8 stimulates autophagy by interacting with LC3 and GABARAP proteins. Autophagy 2012; 8(12): 1724-40.
[http://dx.doi.org/10.4161/auto.21857] [PMID: 22948227]

[7]   Lystad AH, Ichimura Y, Takagi K, *et al.* Structural determinants in GABARAP required for the selective binding and recruitment of ALFY to LC3B-positive structures. EMBO Rep 2014; 15(5): 557-65.
[http://dx.doi.org/10.1002/embr.201338003] [PMID: 24668264]

[8]   Colecchia D, Dapporto F, Tronnolone S, Salvini L, Chiariello M. MAPK15 is part of the ULK complex and controls its activity to regulate early phases of the autophagic process. J Biol Chem 2018; 293(41): 15962-76.
[http://dx.doi.org/10.1074/jbc.RA118.002527] [PMID: 30131341]

[9]   Sou Y, Waguri S, Iwata J, Ueno T, Fujimura T, Hara T, *et al.* The Atg8 Conjugation System Is Indispensable for Proper Development of Autophagic Isolation Membranes in Mice.Subramani S. Mol Biol Cell. 2008; 19: pp. (11)4762-75.
[http://dx.doi.org/10.1091/mbc.e08-03-0309]

[10]   Lamark T, Kirkin V, Dikic I, Johansen T. NBR1 and p62 as cargo receptors for selective autophagy of ubiquitinated targets. Cell Cycle 2009; 8(13): 1986-90.
[http://dx.doi.org/10.4161/cc.8.13.8892] [PMID: 19502794]

[11]   Gatica D, Lahiri V, Klionsky DJ. Cargo recognition and degradation by selective autophagy. Nat Cell Biol 2018; 20(3): 233-42.
[http://dx.doi.org/10.1038/s41556-018-0037-z] [PMID: 29476151]

[12]   Franco LH, Nair VR, Scharn CR, *et al.* The ubiquitin ligase smurf1 functions in selective autophagy of *Mycobacterium tuberculosis* and anti-tuberculous host defense. Cell Host Microbe 2017; 21(1): 59-72.
[http://dx.doi.org/10.1016/j.chom.2016.11.002] [PMID: 28017659]

[13]   Johansen T, Lamark T. Selective autophagy mediated by autophagic adapter proteins. Autophagy 2011; 7(3): 279-96.
[http://dx.doi.org/10.4161/auto.7.3.14487] [PMID: 21189453]

[14]   Pankiv S, Clausen TH, Lamark T, *et al.* p62/SQSTM1 binds directly to Atg8/LC3 to facilitate degradation of ubiquitinated protein aggregates by autophagy. J Biol Chem 2007; 282(33): 24131-45.
[http://dx.doi.org/10.1074/jbc.M702824200] [PMID: 17580304]

[15]   Heath RJ, Goel G, Baxt LA, *et al.* RNF166 determines recruitment of adaptor proteins during antibacterial autophagy. Cell Rep 2016; 17(9): 2183-94.
[http://dx.doi.org/10.1016/j.celrep.2016.11.005] [PMID: 27880896]

[16]   Nozawa T, Aikawa C, Minowa-nozawa A. The intracellular microbial sensor NLRP4 directs Rho-actin signaling to facilitate Group A vacuole formation. Autophagy 2017; 0(0): 1-14.
[http://dx.doi.org/10.1080/15548627.2017.1358343] [PMID: 29099277]

[17]   Choi J, Park S, Biering SB, *et al.* The parasitophorous vacuole membrane of *toxoplasma gondii* is targeted for disruption by ubiquitin-like conjugation systems of autophagy. Immunity 2014; 40(6): 924-35.
[http://dx.doi.org/10.1016/j.immuni.2014.05.006] [PMID: 24931121]

[18]   Harada-Hada K, Harada K, Kato F, *et al.* Phospholipase C-related catalytically inactive protein participates in the autophagic elimination of *Staphylococcus aureus* infecting mouse embryonic fibroblasts. PLoS One 2014; 9(5): e98285.

[http://dx.doi.org/10.1371/journal.pone.0098285] [PMID: 24865216]

[19] Rinchai D, Riyapa D, Buddhisa S, *et al.* Macroautophagy is essential for killing of intracellular *Burkholderia pseudomallei* in human neutrophils. Autophagy 2015; 11(5): 748-55.
[http://dx.doi.org/10.1080/15548627.2015.1040969] [PMID: 25996656]

[20] Tsuchiya M, Ogawa H, Koujin T, *et al.* p62/SQSTM1 promotes rapid ubiquitin conjugation to target proteins after endosome rupture during xenophagy. FEBS Open Bio 2018; 8(3): 470-80.
[http://dx.doi.org/10.1002/2211-5463.12385] [PMID: 29511624]

[21] Birmingham CL, Smith AC, Bakowski MA, Yoshimori T, Brumell JH. Autophagy controls Salmonella infection in response to damage to the Salmonella-containing vacuole. J Biol Chem 2006; 281(16): 11374-83.
[http://dx.doi.org/10.1074/jbc.M509157200] [PMID: 16495224]

[22] Gutierrez MG, Master SS, Singh SB, Taylor GA, Colombo MI, Deretic V. Autophagy is a defense mechanism inhibiting BCG and *Mycobacterium tuberculosis* survival in infected macrophages. Cell 2004; 119(6): 753-66.
[http://dx.doi.org/10.1016/j.cell.2004.11.038] [PMID: 15607973]

[23] World Health Organization Global Report Tuberculosis. 2017.

[24] Sakowski ET, Koster S, Portal Celhay C, *et al.* Ubiquilin 1 promotes IFN-γ-induced xenophagy of *Mycobacterium tuberculosis*. PLoS Pathog 2015; 11(7): e1005076.
[http://dx.doi.org/10.1371/journal.ppat.1005076] [PMID: 26225865]

[25] Manzanillo PS, Ayres JS, Watson RO, *et al.* The ubiquitin ligase parkin mediates resistance to intracellular pathogens. Nature 2013; 501(7468): 512-6.
[http://dx.doi.org/10.1038/nature12566] [PMID: 24005326]

[26] Watson RO, Manzanillo PS, Cox JS. Extracellular *M. tuberculosis* DNA targets bacteria for autophagy by activating the host DNA-sensing pathway. Cell 2012; 150(4): 803-15.
[http://dx.doi.org/10.1016/j.cell.2012.06.040] [PMID: 22901810]

[27] Alonso S, Pethe K, Russell DG, Purdy GE. Lysosomal killing of Mycobacterium mediated by ubiquitin-derived peptides is enhanced by autophagy. Proc Natl Acad Sci USA 2007; 104(14): 6031-6.
[http://dx.doi.org/10.1073/pnas.0700036104] [PMID: 17389386]

[28] Ponpuak M, Davis AS, Roberts EA, *et al.* Delivery of cytosolic components by autophagic adaptor protein p62 endows autophagosomes with unique antimicrobial properties. Immunity 2010; 32(3): 329-41.
[http://dx.doi.org/10.1016/j.immuni.2010.02.009] [PMID: 20206555]

[29] Chong A, Wehrly TD, Child R, *et al.* Cytosolic clearance of replication-deficient mutants reveals *Francisella tularensis* interactions with the autophagic pathway. Autophagy 2012; 8(9): 1342-56.
[http://dx.doi.org/10.4161/auto.20808] [PMID: 22863802]

[30] Ogawa M, Yoshimori T, Suzuki T, Sagara H, Mizushima N, Sasakawa C. Escape of intracellular Shigella from autophagy. Science 2005; 307(5710): 727-31.
[http://dx.doi.org/10.1126/science.1106036] [PMID: 15576571]

[31] Yang A, Pantoom S, Wu Y-W. Elucidation of the anti-autophagy mechanism of the *Legionella* effector RavZ using semisynthetic LC3 proteins. eLife 2017; 6: 1-23.
[http://dx.doi.org/10.7554/eLife.23905] [PMID: 28395732]

[32] Starr T, Child R, Wehrly TD, *et al.* Selective subversion of autophagy complexes facilitates completion of the Brucella intracellular cycle. Cell Host Microbe 2012; 11(1): 33-45.
[http://dx.doi.org/10.1016/j.chom.2011.12.002] [PMID: 22264511]

[33] Duan L, Yi M, Chen J, Li S, Chen W. *Mycobacterium tuberculosis* EIS gene inhibits macrophage autophagy through up-regulation of IL-10 by increasing the acetylation of histone H3. Biochem Biophys Res Commun 2016; 473(4): 1229-34.
[http://dx.doi.org/10.1016/j.bbrc.2016.04.045] [PMID: 27079235]

[34] Dong H, Jing W, Runpeng Z, *et al.* ESAT6 inhibits autophagy flux and promotes BCG proliferation through MTOR. Biochem Biophys Res Commun 2016; 477(2): 195-201.
[http://dx.doi.org/10.1016/j.bbrc.2016.06.042] [PMID: 27317487]

[35] Saini NK, Baena A, Ng TW, *et al.* Suppression of autophagy and antigen presentation by *Mycobacterium tuberculosis* PE_PGRS47. Nat Microbiol 2016; 1(9): 16133.
[http://dx.doi.org/10.1038/nmicrobiol.2016.133] [PMID: 27562263]

[36] Kim JK, Yuk JM, Kim SY, *et al.* MicroRNA-125a Inhibits Autophagy Activation and Antimicrobial Responses during Mycobacterial Infection. J Immunol 2015; 194(11): 5355-65.
[http://dx.doi.org/10.4049/jimmunol.1402557] [PMID: 25917095]

[37] Chen Z, Wang T, Liu Z, *et al.* Inhibition of autophagy by MiR-30A induced by *Mycobacteria tuberculosis* as a possible mechanism of immune escape in human macrophages. Jpn J Infect Dis 2015; 68(5): 420-4.
[http://dx.doi.org/10.7883/yoken.JJID.2014.466] [PMID: 25866116]

[38] Ouimet M, Koster S, Sakowski E, *et al. Mycobacterium tuberculosis* induces the miR-33 locus to reprogram autophagy and host lipid metabolism. Nat Immunol 2016; 17(6): 677-86.
[http://dx.doi.org/10.1038/ni.3434] [PMID: 27089382]

[39] Liu PF, Cheng JS, Sy CL, *et al.* IsaB inhibits autophagic flux to promote host transmission of methicillin-resistant *Staphylococcus aureus.* J Invest Dermatol 2015; 135(11): 2714-22.
[http://dx.doi.org/10.1038/jid.2015.254] [PMID: 26134948]

[40] Miller C, Celli J. Avoidance and subversion of eukaryotic homeostatic autophagy mechanisms by bacterial pathogens. J Mol Biol 2016; 428(17): 3387-98.
[http://dx.doi.org/10.1016/j.jmb.2016.07.007] [PMID: 27456933]

[41] Owen KA, Casanova JE. Salmonella manipulates autophagy to "serve and protect.". Cell Host Microbe 2015; 18(5): 517-9.
[http://dx.doi.org/10.1016/j.chom.2015.10.020] [PMID: 26567504]

[42] Owen KA, Anderson CJ, Casanova JE. Salmonella suppresses the TRIF-dependent type I interferon response in macrophages. MBio 2016; 7(1): e02051-15.
[http://dx.doi.org/10.1128/mBio.02051-15] [PMID: 26884434]

[43] Mitchell G, Cheng MI, Chen C, *et al. Listeria monocytogenes* triggers noncanonical autophagy upon phagocytosis, but avoids subsequent growth-restricting xenophagy. Proc Natl Acad Sci USA 2018; 115(2): E210-7.
[http://dx.doi.org/10.1073/pnas.1716055115] [PMID: 29279409]

[44] Cheng MI, Chen C, Engström P, Portnoy DA, Mitchell G. Actin-based motility allows *Listeria monocytogenes* to avoid autophagy in the macrophage cytosol. Cell Microbiol 2018; 20(9): e12854.
[http://dx.doi.org/10.1111/cmi.12854] [PMID: 29726107]

[45] Gong L, Lai S-C, Treerat P, *et al. Burkholderia pseudomallei* type III secretion system cluster 3 ATPase BsaS, a chemotherapeutic target for small-molecule ATPase inhibitors. Infect Immun 2015; 83(4): 1276-85.
[http://dx.doi.org/10.1128/IAI.03070-14] [PMID: 25605762]

[46] Rolando M, Escoll P, Buchrieser C. *Legionella pneumophila* restrains autophagy by modulating the host's sphingolipid metabolism. Autophagy 2016; 12(6): 1053-4.
[http://dx.doi.org/10.1080/15548627.2016.1166325] [PMID: 27191778]

[47] Valderrama JA, Nizet V, Group A. Group A Streptococcus encounters with host macrophages. Future Microbiol 2018; 13(1): 119-34.
[http://dx.doi.org/10.2217/fmb-2017-0142] [PMID: 29226710]

[48] Lu SL, Kawabata T, Cheng YL, *et al.* Endothelial cells are intrinsically defective in xenophagy of *Streptococcus pyogenes.* PLoS Pathog 2017; 13(7): e1006444.
[http://dx.doi.org/10.1371/journal.ppat.1006444] [PMID: 28683091]

[49]   Zhang L, Hu W, Cho CH, *et al.* Reduced lysosomal clearance of autophagosomes promotes survival and colonization of *Helicobacter pylori*. J Pathol 2018; 244(4): 432-44.
[http://dx.doi.org/10.1002/path.5033] [PMID: 29327342]

[50]   Günther G. Multidrug-resistant and extensively drug-resistant tuberculosis: a review of current concepts and future challenges. Clin Med (Lond) 2014; 14(3): 279-85. [Northfield Il].
[http://dx.doi.org/10.7861/clinmedicine.14-3-279] [PMID: 24889573]

[51]   Carvalho JCT, Perazzo FF, Machado L, Bereau D. Biologic activity and biotechnological development of natural products. BioMed Res Int 2013; 2013: 971745.
[http://dx.doi.org/10.1155/2013/971745] [PMID: 24455743]

[52]   Bombaça ACS, Dossow DV, Barbosa JMC, Paz C, Burgos V, Menna-Barreto RFS. Trypanocidal activity of natural sesquiterpenoids involves mitochondrial dysfunction, ros production and autophagic phenotype in trypanosomacruzi. Molecules 2018; 23(11): 2800.
[http://dx.doi.org/10.3390/molecules23112800] [PMID: 30373326]

[53]   Al Azzaz J, Rieu A, Aires V, *et al.* Resveratrol-Induced Xenophagy Promotes Intracellular Bacteria Clearance in Intestinal Epithelial Cells and Macrophages. Front Immunol 2019; 9: 3149.
[http://dx.doi.org/10.3389/fimmu.2018.03149] [PMID: 30693000]

[54]   Wang Z-Y, Liu J-Y, Yang C-B, *et al.* Neuroprotective Natural Products for the Treatment of Parkinson's Disease by Targeting the Autophagy-Lysosome Pathway: A Systematic Review. Phytother Res 2017; 31(8): 1119-27.
[http://dx.doi.org/10.1002/ptr.5834] [PMID: 28504367]

[55]   Lin S-R, Fu Y-S, Tsai M-J, Cheng H, Weng C-F. Natural Compounds from Herbs that can Potentially Execute as Autophagy Inducers for Cancer Therapy. Int J Mol Sci 2017; 18(7): 1412.
[http://dx.doi.org/10.3390/ijms18071412] [PMID: 28671583]

[56]   Coleman MM, Basdeo SA, Coleman AM, *et al.* All-trans retinoic acid augments autophagy during intracellular bacterial infection. Am J Respir Cell Mol Biol 2018; 59(5): 548-56.
[http://dx.doi.org/10.1165/rcmb.2017-0382OC] [PMID: 29852080]

[57]   O'Connor G, Krishnan N, Fagan-Murphy A, *et al.* Inhalable poly(lactic-co-glycolic acid) (PLGA) microparticles encapsulating all-trans-Retinoic acid (ATRA) as a host-directed, adjunctive treatment for *Mycobacterium tuberculosis* infection. Eur J Pharm Biopharm 2019; 134: 153-65.
[http://dx.doi.org/10.1016/j.ejpb.2018.10.020] [PMID: 30385419]

[58]   Guzmán-Beltrán S, Rubio-Badillo MÁ, Juárez E, Hernández-Sánchez F, Torres M. Nordihydroguaiaretic acid (NDGA) and α-mangostin inhibit the growth of *Mycobacterium tuberculosis* by inducing autophagy. Int Immunopharmacol 2016; 31: 149-57.
[http://dx.doi.org/10.1016/j.intimp.2015.12.027] [PMID: 26735610]

[59]   Arteaga S, Andrade-Cetto A, Cárdenas R. *Larrea tridentata* (Creosote bush), an abundant plant of Mexican and US-American deserts and its metabolite nordihydroguaiaretic acid. J Ethnopharmacol 2005; 98(3): 231-9.
[http://dx.doi.org/10.1016/j.jep.2005.02.002] [PMID: 15814253]

[60]   Al-Massarani SM, El Gamal AA, Al-Musayeib NM, *et al.* Phytochemical, antimicrobial and antiprotozoal evaluation of *Garcinia mangostana* pericarp and α-mangostin, its major xanthone derivative. Molecules 2013; 18(9): 10599-608.
[http://dx.doi.org/10.3390/molecules180910599] [PMID: 24002136]

[61]   Suksamrarn S, Suwannapoch N, Phakhodee W, *et al.* Antimycobacterial activity of prenylated xanthones from the fruits of *Garcinia mangostana*. Chem Pharm Bull (Tokyo) 2003; 51(7): 857-9.
[http://dx.doi.org/10.1248/cpb.51.857] [PMID: 12843596]

[62]   Lü J-M, Nurko J, Weakley SM, *et al.* Molecular mechanisms and clinical applications of nordihydroguaiaretic acid (NDGA) and its derivatives: an update. Med Sci Monit 2010; 16(5): RA93-RA100.

[PMID: 20424564]

[63] Pedraza-Chaverri J, Cárdenas-Rodríguez N, Orozco-Ibarra M, Pérez-Rojas JM. Medicinal properties of mangosteen (*Garcinia mangostana*). Food Chem Toxicol 2008; 46(10): 3227-39.
[http://dx.doi.org/10.1016/j.fct.2008.07.024] [PMID: 18725264]

[64] Hernández-Damián J, Andérica-Romero AC, Pedraza-Chaverri J. Paradoxical cellular effects and biological role of the multifaceted compound nordihydroguaiaretic acid. Arch Pharm (Weinheim) 2014; 347(10): 685-97.
[http://dx.doi.org/10.1002/ardp.201400159] [PMID: 25100573]

[65] Suksamrarn S, Komutiban O, Ratananukul P, Chimnoi N, Lartpornmatulee N, Suksamrarn A. Cytotoxic prenylated xanthones from the young fruit of *Garcinia mangostana*. Chem Pharm Bull (Tokyo) 2006; 54(3): 301-5.
[http://dx.doi.org/10.1248/cpb.54.301] [PMID: 16508181]

[66] Ooi N, Eady EA, Cove JH, O'Neill AJ. Redox-active compounds with a history of human use: antistaphylococcal action and potential for repurposing as topical antibiofilm agents. J Antimicrob Chemother 2015; 70(2): 479-88.
[http://dx.doi.org/10.1093/jac/dku409] [PMID: 25368206]

[67] Tsugawa H, Mori H, Matsuzaki J, Masaoka T, Hirayama T, Nagasawa H, *et al.* Nordihydroguaiaretic acid disrupts the antioxidant ability of *Helicobacter pylori* through the repression of SodB activity in vitro. Biomed Res Int 2015; 2015

[68] Khan N, Pahari S, Vidyarthi A, Aqdas M, Agrewala JN. Stimulation through CD40 and TLR-4 Is an Effective Host Directed Therapy against *Mycobacterium tuberculosis*. Front Immunol 2016; 7: 386.
[http://dx.doi.org/10.3389/fimmu.2016.00386] [PMID: 27729911]

[69] Wu H-M, Wang J, Zhang B, Fang L, Xu K, Liu R-Y. CpG-ODN promotes phagocytosis and autophagy through JNK/P38 signal pathway in *Staphylococcus aureus*-stimulated macrophage. Life Sci 2016; 161: 51-9.
[http://dx.doi.org/10.1016/j.lfs.2016.07.016] [PMID: 27476088]

[70] Ruiz A, Guzmán-Beltrán S, Carreto-Binaghi LE, Gonzalez Y, Juárez E. DNA from virulent *M. tuberculosis* induces TNF-α production and autophagy in M1 polarized macrophages. Microb Pathog 2019; 132(May): 166-77.
[http://dx.doi.org/10.1016/j.micpath.2019.04.041] [PMID: 31054870]

[71] Juárez E, Carranza C, Hernández-Sánchez F, *et al.* NOD2 enhances the innate response of alveolar macrophages to *Mycobacterium tuberculosis* in humans. Eur J Immunol 2012; 42(4): 880-9.
[http://dx.doi.org/10.1002/eji.201142105] [PMID: 22531915]

[72] Juárez E, Carranza C, Hernández-Sánchez F, *et al.* Nucleotide-oligomerizing domain-1 (NOD1) receptor activation induces pro-inflammatory responses and autophagy in human alveolar macrophages. BMC Pulm Med 2014; 14: 152.
[http://dx.doi.org/10.1186/1471-2466-14-152] [PMID: 25253572]

[73] Girardin SE, Boneca IG, Viala J, *et al.* Nod2 is a general sensor of peptidoglycan through muramyl dipeptide (MDP) detection. J Biol Chem 2003; 278(11): 8869-72.
[http://dx.doi.org/10.1074/jbc.C200651200] [PMID: 12527755]

[74] Boyle JP, Mayle S, Parkhouse R, Monie TP. Comparative Genomic and Sequence Analysis Provides Insight into the Molecular Functionality of NOD1 and NOD2. Front Immunol 2013; 4: 317.
[http://dx.doi.org/10.3389/fimmu.2013.00317] [PMID: 24109482]

[75] Inohara N, Chamaillard M, McDonald C, Nuñez G. NOD-LRR proteins: role in host-microbial interactions and inflammatory disease. Annu Rev Biochem 2005; 74(1): 355-83.
[http://dx.doi.org/10.1146/annurev.biochem.74.082803.133347] [PMID: 15952891]

[76] Kanneganti T-D, Lamkanfi M, Núñez G. Intracellular NOD-like receptors in host defense and disease. Immunity 2007; 27(4): 549-59.

[http://dx.doi.org/10.1016/j.immuni.2007.10.002] [PMID: 17967410]

[77]   Divangahi M, Mostowy S, Coulombe F, *et al.* NOD2-deficient mice have impaired resistance to *Mycobacterium tuberculosis* infection through defective innate and adaptive immunity. J Immunol 2008; 181(10): 7157-65.
[http://dx.doi.org/10.4049/jimmunol.181.10.7157] [PMID: 18981137]

[78]   Brooks MN, Rajaram MVS, Azad AK, *et al.* NOD2 controls the nature of the inflammatory response and subsequent fate of *Mycobacterium tuberculosis* and M. bovis BCG in human macrophages. Cell Microbiol 2011; 13(3): 402-18.
[http://dx.doi.org/10.1111/j.1462-5822.2010.01544.x] [PMID: 21040358]

[79]   Rogov V, Dötsch V, Johansen T, Kirkin V. Interactions between autophagy receptors and ubiquitin-like proteins form the molecular basis for selective autophagy. Mol Cell 2014; 53(2): 167-78.
[http://dx.doi.org/10.1016/j.molcel.2013.12.014] [PMID: 24462201]

[80]   Abdulrahman BA, Khweek AA, Akhter A, *et al.* Autophagy stimulation by rapamycin suppresses lung inflammation and infection by Burkholderia cenocepacia in a model of cystic fibrosis. Autophagy 2011; 7(11): 1359-70.
[http://dx.doi.org/10.4161/auto.7.11.17660] [PMID: 21997369]

[81]   Hoang KV, Borteh HM, Rajaram MVS, *et al.* Acetalated dextran encapsulated AR-12 as a host-directed therapy to control Salmonella infection. Int J Pharm 2014; 477(1-2): 334-43.
[http://dx.doi.org/10.1016/j.ijpharm.2014.10.022] [PMID: 25447826]

[82]   Feng FB, Qiu HY. Effects of Artesunate on chondrocyte proliferation, apoptosis and autophagy through the PI3K/AKT/mTOR signaling pathway in rat models with rheumatoid arthritis. Biomed Pharmacother 2018; 102(261): 1209-20.
[http://dx.doi.org/10.1016/j.biopha.2018.03.142] [PMID: 29710540]

[83]   Delong W, Yongling W, Lanying W, Juntao F, Xing Z. Design, synthesis and evaluation of 3-arylidene azetidin-2-ones as potential antifungal agents against Alternaria solani Sorauer. Bioorg Med Chem 2017; 25(24): 6661-73.
[http://dx.doi.org/10.1016/j.bmc.2017.11.003] [PMID: 29137937]

[84]   Schiebler M, Brown K, Hegyi K, *et al.* Functional drug screening reveals anticonvulsants as enhancers of mTOR-independent autophagic killing of *Mycobacterium tuberculosis* through inositol depletion. EMBO Mol Med 2015; 7(2): 127-39.
[http://dx.doi.org/10.15252/emmm.201404137] [PMID: 25535254]

[85]   Konstantinidis T, Kambas K, Mitsios A, *et al.* Immunomodulatory role of clarithromycin in acinetobacter baumannii infection *via* formation of neutrophil extracellular traps. Antimicrob Agents Chemother 2015; 60(2): 1040-8.
[http://dx.doi.org/10.1128/AAC.02063-15] [PMID: 26643338]

[86]   Chiu HC, Kulp SK, Soni S, *et al.* Eradication of intracellular *Salmonella enterica* serovar Typhimurium with a small-molecule, host cell-directed agent. Antimicrob Agents Chemother 2009; 53(12): 5236-44.
[http://dx.doi.org/10.1128/AAC.00555-09] [PMID: 19805568]

[87]   Kim TS, Shin YH, Lee HM, *et al.* Ohmyungsamycins promote antimicrobial responses through autophagy activation *via* AMP-activated protein kinase pathway. Sci Rep 2017; 7(1): 3431.
[http://dx.doi.org/10.1038/s41598-017-03477-3] [PMID: 28611371]

[88]   Ferrari E, Monzani R, Villella VR, *et al.* Cysteamine re-establishes the clearance of *Pseudomonas aeruginosa* by macrophages bearing the cystic fibrosis-relevant F508del-CFTR mutation. Cell Death Dis 2017; 8(1): e2544.
[http://dx.doi.org/10.1038/cddis.2016.476] [PMID: 28079883]

[89]   Dittmar AJ, Drozda AA, Blader IJ. Drug repurposing screening identifies novel compounds that effectively inhibit *toxoplasma gondii* growth. MSphere 2016; 1(2): 1-15.
[http://dx.doi.org/10.1128/mSphere.00042-15] [PMID: 27303726]

[90] Kuo S-Y, Castoreno AB, Aldrich LN, *et al.* Small-molecule enhancers of autophagy modulate cellular disease phenotypes suggested by human genetics. Proc Natl Acad Sci USA 2015; 112(31): E4281-7.
[http://dx.doi.org/10.1073/pnas.1512289112] [PMID: 26195741]

[91] Parihar SP, Guler R, Khutlang R, *et al.* Statin therapy reduces the *Mycobacterium tuberculosis* burden in human macrophages and in mice by enhancing autophagy and phagosome maturation. J Infect Dis 2014; 209(5): 754-63.
[http://dx.doi.org/10.1093/infdis/jit550] [PMID: 24133190]

[92] Bhardwaj M, Paul S, Jakhar R, *et al.* Vitexin confers HSF-1 mediated autophagic cell death by activating JNK and ApoL1 in colorectal carcinoma cells. Oncotarget 2017; 8(68): 112426-41.
[http://dx.doi.org/10.18632/oncotarget.20113] [PMID: 29348836]

[93] Lei GS, Zhang C, Cheng BH, Lee CH. Mechanisms of action of vitamin D as supplemental therapy for *Pneumocystis pneumonia*. Antimicrob Agents Chemother 2017; 61(10): 1-13.
[http://dx.doi.org/10.1128/AAC.01226-17] [PMID: 28760906]

[94] Cilliers P, Seldon R, Smit FJ, Aucamp J, Jordaan A, Warner DF, *et al.* Design, synthesis and antimycobacterial activity of novel ciprofloxacin derivatives. Chem Biol Drug Des 2019; cbdd.13534.
[http://dx.doi.org/10.1111/cbdd.13534]

[95] Baindara P. Host-directed therapies to combat tuberculosis and associated non-communicable diseases. Microb Pathog 2019; 130: 156-68.
[http://dx.doi.org/10.1016/j.micpath.2019.03.003] [PMID: 30876870]

[96] Juárez E, Carranza C, Sánchez G, González M, Chávez J, Sarabia C, *et al.* Loperamide restricts intracellular growth of *Mycobacterium tuberculosis* in lung macrophages. m J Respir Cell Mol Biol 2016; rcmb.2015-.

[97] García-Martínez JM, Wullschleger S, Preston G, *et al.* Effect of PI3K- and mTOR-specific inhibitors on spontaneous B-cell follicular lymphomas in PTEN/LKB1-deficient mice. Br J Cancer 2011; 104(7): 1116-25.
[http://dx.doi.org/10.1038/bjc.2011.83] [PMID: 21407213]

[98] Salabei JK, Balakumaran A, Frey JC, Boor PJ, Treinen-Moslen M, Conklin DJ. Verapamil stereoisomers induce antiproliferative effects in vascular smooth muscle cells *via* autophagy. Toxicol Appl Pharmacol 2012; 262(3): 265-72.
[http://dx.doi.org/10.1016/j.taap.2012.04.036] [PMID: 22627060]

[99] Juárez E, Ruiz A, Cortez O, Sada E, Torres M. Antimicrobial and immunomodulatory activity induced by loperamide in mycobacterial infections. Int Immunopharmacol 2018; 65: 29-36.
[http://dx.doi.org/10.1016/j.intimp.2018.09.013] [PMID: 30268801]

[100] Zecchini S, Proietti Serafini F, Catalani E, *et al.* Dysfunctional autophagy induced by the pro-apoptotic natural compound climacostol in tumour cells. Cell Death Dis 2018; 10(1): 10.
[http://dx.doi.org/10.1038/s41419-018-1254-x] [PMID: 30584259]

[101] Kim H, Lee KI, Jang M, *et al.* Conessine interferes with oxidative stress-induced C2C12 myoblast cell death through inhibition of autophagic flux. PLoS One 2016; 11(6): e0157096.
[http://dx.doi.org/10.1371/journal.pone.0157096] [PMID: 27257813]

[102] Renna M, Schaffner C, Brown K, *et al.* Azithromycin blocks autophagy and may predispose cystic fibrosis patients to mycobacterial infection. J Clin Invest 2011; 121(9): 3554-63.
[http://dx.doi.org/10.1172/JCI46095] [PMID: 21804191]

[103] Andersson AM, Andersson B, Lorell C, Raffetseder J, Larsson M, Blomgran R. Autophagy induction targeting mTORC1 enhances *Mycobacterium tuberculosis* replication in HIV co-infected human macrophages. Sci Rep 2016; 6(May): 28171.
[http://dx.doi.org/10.1038/srep28171] [PMID: 27302320]

[104] Junkins RD, Shen A, Rosen K, McCormick C, Lin TJ. Autophagy enhances bacterial clearance during *P. aeruginosa* lung infection. PLoS One 2013; 8(8): e72263.

[http://dx.doi.org/10.1371/journal.pone.0072263] [PMID: 24015228]

[105] Kimmelman AC, White E. Autophagy and Tumor Metabolism. Cell Metab 2017; 25(5): 1037-43.
[http://dx.doi.org/10.1016/j.cmet.2017.04.004] [PMID: 28467923]

[106] Yang X, Yu D-D, Yan F, *et al.* The role of autophagy induced by tumor microenvironment in different cells and stages of cancer. Cell Biosci 2015; 5(1): 14.
[http://dx.doi.org/10.1186/s13578-015-0005-2] [PMID: 25844158]

CHAPTER 6

Neuro-Immune-Endocrine Interactions During Infections

Montoya-Rosales Alejandra and **Macías-Segura Noé***

Laboratorio de Neuroimunoendocrinología, Departamento de Fisiología y Farmacología, Centro de Ciencias Básicas, Universidad Autónoma de Aguascalientes, 20130 Aguascalientes, Ags., Mexico

Abstract: In recent years, it has been well documented in several studies that there is a close relationship among three of the most important homeostatic-control axes, the nervous, endocrine, and immunologic systems. Clinical and experimental evidence around the world indicates that this physiological phenomenon could be explained as neuro-immune-endocrine interactions (NIEI). The communication between those systems maintains the homeostasis in the presence of stressing stimuli like pathogens (virus, bacteria, fungus, and parasites). Commonly these kinds of stressors generate inflammation processes inside and outside the tissue. Once a pathogen gets into the body, it activates a sensor system through the activation of the innate immune cells such as macrophages and epithelial cells. These cells release cytokines and inflammatory mediators to the circulation such as interleukin-6 (IL-6) and Tumor necrosis factor-alpha (TNF-α), interacting with their specific receptors in different types of cells (local and peripheral cells). In the nervous system, principally in the peripheral nervous system (PNS), there are cytokine receptors to these cytokines, capable to send information from the periphery to the central nervous system (CNS), which is the main control center of the homeostasis. The CNS integrates the information in specific anatomical regions in the brain stem (*e.g.,* a nucleus of the tractus solitarius; NTS) activating hypothalamic cells, which in turn synthesize and secrete hormones to induce more hormones secretion from the pituitary gland and release them into the bloodstream. Some of these hormones travel to stimulate the synthesis and release of anti-inflammatory mediators such as the glucocorticoids, whereas other hormones produce a direct regulatory effect on the immune system through the interaction with its receptor, suppressing or stimulating the immune cells accordingly to the hormones concentration, receptor expression and other molecular, cellular and micro-environmental factors involved. In this chapter, we will review some of the principal molecular and cellular mediators involved in the homeostasis control by the NIE system during the infection with some kind of pathogens.

---

* **Corresponding author Macías-Segura Noé:** Neuroimmune-endocrinology laboratory, Physiology and Pharmacology department, Basic Sciences Centre, Universidad Autónoma de Aguascalientes, Aguascalientes, 20130 Aguascalientes, Ags., Mexico; Tel: 4499107400, Ext. 51257;
E-mail: nmsegura@correo.uaa.mx

Keywords: Bacterial Infections, Cytokines, Fungal Infections, Homeostasis, Hormones, Neurotransmitters, Neuro-Immune Biology, Neuro-Endocrine System, Parasite Infections, Viral Infections.

STRESS AND HOMEOSTASIS

Inflammation is commonly a defense response induced by specific injuries or infections [1]. Inflammation can be represented as an exacerbation of the immune system (IS), which disrupts the homeostasis generating a pathological feature. Inflammatory products are considered stress inductors in which several molecules and cells are involved [2]. Whether homeostasis is fundamentally the control mechanism of stress in the body. It maintains the key regulatory variables at different levels, whole body, specific tissues, and inside each cell. Within the tissues, all cells can maintain the homeostasis by intrinsic and extrinsic mechanisms to control systemic variables as blood ions concentration, glucose levels, pH, oxygen, osmolarity, and others [3]. All these variables are successfully controlled principally through the interaction of the endocrine and autonomic nervous systems.

Tissue homeostasis is characterized by the regulation of cell number, architecture, proliferation, infiltration of the resident cells, *etc.* The homeostasis regulates the mechanisms of stress control [4]. These mechanisms of stress control could be divided into two different responses: stress control response and defense response. The first stress control response is mediated by receptors or channels that sense metabolic changes, pH, hypoxia, DNA damage, *etc* [5]. The referred changes modify the transcriptional signature inside the cell, activating several intrinsic mechanisms of stress control. An example is the cell response to hypoxia and the stimulation and activation of molecules such as the activation of vascular epithelial grow factor (VEGF) by macrophages to increase vascularization and improve the oxygenation in the stressed tissue [6]. Another example of the mechanism is the defense response to injuries and inflammation mediated by pathogens. This mechanism is regulated by resident cells of the connective tissue (*e.g.,* macrophages and mast cells). Resident cells detect the presence of disturbances caused by specific pattern recognition receptors (PRRs) that detect damage-associated molecular patterns (DAMPs) [7] or pathogen-associated molecular patterns (PAMPs) [3, 8]. Identification of any of the DAMPs or PAMPs initiates the release of endocrine, paracrine, and exocrine molecules which in turn stimulate the stress center in the central nervous system, directly through cytokines release or indirectly by the activation of paraganglion cells. Then, the central nervous system activates cells at the hypothalamus level, releasing hormones capable to limit or induce cell proliferation and cell differentiation depending on the stimuli in the target tissue or organ [8, 9].

Hormones released by the hypothalamic-pituitary axis regulate cells directly and indirectly from the immune system through several mechanisms, described below in this chapter (Fig. **1**).

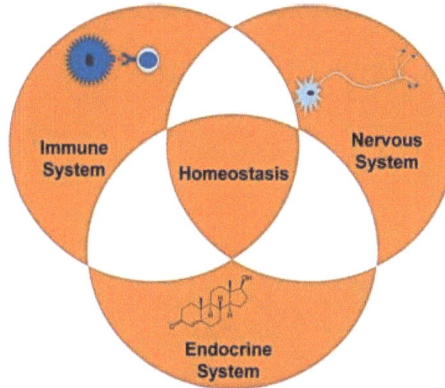

Fig. (1). Interactions between nervous, endocrine and immune systems initiate several homeostatic mechanisms through the release of neurotransmitters, hormones and cytokines in response to injury.

NEURO-IMMUNE-ENDOCRINE SYSTEM DURING INFECTION.

The neuroendocrine system is the major homeostatic system that senses and responds against stressors throughout the synthesis and releases of neurotransmitters and hormones. Furthermore, the immune system is capable to stimulate the nervous and the endocrine systems through the release of cytokines, chemokines, and other inflammatory mediators. In addition, the immune system initiates phagocytosis and cell lysis by specialized cells to eliminate stressors, such as pathogens [9, 10]. The neuroimmune-endocrine interactions across the body can initiate the homeostasis (Fig. **2**), controlling the entrance and clearance of pathogens [3, 11].

Once a pathogen gets inside the body, it activates the innate immune system, initiating the homeostasis reestablishment. At the beginning of an infection, some cells and mediators exert natural immunity (innate immunity) [12]. Monocyte/macrophages, granulocytes, a subset of B lymphocytes producing natural antibodies, γδ T cells, and natural killer cells play a major role in the innate immune response (IIR) with the clearance of a pathogen [13]. If the innate immune response is not enough to eliminate the pathogen, the adaptive immune response is activated. This response is based on specialized cell proliferation and is susceptible to senescence and multiple factors that affect cell differentiation and growth. IIR gives an initial defense against pathogens, whereas the adaptive immunity is the late, strongest, and most sustained response. The adaptive immune response (AIR) involves the gene recombination and clonal selection for the antigen receptor repertoire of specific antigen determinants (epitopes). All these epitopes help the immune system cells to recognize specific foreign antigens, driving a selection process, ensuring that mature cells release to the circulation and eliminate the antigen [14 - 16].

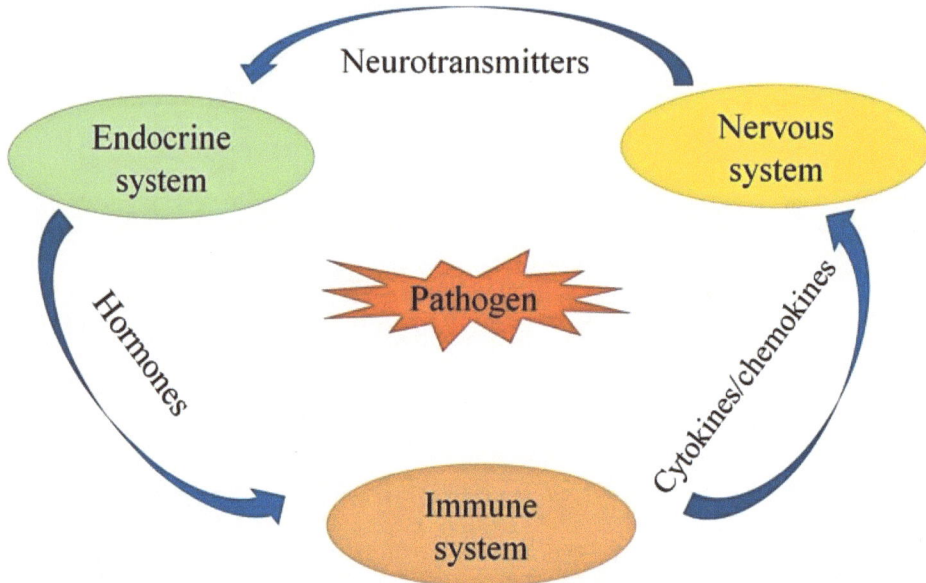

Fig. (2). The regulation mechanism of the neuroimmune-endocrine system is defined by the synthesis and release of neurotransmitters, hormones and cytokines. The cell expression of neurotransmitters, hormones and cytokines receptors can respond against pathogens and regulate the homeostasis.

To pass from IIR to AIR, it is necessary to activate several signal pathways across the human body. In particular, through the circulation and in response to bacterial lipopolysaccharide (LPS), cytokines are produced and released from immune cells *e.g.,* interleukin-6 (IL-6), IL-1β, and tumor necrosis factor-alpha (TNF-α). These cytokines can directly act on the hypothalamus through afferent nerves or bloodstream to activate the hypothalamic-pituitary-adrenal axis (HPA) [15, 17, 18]. When this axis is activated by the hypothalamus, the corticotropin-released hormone is secreted and acts on the anterior pituitary gland to stimulate the synthesis of adrenocorticotropic hormone (ACTH). Then, the ACTH stimulates the secretion of glucocorticoids (GC; corticosteroid hormones, cortisol in humans and corticosterone in rodents) into the bloodstream by the adrenal cortex. These hormones exert multiple effects when they bind to their receptor in nucleated cells [19, 20].

When IIR eliminates a pathogen, the level of cortisol becomes low and the hormone returns to basal levels. [20, 21]. However, when AIR maintains a pathogen stimulus for a long period, it becomes a chronic phenomenon with high levels of cortisol. This generates alterations in the neuroendocrine system and the immune response, with a deregulation of the NIEI and predisposition to disease [22, 23].

Neurotransmitters, hormones, and cytokines are the molecules responsible to interconnect the nervous system and the immune response and to establish a communication process that can regulate several physiological functions. The communication among nervous, endocrine and immune systems regulates multiple physiological processes. This affects the peripheral inflammation which is the most studied process in the NIE communication and has two principal mechanisms; neural and humoral [24, 25].

The neural mechanism of NIEI involves the activation of sensory fibers from the afferent vagal nerve to the CNS, indicating that the inflammatory process is mediated by a pathogen [26]. Cytokines from resident cells such as fibroblasts, epithelial cells, dendritic cells, macrophages, natural killer cells or other innate lymphoid cells (ILC), activate chemoreceptors on cells associated with paraganglion. One example from those cytokines is the release of interleukin 1 beta (IL1-β), which is secreted by dendritic cells (DC) and macrophages (MΦ). In this case, when animals are injected intraperitoneally with LPS, then DCs and MΦs are found near the vagal nerve [27]. Then, vagal paraganglion cells activate the vagal afferent fibers when IL1-β interacts with IL-1 receptor (type I) [28, 29].

The vagal afferent fibers end inside the spinal bulb (medulla oblongata), in which the following regions are found: the dorsal vagal complex (DVC), the nucleus of the tractus solitarius (NTS), the nucleus of the dorsal motor vagus (DMV) and the area postrema (AP) [30, 31]. All these anatomical regions in the spinal bulb have important neuronal interconnections among themselves, and they are activated at the same time when a stimulus arrives. In the DMV, there are cells that receive efferent preganglionic fibers from the vagus, which generate an anti-inflammatory response mediated by the vagus. The AP does not have a blood-brain barrier and is an important circumventricular organ for humoral communication between the immune and nervous systems [32].

Most of the sensory information that arrives at the spinal bulb activates the NTS, which stimulates and coordinates autonomic functions and interacts directly with the endocrine system. NTS cells have multiple projections in the spinal bulb, they send projections to the magnocellular and parvocellular cells in the paraventricular nucleus in the hypothalamus [33]. When parvocellular cells are activated they respond to stress, and they participate in the secretion and synthesis of corticotrophin-released hormone [34, 35]. Furthermore, this hormone stimulates cells in the adenohypophysis (anterior pituitary lobe) and activates the

HPA axis. On the other side, the stimuli of the magnocellular cells release arginine vasopressin (AVP) and oxytocin (OXY) into the bloodstream by the neurohypophysis (posterior pituitary lobe) [36, 37]. Both hormones are recognized as direct immune regulators in macrophages, dendritic cells and lymphocytes [38, 39].

Communication between the immune and nervous systems travels from the vagus nerve, and depends on the intensity of the stimulus, the degree of damage and/or psychological stress. Also, this communication is proportional to the peripheral concentration of cytokines [40].

Neural pathways of vagal afferences have critical participation in inflammatory modulation on peripheral, acute, chronic and intense immune responses which can stimulate the CNS by humoral mechanisms. In all cases, a minimal cytokine concentration of approximately 10 nM to activate humoral mechanisms is necessary [41].

Several experimental pieces of evidence support the importance of humoral mechanisms of communication between the IS and the CNS. During infectious challenges, the immune cells release cytokines like TNF-α, IL-1β and IL-6, and they interact directly and indirectly with the CNS [42].

Direct communication between peripheral cytokines and the CNS occurs in circumventricular sites, like the AP. Blood-brain barrier is absent in AP and is located on the dorsal surface of the medulla oblongata at the caudal end of the fourth ventricle, where dendritic ends of the NTS and DMN cells get into the AP. Interactions among these cells represent the principal connection between the sympathetic nervous system (SNS) and the HPA axis.

A high concentration of peripheral cytokines travels into the blood-brain barrier and arrives in the cerebrospinal fluid and spinal cord, this process is subject to the concentration of transporter-dependent. In addition to this process, endothelial cells produce IL-1α and IL-β, and vascular smooth muscle cells produce TNF-α, IL-1β and IL-1α. These cytokines interact directly with endothelial vascular cells' surface in the brain, increasing the synthesis and release of prostaglandins (PG) and nitric oxide (NO) [43]. PG and NO interact with other neurons at the CNS level, suggesting a relation with fever and activation of the HPA axis.

COMMUNICATION BETWEEN BRAIN AND IMMUNE SYSTEM

The immune system can be regulated in three ways: a) the immune cells *per se,* b) through the sympathetic nervous system, and c) indirectly by the HPA axis. This HPA axis is a neuro-hormonal pathway. Principal components of this HPA axis are: hypothalamus, PVN, the anterior lobe of the pituitary gland, and the adrenal cortex. Some neurons in the PVN synthesize the corticotropin-releasing hormone (CRH), which is released in the portal vein system inducing the secretion of the adrenocorticotropic hormone (ACTH) by the anterior pituitary lobe. ACTH is the principal stimulator for the release and synthesis of GC by the adrenal cortex, such as: cortisol and dehydroepiandrosterone (DHEA) [44, 45]. Cortisol is synthetized and released in high concentration into the bloodstream and interacts with a glucocorticoid receptor (CR) located in the cytoplasm of several cell types, a nuclear receptor subfamily 3, group C and member 1 (NR3C1). In turn, NR3C1 is translocated into the nucleus to up-regulate the transcription of anti-inflammatory cytokines (*e.g.* IL-10) and to down-regulate the inflammatory cytokines (*e.g.* IL-6 and IL-8) [46]. The secretion of GCs in response to injury by the adrenal glands first stimulates the immune response (IR) with low concentration, and later suppresses the IR with high concentration.

Then, the HPA axis is regulated by GC´s negative feedback. The hypothalamus-pituitary axis is mainly regulated by neurotransmitters such as acetylcholine (ACh), catecholamines, Gamma aminobutyric acid (GABA), serotonin and histamine. In contrast, the GCs act directly on their intracellular receptors activating or inactivating the transcription of specific genes depending on the GC concentration [47]. Also, IL-1β and IL-6 can change the peripheral effects of GC when interact with their receptors (IL-1R and IL-6R) [48].

The negative immune regulation mediated by GCs is associated with the suppression of the activation of nuclear factors, such as the nuclear factor kappa B (Nf-κB). Nf-κB regulates the transcription of proinflammatory cytokines that include IL-18, Il-12, TNF-α, Il-1β, and IFN-γ. These GCs also activate anti-inflammatory molecules such as, Il-10 and IL-4. Furthermore, they inhibit the proliferation of immune cells and the expression of adhesion molecules (Fig. **3**) [49, 50].

SNS has a critical role in the tissue inflammatory regulation and during the infection, it can activate the IR. The locus coeruleus (LC) and the rostral ventral medulla (RVM) send cholinergic preganglionic neurons through the spinal cord to finally arrive at secondary and primary lymphoid organs. These innervations in secondary and primary lymphoid organs are direct communication between CNS and IS [39, 51]. When innervated cells are activated by sympathetic preganglionic neurons it can induce the release of catecholamines into the bloodstream that may act as hormones. Then, the SNS acts similarly to an endocrine regulation and releases the catecholamines in the adrenal cortex. In the adrenal glands, the SNS regulates the GC synthesis, this interaction is an important regulatory component of the IS [52, 53].

Many of the mechanisms, molecules and anatomical structures mentioned above are shared during the pathogen-mediated injury, but some differences are contingent of the pathogen: mechanisms of infection, immune competence, and pathogen-associated virulence.

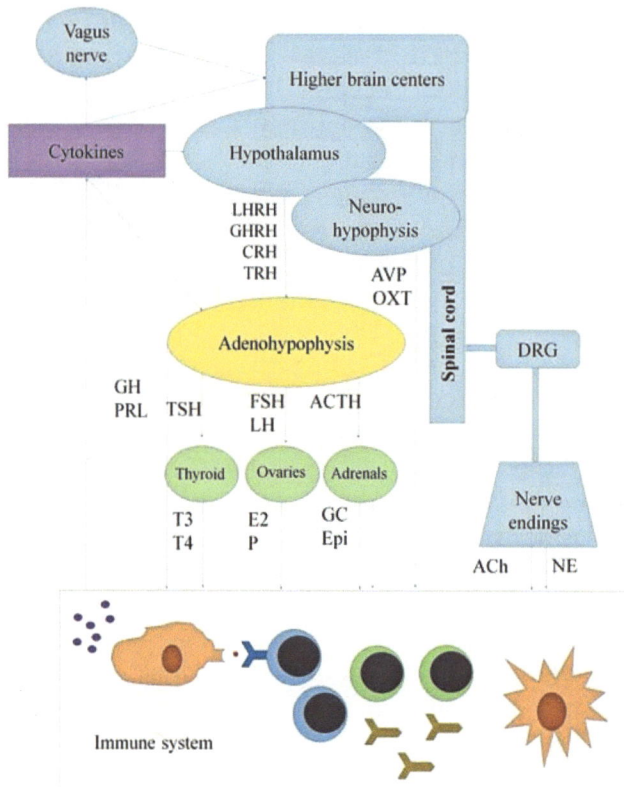

Fig. (3). The immune system is an example of the initiation of a response mediated by pathogen antigens. This figure represents the immune synapsis between antigen-presenting cells and lymphoid cells, and the subsequent activation of the humoral response, cytokines release and cell migration. Lymphoid organs can be directly or indirectly modulated by dorsal root ganglion-derived nerve endings and several hormones and neuropeptides. Ach = Acetylcholine; AVP = arginine vasopressin; DRG = dorsal root ganglion; E2 = estradiol; Epi = epinephrine; FSH = follicle stimulant hormone; GHRH = GH releasing hormone; LH = luteinizing hormone; LHRH = LH releasing hormone; NE = norepinephrine; OT = oxytocin; P = progesterone; T3 = triiodothyronine; T4 = thyroxin; TRH = Thyrotropin-releasing hormone; TSH = thyroid-stimulating hormone. Modified from Savino W, 2017 [39].

INIE DURING BACTERIAL INFECTIONS

Bacterial infections are highly prevalent among humans and several INIE mechanisms are involved during the infection process. Additionally, bacterial infections can be caused by both extracellular and intracellular pathogens. These microorganisms can generate strong inflammation that could drive local tissue destruction and high toxins concentration with systemic damage effects. Then, the innate immune response against extracellular bacteria is taken by the complement system. For example, the response against peptidoglycan contained in the cell wall of gram-negative bacteria activates the alternative complement pathway inducing the formation of C3-convertase [54]. Another example is that the LPS from the cell wall of gram-negative bacteria activates the complement alternative pathway without antibodies. Once the complement is activated it can opsonize and potentiate the phagocytosis of the bacteria. In addition, the membrane attack complex kills the bacteria, lysing the cell into fragments and initiating the inflammatory responses which attract and activate leukocytes [55, 56]. The phagocytosis effect of macrophages and dendritic cells is initiated through recognition receptors of mannose, scavenger and complement. Other receptors like the toll-like receptors (TLR) identify pathogen-associated molecular patterns (PAMPs) and activate phagocytosis. Then, the phagocytosis promotes the expansion of IR, the release of inflammatory cytokines and the arrival of leukocytes at the site of infection [57]. The macrophages at the site of infection present extracellular and intracellular antigens to B and T cells through the major histocompatibility complex (MHC) class II or class I, respectively [58]. When the infection persists at the site, then the humoral immune response (HIR) mediated by antibodies initiates the AIR to eliminate the pathogen (*e.g.* encapsulated bacteria rich in polysaccharides). HIR promotes bacterial particles opsonization, phagocytosis, neutralization, and activates the classic complement pathway [59]. Bacterial neutralization is mediated by IgG and IgA isotypes. Subtypes of IgG mediates opsonization, complement activation, and releases IgM. Protein antigens from bacteria activate T CD4+ cells which release pro-inflammatory cytokines that promote the synthesis and secretion of antibodies, local inflammation and phagocytosis. The release of IFN-γ from T cells promotes the activation of macrophages that release TNF-α to initiate inflammation. In addition, the release of IL-17 by Th17 cells is responsible for neutrophils mediated-inflammation which is critical for bacterial clearance [60].

During intracellular bacterial infection, natural killer cells (NK) are responsible for microorganisms' clearance in recognition of infected antigen-presenting cells (APCs). APCs are a heterogeneous group of immune cells that present intracellular antigens to NK or cytotoxic CD8+ T cells through the MHC class I. Immunologic synapses between APC and NK stimulate the release of inflammatory cytokines including TNF-α and IL-12 by APCs. Then, TNF-α and IL-12 induce chemotaxis and proliferation of NK cells. NK cells release IFN-γ and activate more APCs to eliminate the pathogen. Animals without T and B cells are capable to respond against intracellular bacteria when NK cells release IFN-γ [61]. In this context, the killing of the intracellular pathogen by innate immune response alone is not always enough, so the participation of the adaptive immune response is necessary for efficient pathogen clearance.

Inflammation mediated by bacterial infection is crucial for the survival of the infected host. This inflammation is a clinical sign and a consequence of mortality in infected patients. Patients who are diagnosed with tuberculosis (TB), infection mediated by *Mycobacterium tuberculosis* (Mtb), show a high concentration of IL-10, IL-6, IFN-γ and cortisol, and low levels of DHEA [62]. DHEA is an anti-inflammatory hormone that could inhibit the transcription factor NK-κB and enhance IL-2 transcription. This transcription factor NK-κB is responsible for activating cytokine expression (*e.g.* IL-6 and IFN-γ) and has an important role in inflammatory responses. Through the interaction of the DHEA with estrogen (ER) and androgen receptors (AR), DHEA binds to monocytes and T cells and reduces the inflammatory response. TNF-α, IL-6 and IFN-γ activate the HPA axis which is associated with inflammatory processes with high levels of cortisol and DHEA and supports the negative neuro-immune-endocrine feedback [63]. Some studies indicate low levels of DHEA in fluids of TB patients and support that DHEA could be an important regulator for inflammation in TB. In one study, supernatants from *Mtb*-stimulated peripheral blood mononuclear cells obtained from TB patients, show the inhibition of DHEA in a human adrenal cell line. This inhibition of DHEA indicates endocrine changes that could be mediated by endogenous cytokines. Another study indicated that deficient DHEA/cortisol ratio in *Mtb* infection is related to a deficient control of inflammation in TB patients, this could explain the deficient process to control inflammation [45, 64].

The reduction of testosterone levels in TB patients suggests that the HPA axis is affected. For example, some authors proposed that changes in testosterone concentration and the presence of inflammatory cytokines are associated with aromatase-mediated conversion into proinflammatory estrogens. Furthermore, other authors found high levels and positive correlation of estradiol and IL-6 in TB patients. TB patients exhibit a high concentration of cortisol, estradiol, prolactin, and thyroid hormone, and low concentration of DHEA and testosterone [65, 66]. These studies suggested endocrine deregulation associated with inflammation in *Mtb* infection.

As stated previously, the HPA axis is not the only pathway that releases hormones and is associated with immune regulation. A high concentration of TNF-α, IFN-γ and IL-6 activates the NTS and the PVN in the hypothalamus, sending nerve signals to the posterior lobe of the hypophysis which is followed by the secretion of the AVP and OXT into the bloodstream. Elimination of the posterior lobe of the hypophysis shows low levels of immunoglobulins mediated by *Salmonella* infection. These immunoglobulins level is restored when an AVP V2 receptor agonist is injected intraperitoneally. In addition, OXT reduces efficiently the concentration of TNF-α in several infected and non-infected models. This suggests that AVP could be pro-inflammatory and OXT anti-inflammatory [67].

Some studies indicate that the release of microbial metabolites from the gut microbiota is capable to regulate cytokines and cell profiles and polarize the peripheral concentration of pro-inflammatory or anti-inflammatory mediators. These cytokines travel from the intestine to the CNS where they can regulate brain development, function and behavior. Some specific gut microbiota species profiles are associated with neuroinflammatory conditions (*e.g.* multiple sclerosis disease; MS). A gut microbiota species profile has been associated with MS, which includes high counts of Streptococcusand Eggerthella,and low counts of Clostridia clusters XIVa and IV, Bacteroidetes and *Faecalibacterium*. This gut microbiota profile creates important changes in the gut microbiota and modulates the T-cell profiles through the release and interaction with polysaccharides A (PSA) and short-chain fatty acids (SCFAs; primary products of bacterial fermentation). PSA and SCFAs activate T-cells and differentiate into Th-17, to release IL-17A and reduce the numbers of T-reg cells. In a mouse model of experimental autoimmune encephalomyelitis (EAE), with a gut microbiota profile characterized by high numbers of *Streptococcus* and low numbers of *Bacteroides fragilis* induce an exacerbation of Th17 cells in the small intestine. This profile increases the neuroinflammation and promotes the disease. This and other profiles indicate that gut microbiota interacts with the CNS and modulates the immune cells profiles, thus, reduces or increases the neuroinflammation [68].

INIE DURING VIRAL INFECTIONS

Viruses are obligated intracellular microorganisms and capable of infecting a wide variety of cell types through surface receptors on the cells [69]. Inside the cell, the virus´ units use nuclei acids and the protein synthesis machinery to replicate and generate several histolytic damages and deficient synthesis of cell proteins that affect various cellular mechanisms. Furthermore, viruses can induce latent infections where the viral genetic material stays permanently in host cells and synthesizes proteins that can affect the normal cell functions. The latency is frequently a balance between the immune system and the persistent infection in which the immune cells control the infection but do not eliminate the pathogen [49].

The IIR against viruses is mediated by the antiviral response of the type I interferons (IFN-α/β) and the lytic effect of natural killer cells (NK). In contrast, AIR is mainly mediated by antibodies, T helper cells (CD4+) and cytotoxic T cells (CD8+). In this context, the neuroendocrine system is responsible for a regulated activation of the IIR and AIR against viruses [49, 50].

A viral infection is associated with the release of type I interferons by infected cells like plasmacytoid dendritic cells (DC) [49]. The pathways that activate the synthesis and the release of these interferons are correlated with the expression of toll-like receptors (TLRs) that recognize viral RNA and DNA. Other cytokines like TNF-α, IL-1, and IL-6 are also released by many cell types during IIR. These cell types include phagocytes such as macrophages and their CNS counterparts' microglial cells, vascular endothelial cells, fibroblast and neurons. Other significant types of cytokines involved in the defense against viral infections are IL-2 and IFN-γ, which are released by T cells and mediate the late response of AIR. As stated earlier, some of these cytokines activate the HPA axis that results in the release of GCs from the adrenal gland. These GCs regulate negatively the immune cells to suppress the release and synthesis of cytokines, to protect the host's detrimental consequences from the anti-viral inflammatory process (*e.g.*, septic shock, organ and tissue damage, autoimmunity, and depression) [70].

The release of type I interferons and IL-12 activates immune cells like NK cells which generate a cytotoxic mediated response to eliminate the infected cells through the interaction with the MHC class I molecule in the antigen-presenting cells (APCs). This communication induces the release of IFN-γ and is crucial to control infections before the activation of T cells to produce more IFN-γ. In the presence of IFN-γ and IL-12, CD4+ T cells initiate an inflammatory process (Th1) characterized by cell proliferation and differentiation, that promote the cellular immunity mediated by macrophages (*via* IFN-γ release) and CD8+ T cells (*via* IL-2 release) [49, 71].

The connection of the cytokine's mechanisms with the HPA axis during a viral infection is critical to recognize as there is a pleiotropic effect of cytokines that are redundant, causing an effect on the release of other cytokines (*e.g.*, TNF-α →IL-1 → IL-6, while IL-6 inhibits TNF-α and IL-1 synthesis). These cytokines often modify the action of other cytokines (IL-6, IL-1 and TNF-α act in synergy). Studies showed that the effect of the HPA axis by inflammatory cytokines can control the body's homeostasis during infections. For example, the levels of CRH are much greater during the administration of LPS in peritoneal macrophages as compared to the administration of IL-6 or TNF-α in the same cells. Also, the evidence showed that the synergy of these cytokines strongly activates the release of ACTH as compared to their actions alone [16, 22, 72, 73].

To study the neuroimmune-endocrine interactions mediated by viruses, some researchers use the polyinosinic polcytidilic acid (poly I:C), a synthetic double-stranded RNA and the Newcastle disease virus (NDV). The use of poly I:C and NDV does not actively infect the host. Poly I:C has been used to mimic a viral infection that rapidly activates the HPA axis IL-6-dependent (with the release of CRH). For example, a study with IL-6 KO mice treated with poly I:C exhibited a reduced corticosterone response (opposite to the significantly low levels shown in LPS infection) and no changes in stressed mice. This study demonstrated that the glucocorticoid release in response to IL-6 can be dependent on the virus-type stimuli [49].

The infection with NDV produced elevated levels of ACTH and corticosterone in the first two hours post-injection (p/i) in mice and rats. Also, the two hours p/i of NDV showed elevated levels of 3-Methoxy-4-hydroxyphenylglycol (MHPG), a norepinephrine catabolite and eight hours p/i of NDV showed the elevated levels of tryptophan and serotonin catabolite 5-hydroxyindoleacetic acid (5-HIAA). The increased levels of ACTH/corticosterone were also observed in animals injected with virus-free supernatants derived from cultures of leukocytes infected with NDV. This suggests that the stimulation of the HPA axis is mediated by products of leukocytes, but not by the virus itself [74, 75]. Furthermore, IL-1 was reported as the principal factor in the activation of the HPA axis during the infection with NDV. This is supported due to the inactivation of this cytokine by an anti-IL-1 antibody that can stopped the stimulatory effect in the HPA axis. Also, hypophysectomized mice infected with NDV did not activate the HPA axis and exhibited low levels of corticosterone [74].

Studies in an infected model with murine cytomegalovirus (MCMV) show that IL-6 and IL-1α are responsible for the release of corticosterone. These GCs reduce the proinflammatory cytokine levels and down-regulate the inflammatory response in MCMV infection. The levels of IL-12, IFN-γ, TNF-α, and IL-6 increased in animals with adrenalectomy and infected with MCMV can cause septic shock and death. The supplementation of corticosterone or TNF-antisera in these MCMV infected mice can restore the survival [76, 77].

The acquired immune deficiency syndrome (AIDS) is an infection caused by the human immunodeficiency virus (HIV) characterized by low counts of CD4+ T cells, neuroendocrine disturbances and impairment of the HPA axis. Reports indicated that HIV-positive patients, both symptomatic and asymptomatic, have increased basal levels of ACTH/cortisol levels, but blunt ACTH and cortisol responses to stress. However, the administration of viral products in animals increases the levels of ACTH and corticosterone and correlates positively with inflammatory mediators like prostaglandins or IL-1. In addition, the overexpression of pg-120 (an envelope protein of HIV) in transgenic mice showed high levels of peripheral ACTH and corticosterone. The gp-120 administration in murine hypothalamic explants increased the levels of CRH (intrahypothalamic and soluble) and AVP and increased the transcription of *Crh* mRNA. Some of these interactions are mediated by nitric oxide synthase (NOs) and showed the important role of IIR in endocrine regulation during viral infections [49, 78].

Pathological inflammatory mechanisms in viral infections are regulated by the HPA axis and this regulation depends on the type of virus and the peripheral concentration of inflammatory cytokines. These inflammatory cytokines like IL-1 or IL-6 activate the HPA axis and increase GCs levels. This HPA axis activation induces the release of the DHEA, another steroid hormone capable to regulate the IR and GCs. Lastly, high or low concentration of steroid hormones in viral infections may result in pathological outcomes with a deficient immune response against the microorganism.

NIEI DURING PARASITIC AND FUNGAL INFECTIONS

Parasitic and fungal infectious diseases are produced by eukaryotic opportunistic microbes. Parasites that can cause infectious diseases include protozoa, helminths and ectoparasites; and fungal diseases include yeasts and molds. Parasites are responsible for high morbidity and mortality rates compared to other microorganisms, particularly in developing countries. Furthermore, parasites can develop complex vital cycles in humans or vertebrates. The life cycle of parasites in humans or vertebrates depends on intermediate hosts like mosquitos, ticks and snails. In particular, humans can be infected by mosquitos' bites, other intermediate hosts, or by accidentally eating contaminated food. For example, parasites in malaria and trypanosomiasis are transferred into humans through insects' bites, and parasites in schistosomiasis are transferred from infected water.

Most of parasitic chronic diseases are caused by weak immunity, immune-deficiencies or parasite immune evasion. Many anti-parasitic antibiotics do not permanently eliminate these microorganisms, extend their reproduction in the host and cause chronic diseases. Studies indicate that intracellular parasitic agents initiate a defensive immune response mediated by cytokines released from macrophages [79].

As stated above, the release of TNF-α, IFN-γ and IL-1β stimulates the HPA axis and increases plasma levels of GC and DHEA. This HPA axis is the common immune-endocrine pathway that controls inflammation; and the HPA axis' deregulation is associated with pathophysiological mechanisms. The complex network of immunoendocrine interactions has control during a parasitic infection, which depends on the pathogen nature, the temporality of illness and the nature of the infected host. For example, high levels of corticosterone and a preserved adrenal cortex activity occur during the acute infection caused by *Trypanosoma cruzi* [39]. The activation of the adrenal gland in the *T. cruzi* infection positively correlates with high levels of TNF-α, IFN-γ and IL-6. However, a disconnection between the cytokine levels and the HPA axis was identified. Studies showed that in some parasitic infections, the peripheral corticosterone levels are high, the content of CRH in the hypothalamus is low and ACTH circulating level is unaltered. Similarly, in chagasic infection, mice with higher basal levels of GCs showed better disease progress and faster development of the GCs response. This HPA-independent pathway suggests an increase of the GC secretion and these GCs do not associate with levels of inflammatory cytokines.

Through the regulation of stress response, the HPA axis function is essential for physiological adaptation and homeostasis control during critical illness. In baboons with primary schistosomiasis infection, worm recovery and oviposition rates were high and hepatic schistosome egg granulomas were large. As infection progressed, primary infected baboons showed to have decreased levels of CRH, ACTH, DHEA, and cortisol, as compared to both uninfected and reexposed baboons [80]. In contract to schistosome, primary and secondary adrenal insufficiency are shown in patients with severe malaria infection, but it can be ameliorated by the increment of circulating IL-6. However, adrenalectomy in different models of malaria demonstrated that the adrenal hormones conferred disease tolerance and early mortality rates reduction independently of the parasitemia. Also, AVP is another hormone associated with malarial infection beyond the HPA axis. AVP secretion is mediated by the hypothalamus when proinflammatory cytokines like IL-6, TNFα and IL-1β are increased, and then released by the neurohypophysis. Levels of circulating AVP are increased in severe infection with malaria, especially with cerebral malaria. The increment of circulating AVP is also positively associated with hyponatraemia and negatively associated with C-reactive protein, this suggests an important role of the hormone during malarial infection [81].

As stated earlier, the role of the vagus nerve is critical during an infection. Once the vagus nerve is activated by inflammatory mediators, it sends afferences to the NTS and then the nucleus sends back the response through the sympathetic or parasympathetic nervous systems. The released neurotransmitters can activate or inactivate the immune system. Mice infected with *Plasmodium yoelii* and treated with adrenaline showed a reduction in their parasitemia. This treatment with adrenaline suggested the critical role of neurotransmitters to control the infection. Other experiments demonstrated the importance of the activation of the SNS and PNS in parasitic infections. Vagotomized rats with *Entamoeba histolytica* infection had low levels of macrophages, neutrophils and NK around the amoeba. This experiment revealed the importance of the interaction between the PNS and CNS with IIR in parasitic infections [82].

The fungal infections are characterized by opportunistic mycosis in immunocompromised patients. Specifically, patients with AIDS are susceptible to acquire a co-infection with *Pneumocistis jiroveci* and can develop pneumonia. Several fungi can live and reproduce on extracellular spaces within the tissues or inside phagocytes. In this context, the IR against fungus is highly activated mainly in co-infections with bacteria or virus.

In mycosis, the innate immune mediators are physical barriers, mucous membranes of the respiratory, gastrointestinal and genitourinary tracts. Mucous barriers and skin are the principal physical barriers that protect the host against fungal infections. These barriers have several antimicrobial substances on their surface that are released by epithelial and endothelial cells. In humans, the lungs are the most common sites of mycotic infection by *Aspergillus*. *A. fumigatus* conidia is eliminated by the action of cilia of the pseudo-stratified ciliated cylindrical epithelium on the upper part of the tracheobronchial tree [83]. The fungus releases and synthetizes gliotoxin, fumagilina and helvolic acid that can inhibit the ciliary movement. The endothelial and the epithelial cells are able to internalize conidia which may facilitate the fungal infection. Also, the airway mucus is one of the most effective physical barriers against fungus because the secretion of glycoproteins, proteoglycans, lipids, lysozyme and surfactants facilitates the killing of fungal conidia [84].

Other participants against fungal infections are leukocytes from the immune system, such as neutrophils and macrophages. Patients with low levels of leukocytes are most susceptible to acquire an opportunistic fungal infection. The neutrophils are important immune regulators during mycosis, since neutrophils release nitric oxygen species and lysosomic enzymes, and engulf the fungus. Neutrophils react to pattern recognition receptors (PRRs) such as lung surfactant proteins A and D (SP-A and SP-D), mannan-binding lectin (MBL) and TLRs, which also strengthen the IIR. The activation of PRRs with the Granulocyte-macrophages colony-stimulator factor (GM-GSF) prime macrophages releases pro-inflammatory mediators like IL-1 and TNF-α. TNF-α stimulates neutrophils to phagocyte conidia, augments neutrophil oxidative respiratory burst and induces degranulation by opsonized fungi. Besides, IL-6 is rapidly released by NK cells after intranasal infection with *A. fumigatus*, and it could have an immunomodulatory role in pulmonary host defense in response to fungus injury [85].

The role of the pituitary gland in mycosis has been demonstrated by several observations. One example is the infection with *Lysteria monocytogenes* in which the reduction of prolactin levels with bromocriptine increases mortality rates in infected subjects, while the exogenous administration of this hormone reduces its susceptibility [86]. Additionally, another study demonstrated that the pituitary gland has CD4 and some PRRs (*e.g.* TLR4) that interact with glucans. These glucans are (1→3)-ß-linked linear and branched polymers containing anhydroglucose repeating units. Furthermore, glucans are the major portions of the cell wall of saprophytic and pathogenic fungi. Direct stimulation with glucans in corticotropic cells in the pituitary anterior lobe promotes the release of prolactin, which suggests that glucans from fungi can promote prolactin secretion and reduce the susceptibility to infection [83, 87]. Also, in infection with *C. albicans*, it is evident that infected Wistar rats have high ACTH and corticosterone levels where livers were heavily colonized by the fungi, but did not colonize the thymus [83, 88]. Also, at the systemic level, these Wistar rats exhibited TNF-α and IL-6 reduction, poorly developed granulomas, different types and localizations of steatosis and severe liver injury. Also, at the site of fungal infection, they showed lower cell recruitment, reduced colonization index and higher fungal load [89, 90]. These data suggested that different hormonal regulation mechanisms exist in the pituitary gland that depend on the microbial characteristics and the type of activation of the corticotropic cells (direct or indirect).

CONCLUDING REMARKS

There are many lines of evidence that demonstrate that the neuroimmune endocrine system is mediated in the beginning by the release of proinflammatory cytokines like TNF-α, IFN-γ, IL-6 and IL-1β. These cytokines stimulate vagal afferences and efferences by neurotransmitters and directly activate the CNS through the interaction with the PA in the medulla oblongata. The PVN in the hypothalamus activates the HPA and HPG axis which stimulates the release of DHEA and glucocorticoids to induce a negative regulation of the immune system and to control inflammation. Another parallel pathway in the PVN activates the release of AVP and OXT from the posterior pituitary lobe, which induce immune regulation through the direct interaction with immune cells. Other hormones have been reported as immune regulators like estrogen, prolactin and testosterone, and some neurotransmitters as epinephrine and acetylcholine have also been reported to regulate the immune response during infections.

ABBREVIATIONS

5-HIAA   5-hydroxyindoleacetic acid

Ach   acetylcholine

ACTH   adrenocorticotropic hormone

AIDS   Acquired Immune Deficiency Syndrome

AIR	adaptive immune response
AP	area postrema
APC´s	antigen-presenting cells
AVP	arginine vasopressin
CNS	central nervous system
CRH	corticotrophin-releasing hormone
DAMPs	Damage associated molecular patterns
DC	dendritic cells
DHEA	dehydroepiandrosterone
DMV	dorsal motor vagus
DNA	Deoxyribonucleic acid
DVC	dorsal vagal complex
GABA	gamma-aminobutyric acid
GC	glucocorticoids
HIV	human immunodeficiency virus
HPA	hypothalamic-pituitary-adrenal axis
IFN-γ	Interferon gamma
IgA	Immunoglobulin A
IgG	Immunoglobulin G
IgM	Immunoglobulin M
IIR	innate immune response
IL-1 β	interleukin 1 beta
IL-10	Interleukin 10
IL-12	Interleukin 12
IL-17	interleukin 17
IL-18	Interleukin 18
IL-4	Interleukin 4
IL-6	Interleukin 6
ILC	innate lymphoid cells
KO	Knockout
LC	locus coeruleus
LPS	lipopolysaccharide
MCMV	murine cytomegalovirus
MHC	Major histocompatibility complex
MHPG	4-hydroxyphenylethyleneglycol

Mtb	*Mycobacterium tuberculosis*
NDV	Newcastle disease virus
Nf-κB	Nuclear factor kappa-light-chain-enhancer of activated B cells
NIEI	neuro-immune-endocrine interactions
NK	natural killer cells
NO	nitric oxide
NOs	nitric oxide synthase
NTS	nucleus of the tractus solitarius
OXY	oxytocin
PAMPs	pathogen-associated molecular patterns
PNS	Peripheral nervous system
PRRs	Pattern recognition receptors
PVN	paraventricular nucleus
RVM	rostral ventral medulla
SNS	sympathetic nervous system
SP-A	surfactant proteins A
SP-D	surfactant proteins D
Tb	Tuberculosis
TLR	Toll-like receptors
TNF-a	Tumor necrosis factor alfa
VEGF	Vascular Endothelial Growth Factor

CONSENT FOR PUBLICATION

Not applicable.

CONFLICT OF INTEREST

The authors confirm that the content of this chapter has no conflict of interest.

ACKNOWLEDGEMENTS

Declared none.

REFERENCES

[1]   Chen L, Deng H, Cui H, *et al.* Inflammatory responses and inflammation-associated diseases in organs. Oncotarget 2017; 9(6): 7204-18.
[http://dx.doi.org/10.18632/oncotarget.23208] [PMID: 29467962]

[2]   Solleiro-Villavicencio H, Rivas-Arancibia S. Effect of chronic oxidative stress on neuroinflammatory response mediated by CD4$^+$T cells in neurodegenerative diseases. Front Cell Neurosci 2018; 12: 114.

[http://dx.doi.org/10.3389/fncel.2018.00114] [PMID: 29755324]

[3]   Chovatiya R, Medzhitov R. Stress, inflammation, and defense of homeostasis. Mol Cell 2014; 54(2): 281-8.
        [http://dx.doi.org/10.1016/j.molcel.2014.03.030] [PMID: 24766892]

[4]   Biteau B, Hochmuth CE, Jasper H. Maintaining tissue homeostasis: dynamic control of somatic stem cell activity. Cell Stem Cell 2011; 9(5): 402-11.
        [http://dx.doi.org/10.1016/j.stem.2011.10.004] [PMID: 22056138]

[5]   Tabas I, Glass CK. Anti-inflammatory therapy in chronic disease: challenges and opportunities. Science 2013; 339(6116): 166-72.
        [http://dx.doi.org/10.1126/science.1230720] [PMID: 23307734]

[6]   Benemei S, Patacchini R, Trevisani M, Geppetti P. TRP channels. Curr Opin Pharmacol 2015; 22: 18-23.
        [http://dx.doi.org/10.1016/j.coph.2015.02.006] [PMID: 25725213]

[7]   Roh JS, Sohn DH. Damage-associated molecular patterns in inflammatory diseases. Immune Netw 2018; 18(4)e27.
        [http://dx.doi.org/10.4110/in.2018.18.e27] [PMID: 30181915]

[8]   Taghavi M, Khosravi A, Mortaz E, Nikaein D, Athari SS. Role of pathogen-associated molecular patterns (PAMPS) in immune responses to fungal infections. Eur J Pharmacol 2017; 808: 8-13.
        [http://dx.doi.org/10.1016/j.ejphar.2016.11.013] [PMID: 27851904]

[9]   Odegaard JI, Chawla A. The immune system as a sensor of the metabolic state. Immunity 2013; 38(4): 644-54.
        [http://dx.doi.org/10.1016/j.immuni.2013.04.001] [PMID: 23601683]

[10]   Navab M, Gharavi N, Watson AD. Inflammation and metabolic disorders. Curr Opin Clin Nutr Metab Care 2008; 11(4): 459-64.
        [http://dx.doi.org/10.1097/MCO.0b013e32830460c2] [PMID: 18542007]

[11]   Haddad JJ, Saadé NE, Safieh-Garabedian B. Cytokines and neuro-immune-endocrine interactions: a role for the hypothalamic-pituitary-adrenal revolving axis. J Neuroimmunol 2002; 133(1-2): 1-19.
        [http://dx.doi.org/10.1016/S0165-5728(02)00357-0] [PMID: 12446003]

[12]   Kumar H, Bot A. Innate immunity and infectious diseases-an update. Int Rev Immunol 2017; 36(2): 55-6.
        [http://dx.doi.org/10.1080/08830185.2017.1307021] [PMID: 28333564]

[13]   Tosi MF. Innate immune responses to infection. J Allergy Clin Immunol 2005; 116(2): 241-9.
        [http://dx.doi.org/10.1016/j.jaci.2005.05.036] [PMID: 16083775]

[14]   Chaplin DD. Overview of the immune response. J Allergy Clin Immunol 2010; 125(2) (Suppl. 2): S3-S23.
        [http://dx.doi.org/10.1016/j.jaci.2009.12.980] [PMID: 20176265]

[15]   Besedovsky HO, del Rey A. Central and peripheral cytokines mediate immune-brain connectivity. Neurochem Res 2011; 36(1): 1-6.
        [http://dx.doi.org/10.1007/s11064-010-0252-x] [PMID: 20820913]

[16]   Anisman H, Baines MG, Berczi I, *et al.* Neuroimmune mechanisms in health and disease: 2. Disease. CMAJ 1996; 155(8): 1075-82.
        [PMID: 8873636]

[17]   Del Rey A, Roggero E, Randolf A, *et al.* IL-1 resets glucose homeostasis at central levels. Proc Natl Acad Sci USA 2006; 103(43): 16039-44.
        [http://dx.doi.org/10.1073/pnas.0607076103] [PMID: 17035503]

[18]   del Rey A, Balschun D, Wetzel W, Randolf A, Besedovsky HO. A cytokine network involving brain-borne IL-1β, IL-1ra, IL-18, IL-6, and TNFα operates during long-term potentiation and learning. Brain

Behav Immun 2013; 33: 15-23.
[http://dx.doi.org/10.1016/j.bbi.2013.05.011] [PMID: 23747799]

[19] Besedovsky HO, Del Rey A, Sorkin E, Lotz W, Schwulera U. Lymphoid cells produce an immunoregulatory glucocorticoid increasing factor (GIF) acting through the pituitary gland. Clin Exp Immunol 1985; 59(3): 622-8.
[PMID: 2985305]

[20] Berkenbosch F, van Oers J, del Rey A, Tilders F, Besedovsky H. Corticotropin-releasing factor-producing neurons in the rat activated by interleukin-1. Science 1987; 238(4826): 524-6.
[http://dx.doi.org/10.1126/science.2443979] [PMID: 2443979]

[21] del Rey A, Besedovsky H, Sorkin E. Endogenous blood levels of corticosterone control the immunologic cell mass and B cell activity in mice. J Immunol 1984; 133(2): 572-5.
[PMID: 6610705]

[22] del Rey A, Besedovsky HO. Immune-neuro-endocrine reflexes, circuits, and networks: Physiologic and evolutionary implications. Front Horm Res. Karger Publishers 2017; 48: pp. 1-18.
[http://dx.doi.org/10.1159/000452902]

[23] Perez de la Hoz RA, Swieszkowski SP, Cintora FM, *et al.* Neuroendocrine system regulatory mechanisms: Acute coronary syndrome and stress hyperglycaemia. Eur Cardiol 2018; 13(1): 29-34.
[http://dx.doi.org/10.15420/ecr.2017:19:3] [PMID: 30310467]

[24] Dantzer R. Neuroimmune interactions: From the brain to the immune system and vice versa. Physiol Rev 2018; 98(1): 477-504.
[http://dx.doi.org/10.1152/physrev.00039.2016] [PMID: 29351513]

[25] Procaccini C, Pucino V, De Rosa V, Marone G, Matarese G. Neuro-endocrine networks controlling immune system in health and disease. Front Immunol 2014; 5: 143.
[http://dx.doi.org/10.3389/fimmu.2014.00143] [PMID: 24778633]

[26] Breit S, Kupferberg A, Rogler G, Hasler G. Vagus nerve as modulator of the brain-Gut axis in psychiatric and inflammatory disorders. Front Psychiatry 2018; 9: 44.
[http://dx.doi.org/10.3389/fpsyt.2018.00044] [PMID: 29593576]

[27] Goehler LE, Gaykema RP, Nguyen KT, *et al.* Interleukin-1beta in immune cells of the abdominal vagus nerve: a link between the immune and nervous systems? J Neurosci 1999; 19(7): 2799-806.
[http://dx.doi.org/10.1523/JNEUROSCI.19-07-02799.1999] [PMID: 10087091]

[28] Quintanar-Stephano A, Viñuela-Berni A, Kovacs K, Berczi I. The Neuroimmune Biology of Phagocytosis. Adv Neuroimmune Biol 2017; 6(3-4): 117-30.
[http://dx.doi.org/10.3233/NIB-150104]

[29] Dantzer R, O'Connor JC, Freund GG, Johnson RW, Kelley KW. From inflammation to sickness and depression: when the immune system subjugates the brain. Nat Rev Neurosci 2008; 9(1): 46-56.
[http://dx.doi.org/10.1038/nrn2297] [PMID: 18073775]

[30] Swartz EM, Holmes GM. Gastric vagal motoneuron function is maintained following experimental spinal cord injury. Neurogastroenterol Motil 2014; 26(12): 1717-29.
[http://dx.doi.org/10.1111/nmo.12452] [PMID: 25316513]

[31] Momose-Sato Y, Kinoshita M, Sato K. Development of vagal afferent projections circumflex to the obex in the embryonic chick brainstem visualized with voltage-sensitive dye recording. Neuroscience 2007; 148(1): 140-50.
[http://dx.doi.org/10.1016/j.neuroscience.2007.05.032] [PMID: 17629626]

[32] Pavlov VA, Wang H, Czura CJ, Friedman SG, Tracey KJ. The cholinergic anti-inflammatory pathway: a missing link in neuroimmunomodulation. Mol Med 2003; 9(5-8): 125-34.
[http://dx.doi.org/10.1007/BF03402177] [PMID: 14571320]

[33] Kawai Y. Differential ascending projections from the male rat caudal nucleus of the tractus solitarius: an interface between local microcircuits and global macrocircuits. Front Neuroanat 2018; 12: 63.

[http://dx.doi.org/10.3389/fnana.2018.00063] [PMID: 30087599]

[34]   Herman JP, McKlveen JM, Ghosal S, *et al.* Regulation of the hypothalamic-pituitary-adrenocortical stress response. Compr Physiol 2016; 6(2): 603-21.
       [http://dx.doi.org/10.1002/cphy.c150015] [PMID: 27065163]

[35]   Brunson KL, Avishai-Eliner S, Hatalski CG, Baram TZ. Neurobiology of the stress response early in life: evolution of a concept and the role of corticotropin releasing hormone. Mol Psychiatry 2001; 6(6): 647-56.
       [http://dx.doi.org/10.1038/sj.mp.4000942] [PMID: 11673792]

[36]   Ohbuchi T, Haam J, Tasker JG. Regulation of Neuronal Activity in Hypothalamic Vasopressin Neurons. Interdiscip Inf Sci 2015; 21(3): 225-34.
       [http://dx.doi.org/10.4036/iis.2015.B.07] [PMID: 28035187]

[37]   Brownstein MJ, Russell JT, Gainer H. Synthesis, transport, and release of posterior pituitary hormones. Science 1980; 207(4429): 373-8.
       [http://dx.doi.org/10.1126/science.6153132] [PMID: 6153132]

[38]   Urbanski A, Rosinski G. Role of neuropeptides in the regulation of the insect immune system - current knowledge and perspectives. Curr Protein Pept Sci 2018; 19(12): 1201-13.
       [http://dx.doi.org/10.2174/1389203719666180809113706] [PMID: 30091409]

[39]   Savino W. Endocrine immunology of Chagas disease. In: Savino W, Guaraldi F, Eds. Endocrine Immunology. Front Horm Res. Basel, Karger, 2017, vol 48, pp 160-75.
       [http://dx.doi.org/10.1159/000452914]

[40]   Howland RH. Vagus nerve stimulation. Curr Behav Neurosci Rep 2014; 1(2): 64-73.
       [http://dx.doi.org/10.1007/s40473-014-0010-5] [PMID: 24834378]

[41]   Kaniusas E, Kampusch S, Tittgemeyer M, *et al.* Current directions in the auricular vagus nerve stimulation I - A physiological perspective. Front Neurosci 2019; 13: 854.
       [http://dx.doi.org/10.3389/fnins.2019.00854] [PMID: 31447643]

[42]   Miller AH, Haroon E, Raison CL, Felger JC. Cytokine targets in the brain: impact on neurotransmitters and neurocircuits. Depress Anxiety 2013; 30(4): 297-306.
       [http://dx.doi.org/10.1002/da.22084] [PMID: 23468190]

[43]   Sprague AH, Khalil RA. Inflammatory cytokines in vascular dysfunction and vascular disease. Biochem Pharmacol 2009; 78(6): 539-52.
       [http://dx.doi.org/10.1016/j.bcp.2009.04.029] [PMID: 19413999]

[44]   Berczi I, Quintanar-Stephano A, Kovacs K. Neuroimmune regulation in immunocompetence, acute illness, and healing. Ann N Y Acad Sci 2009; 1153: 220-39.
       [http://dx.doi.org/10.1111/j.1749-6632.2008.03975.x] [PMID: 19236345]

[45]   Rey AD, Mahuad CV, Bozza VV, *et al.* Endocrine and cytokine responses in humans with pulmonary tuberculosis. Brain Behav Immun 2007; 21(2): 171-9.
       [http://dx.doi.org/10.1016/j.bbi.2006.06.005] [PMID: 16890403]

[46]   Castro R, Zou J, Secombes CJ, Martin SA. Cortisol modulates the induction of inflammatory gene expression in a rainbow trout macrophage cell line. Fish Shellfish Immunol 2011; 30(1): 215-23.
       [http://dx.doi.org/10.1016/j.fsi.2010.10.010] [PMID: 20965252]

[47]   Spies CM, Straub RH, Cutolo M, Buttgereit F. Circadian rhythms in rheumatology--a glucocorticoid perspective. Arthritis Res Ther 2014; 16(2) (Suppl. 2): S3.
       [http://dx.doi.org/10.1186/ar4687] [PMID: 25608777]

[48]   Ehrchen JM, Roth J, Barczyk-Kahlert K. More than suppression: glucocorticoid action on monocytes and macrophages. Front Immunol 2019; 10: 2028.
       [http://dx.doi.org/10.3389/fimmu.2019.02028] [PMID: 31507614]

[49]   Silverman MN, Pearce BD, Biron CA, Miller AH. Immune modulation of the hypothalamic-pituitar-

-adrenal (HPA) axis during viral infection. Viral Immunol 2005; 18(1): 41-78.
[http://dx.doi.org/10.1089/vim.2005.18.41] [PMID: 15802953]

[50]   Gordon S, Taylor PR. Monocyte and macrophage heterogeneity. Nat Rev Immunol 2005; 5(12): 953-64.
[http://dx.doi.org/10.1038/nri1733] [PMID: 16322748]

[51]   Muto Y, Sakai A, Sakamoto A, Suzuki H. Activation of NK₁ receptors in the locus coeruleus induces analgesia through noradrenergic-mediated descending inhibition in a rat model of neuropathic pain. Br J Pharmacol 2012; 166(3): 1047-57.
[http://dx.doi.org/10.1111/j.1476-5381.2011.01820.x] [PMID: 22188400]

[52]   McCorry LK. Physiology of the autonomic nervous system. Am J Pharm Educ 2007; 71(4): 78.
[http://dx.doi.org/10.5688/aj710478] [PMID: 17786266]

[53]   Sharara-Chami RI, Joachim M, Pacak K, Majzoub JA. Glucocorticoid treatment--effect on adrenal medullary catecholamine production. Shock 2010; 33(2): 213-7.
[http://dx.doi.org/10.1097/SHK.0b013e3181af0633] [PMID: 19503019]

[54]   Heesterbeek DAC, Angelier ML, Harrison RA, Rooijakkers SHM. Complement and bacterial infections: from molecular mechanisms to therapeutic applications. J Innate Immun 2018; 10(5-6): 455-64.
[http://dx.doi.org/10.1159/000491439] [PMID: 30149378]

[55]   Sprong T, Møller AS, Bjerre A, *et al.* Complement activation and complement-dependent inflammation by *Neisseria meningitidis* are independent of lipopolysaccharide. Infect Immun 2004; 72(6): 3344-9.
[http://dx.doi.org/10.1128/IAI.72.6.3344-3349.2004] [PMID: 15155639]

[56]   Merle NS, Noe R, Halbwachs-Mecarelli L, Fremeaux-Bacchi V, Roumenina LT. Complement System Part II: Role in Immunity. Front Immunol 2015; 6: 257.
[http://dx.doi.org/10.3389/fimmu.2015.00257] [PMID: 26074922]

[57]   Mogensen TH. Pathogen recognition and inflammatory signaling in innate immune defenses. Clin Microbiol Rev 2009; 22(2): 240-73.
[http://dx.doi.org/10.1128/CMR.00046-08] [PMID: 19366914]

[58]   Hoshino K, Kaisho T, Iwabe T, Takeuchi O, Akira S. Differential involvement of IFN-β in Toll-like receptor-stimulated dendritic cell activation. Int Immunol 2002; 14(10): 1225-31.
[http://dx.doi.org/10.1093/intimm/dxf089] [PMID: 12356687]

[59]   Henneke P, Takeuchi O, Malley R, *et al.* Cellular activation, phagocytosis, and bactericidal activity against group B streptococcus involve parallel myeloid differentiation factor 88-dependent and independent signaling pathways. J Immunol 2002; 169(7): 3970-7.
[http://dx.doi.org/10.4049/jimmunol.169.7.3970] [PMID: 12244198]

[60]   Arango Duque G, Descoteaux A. Macrophage cytokines: involvement in immunity and infectious diseases. Front Immunol 2014; 5: 491.
[http://dx.doi.org/10.3389/fimmu.2014.00491] [PMID: 25339958]

[61]   Woolard MD, Hudig D, Tabor L, Ivey JA, Simecka JW. NK cells in gamma-interferon-deficient mice suppress lung innate immunity against Mycoplasma spp. Infect Immun 2005; 73(10): 6742-51.
[http://dx.doi.org/10.1128/IAI.73.10.6742-6751.2005] [PMID: 16177352]

[62]   Bongiovanni B, Mata-Espinosa D, D'Attilio L, *et al.* Effect of cortisol and/or DHEA on THP1-derived macrophages infected with *Mycobacterium tuberculosis*. Tuberculosis (Edinb) 2015; 95(5): 562-9.
[http://dx.doi.org/10.1016/j.tube.2015.05.011] [PMID: 26099547]

[63]   Besedovsky HO, del Rey A. The cytokine-HPA axis feed-back circuit. Z Rheumatol 2000; 59: II26-30.
[http://dx.doi.org/10.1007/s003930070014]

[64]   Zetter M, Barrios-Payán J, Mata-Espinosa D, Marquina-Castillo B, Quintanar-Stephano A,

Hernández-Pando R. Involvement of vasopressin in the pathogenesis of pulmonary tuberculosis: a new therapeutic target? Front Endocrinol (Lausanne) 2019; 10: 351.
[http://dx.doi.org/10.3389/fendo.2019.00351] [PMID: 31244771]

[65] Oyola MG, Handa RJ. Hypothalamic-pituitary-adrenal and hypothalamic-pituitary-gonadal axes: sex differences in regulation of stress responsivity. Stress 2017; 20(5): 476-94.
[http://dx.doi.org/10.1080/10253890.2017.1369523] [PMID: 28859530]

[66] Oyola MG, Thompson MK, Handa AZ, Handa RJ. Distribution and chemical composition of estrogen receptor β neurons in the paraventricular nucleus of the female and male mouse hypothalamus. J Comp Neurol 2017; 525(17): 3666-82.
[http://dx.doi.org/10.1002/cne.24295] [PMID: 28758220]

[67] Qin C, Li J, Tang K. The paraventricular nucleus of the hypothalamus: development, function, and human diseases. Endocrinology 2018; 159(9): 3458-72.
[http://dx.doi.org/10.1210/en.2018-00453] [PMID: 30052854]

[68] Fung TC, Olson CA, Hsiao EY. Interactions between the microbiota, immune and nervous systems in health and disease. Nat Neurosci 2017; 20(2): 145-55.
[http://dx.doi.org/10.1038/nn.4476] [PMID: 28092661]

[69] Carrasco L. The inhibition of cell functions after viral infection. A proposed general mechanism. FEBS Lett 1977; 76(1): 11-5.
[http://dx.doi.org/10.1016/0014-5793(77)80110-5] [PMID: 852597]

[70] Sheridan JF, Stark JL, Avitsur R, Padgett DA. Social disruption, immunity, and susceptibility to viral infection. Role of glucocorticoid insensitivity and NGF. Ann N Y Acad Sci 2000; 917(1): 894-905.
[http://dx.doi.org/10.1111/j.1749-6632.2000.tb05455.x] [PMID: 11270350]

[71] Bertoletti A, Gehring AJ. The immune response during hepatitis B virus infection. J Gen Virol 2006; 87(Pt 6): 1439-49.
[http://dx.doi.org/10.1099/vir.0.81920-0] [PMID: 16690908]

[72] Pérez AR, Bottasso O, Savino W. The impact of infectious diseases upon neuroendocrine circuits. Neuroimmunomodulation 2009; 16(2): 96-105.
[http://dx.doi.org/10.1159/000180264] [PMID: 19212129]

[73] Bunn SJ, Ait-Ali D, Eiden LE. Immune-neuroendocrine integration at the adrenal gland: cytokine control of the adrenomedullary transcriptome. J Mol Neurosci 2012; 48(2): 413-9.
[http://dx.doi.org/10.1007/s12031-012-9745-1] [PMID: 22421803]

[74] Dunn AJ, Powell ML, Moreshead WV, Gaskin JM, Hall NR. Effects of Newcastle disease virus administration to mice on the metabolism of cerebral biogenic amines, plasma corticosterone, and lymphocyte proliferation. Brain Behav Immun 1987; 1(3): 216-30.
[http://dx.doi.org/10.1016/0889-1591(87)90024-9] [PMID: 3509812]

[75] Smith EM, Meyer WJ, Blalock JE. Virus-induced corticosterone in hypophysectomized mice: a possible lymphoid adrenal axis. Science 1982; 218(4579): 1311-2.
[http://dx.doi.org/10.1126/science.6183748] [PMID: 6183748]

[76] Price P, Olver SD, Silich M, Nador TZ, Yerkovich S, Wilson SG. Adrenalitis and the adrenocortical response of resistant and susceptible mice to acute murine cytomegalovirus infection. Eur J Clin Invest 1996; 26(9): 811-9.
[http://dx.doi.org/10.1046/j.1365-2362.1996.2210562.x] [PMID: 8889445]

[77] Orange JS, Salazar-Mather TP, Opal SM, Biron CA. Mechanisms for virus-induced liver disease: tumor necrosis factor-mediated pathology independent of natural killer and T cells during murine cytomegalovirus infection. J Virol 1997; 71(12): 9248-58.
[http://dx.doi.org/10.1128/JVI.71.12.9248-9258.1997] [PMID: 9371583]

[78] Verges B, Chavanet P, Desgres J, *et al.* Adrenal function in HIV infected patients. Acta Endocrinol (Copenh) 1989; 121(5): 633-7.

[http://dx.doi.org/10.1530/acta.0.1210633] [PMID: 2555993]

[79]   Schmid-Hempel P. Evolutionary parasitology: the integrated study of infections, immunology, ecology, and genetics. Oxford University Press 2011.

[80]   Morales-Montor J, Newhouse E, Mohamed F, Baghdadi A, Damian RT. Altered levels of hypothalamic-pituitary-adrenocortical axis hormones in baboons and mice during the course of infection with Schistosoma mansoni. J Infect Dis 2001; 183(2): 313-20.
[http://dx.doi.org/10.1086/317919] [PMID: 11110642]

[81]   Sowunmi A, Newton CR, Waruiru C, Lightman S, Dunger DB. Arginine vasopressin secretion in Kenyan children with severe malaria. J Trop Pediatr 2000; 46(4): 195-9.
[http://dx.doi.org/10.1093/tropej/46.4.195] [PMID: 10996978]

[82]   Sánchez-Alemán E, Quintanar-Stephano A, Escobedo G, Campos-Esparza MdelR, Campos-Rodríguez R, Ventura-Juárez J. Vagotomy induces deregulation of the inflammatory response during the development of amoebic liver abscess in hamsters. Neuroimmunomodulation 2015; 22(3): 166-80.
[http://dx.doi.org/10.1159/000362240] [PMID: 24819982]

[83]   Rodríguez-Galán MC, Sotomayor CE, Cano R, *et al.* Immune neuroendocrine interactions during a fungal infection in immunocompetent or immunosuppressed hosts. Neuroimmunomodulation 2010; 17(3): 188-91.
[http://dx.doi.org/10.1159/000258720] [PMID: 20134199]

[84]   Blanco JL, Garcia ME. Immune response to fungal infections. Vet Immunol Immunopathol 2008; 125(1-2): 47-70.
[http://dx.doi.org/10.1016/j.vetimm.2008.04.020] [PMID: 18565595]

[85]   Bouzani M, Ok M, McCormick A, *et al.* Human NK cells display important antifungal activity against Aspergillus fumigatus, which is directly mediated by IFN-γ release. J Immunol 2011; 187(3): 1369-76.
[http://dx.doi.org/10.4049/jimmunol.1003593] [PMID: 21697457]

[86]   Bernton EW, Bryant HU, Holaday JW. Prolactin and immune function. In: Psychoneuroimmunology. London: Academic Press 1991; pp. 403-28.

[87]   Breuel KF, Kougias P, Rice PJ, *et al.* Anterior pituitary cells express pattern recognition receptors for fungal glucans: implications for neuroendocrine immune involvement in response to fungal infections. Neuroimmunomodulation 2004; 11(1): 1-9.
[http://dx.doi.org/10.1159/000072963] [PMID: 14557673]

[88]   Louria DB, Browne HG. The effects of cortisone on experimental fungus infections. Ann N Y Acad Sci 1960; 89(1): 39-46.
[http://dx.doi.org/10.1111/j.1749-6632.1960.tb20128.x] [PMID: 13763696]

[89]   Rodriguez-Galán MC, Correa SG, Cejas H, Sotomayor CE. Impaired activity of phagocytic cells in *Candida albicans* infection after exposure to chronic varied stress. Neuroimmunomodulation 2001; 9(4): 193-202.
[http://dx.doi.org/10.1159/000049026] [PMID: 11847481]

[90]   Rodriguez-Galán MC, Sotomayor C, Costamagna ME, *et al.* Immunocompetence of macrophages in rats exposed to *Candida albicans* infection and stress. Am J Physiol Cell Physiol 2003; 284(1): C111-8.
[http://dx.doi.org/10.1152/ajpcell.00160.2002] [PMID: 12388114]

CHAPTER 7

Regulation of Haemoglobin, Haem Uptake by FrpB Family Proteins in *Helicobacter pylori*

José de Jesús Olivares Trejo[1,*] and Juan Mosqueda[2]

[1] *Universidad Autónoma de la Ciudad de México, Posgrado en Ciencias Genómicas San Lorenzo 290, C.P. 03100, Ciudad de México, México*

[2] *Facultad de Ciencias Naturales, Universidad Autónoma de Querétaro, 76230 Juriquilla, Qro., Mexico*

Abstract: *Helicobacter pylori* is a Gram-negative spiral bacteria that has been associated with peptic ulcers, gastritis, duodenitis and it is believed to be the causative agent of gastric cancer and anemia. Its iron requirements when it infects its human host are high, therefore this bacterium has developed mechanisms to obtain iron from human sources. This human pathogen can grow in broth media using as iron source human proteins such as lactoferrin (Lf), haem and haemoglobin (Hb). However, it is still not fully understood how the process of iron acquisition occurs. An *in silico* analysis has shown that *H. pylori* has a family of three outer membrane proteins regulated by iron termed FrpB (Iron-regulated outer membrane protein). Two of them: FrpB1 and FrpB2 bind haem and FrpB1 also binds Hb. The last protein, FrpB3 has the capacity of haem-binding. The analysis by 3D model showed that three proteins are structurally conserved with the typical barrel structure inserted into the membrane. Moreover, the necessary motifs for Hb-binding have been identified. Each gene is regulated by the presence of an iron source, for instance *FrpB1* is overexpressed if haem is present, while *FrpB2* was induced in the presence of haem and Hb. In the case of FrpB3, it is overexpressed in the presence of free iron. It is believed that there are other proteins implicated in iron acquisition that have not been investigated yet. In summary, *H. pylori* secretes proteins to support the extreme environment present in the stomach. Perhaps iron helps the bacterium to resist the acidic environment of the human stomach and this mechanism is vital for *H. pylori* during the infection process.

Keywords: Gene Regulation, *Helicobacter pylori*, Haemoglobin, Haem, 3D Model.

INTRODUCTION

Iron is necessary for all organisms because it participates in several cellular

---

* **Corresponding author José de Jesús Olivares Trejo:** Universidad Autónoma de la Ciudad de México, Posgrado en Ciencias Genómicas. San Lorenzo 290, C.P. 03100, Ciudad de México, México; Tel: +525554886661 Ext. 15309; E-mail:olivarestrejo@yahoo.com

pathways, for instance, the respiratory chain [1]. Free iron is toxic because it can induce the production of reactive oxygen species (ROS), for this reason, in the human body it must be stored in proteins such as Hb or haem [2]. When pathogens infect humans, they obtain iron from human sources using two mechanisms [3]: 1) A direct mechanism; consists in the expression of receptors, which are membrane proteins that can bind an iron source directly. 2) An indirect mechanism; consists in the secretion of molecules (siderophores or haemophores), which scavenge iron [4]. The iron source is then carried towards the surface of the cell, where a specific receptor protein [5] awaits [2, 6, 7]. These two mechanisms obtain their energy using the TonB system [8], TonB-dependent regulatory systems consist of six proteins. This system interacts with outer membrane receptor proteins to carry out high-affinity and energy-dependent uptake of specific substrates into the periplasmic space [3], those substrates are either poorly transported through non-specific porin channels are encountered at very low concentrations. In the absence of TonB, these receptors bind their substrates but do not carry out active transport. TonB-dependent receptors include a plug domain, an independently folding subunit that acts as the channel gate, blocking the pore until the channel is bound by ligand. At this point, it undergoes conformational changes, opening the channel.

H. pylori is a human pathogen, this bacterium infects half of the human population worldwide, however, not all the individuals develop helicobacteriosis. Permanent colonization of the human stomach by *H. pylori* is associated with asymptomatic gastric inflammation (gastritis) and an increased risk of duodenal ulceration, gastric ulceration and non-cardia gastric cancer [9]. Persistent, chronic infections caused by this pathogen could induce anemia [10 - 12] due to iron depletion, suggesting that this pathogen requires high concentration of iron. For all above *H. pylori* needs to express several genes that allow this pathogen to obtain iron from human sources [13]. *H. pylori* can support its cellular growth, using human sources such as Tf, Hb or haem when free iron is eliminated by a chelant.

When *H. pylori* is cultivated under iron starvation, the bacterium increases the expression of three outer membrane proteins that bind haem, showing that they are regulated by iron [14]. However, their identities remain undetermined. Therefore, investigating the mechanism by which *H. pylori* obtains iron from human sources could be useful in understanding how this bacterium survives in the stomach.

H. pylori SUPPORTS ITS CELLULAR GROWTH USING HUMAN IRON SOURCES LIKE HB, HAEM AND FREE IRON

H. pylori has the capacity to grow in Casman agar medium at 37 °C, under microaerophilic conditions for 24 h. In order to test human sources bacteria have to be cultivated in Casman medium after they are collected and washed three times. Then, the biomass is transferred into Brucella medium and cultivated under microaerobic conditions for 24 h. During this period, the optical density has to be monitored to obtain several phases of growth. Bacteria are collected at an exponential phase. At this time, bacteria are washed three times after it is resuspended in iron free (-Fe)-Brucella broth. Iron must be chelated and 3 h later the culture medium is supplemented with Hb or ferric ammonium citrate. Additionally, a control without supplementation is included. As shown in Fig. (**1**), *H. pylori* can support its cellular growth using Hb (triangles) or iron (circles) as the only iron source. However, a control without supplementation (squares) can not. This graphic shows that *H. pylori* has the capacity of supporting its cellular growth using Hb or free iron as the only iron source [15].

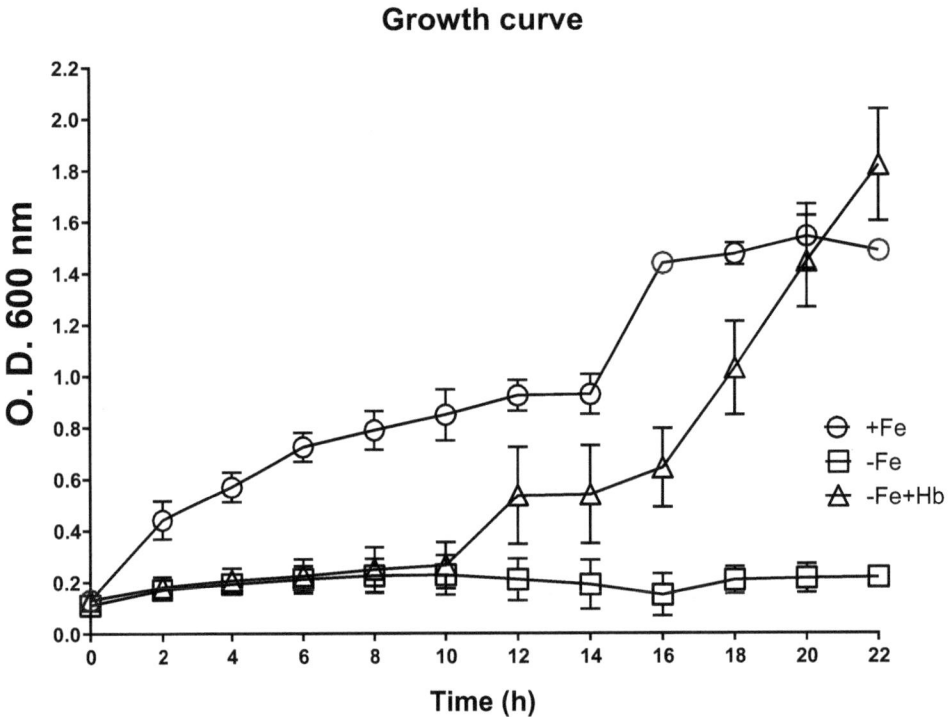

Fig. (1). *H. pylori* grows using Hb or free iron as an iron source. Samples of *H. pylori* were collected in its exponential phase of cellular growth. Subsequently, after 3 h, 10 mM Hb (triangles) or 10 mM ferric ammonium citrate (circles) were added to analyze its growth. Negative control with only a chelating agent (squares) was performed. Optical density was monitored every 2 h. The graphic shows the standard deviation of three independent biological experiments.

FERRIC REGULATED PROTEIN FAMILY (FrpB)

H. pylori has three genes *FrpB* (ferric regulated protein) that codify for proteins named FrpB1, FrpB2 and FrpB3, which are annotated in the *H. pylori* data base [16]. FrpB3 is expressed under haem and Hb, this receptor can bind haem [15]. It is hypothesized that this gene is expressed constitutively in order to obtain iron from haem in the presence of free iron because the necessity of iron is imperative, therefore, this receptor is ready when haem is available. FrpB2 is expressed under iron starvation and when the medium is supplemented with haem. In fact, this gene restores the cellular growth of *Escherichia coli* (without Hb-receptor) when the gene is overexpressed and the cellular growth is supplemented with haem. These observations support the idea that *FrpB2* is regulated by haem.

The *FrpB1* gene [17] increases its mRNA levels when the iron is chelated from the media broth and is supplemented with Hb. In addition, this gene is capable of supporting the cellular growth of *E. coli* when the free iron is chelated from the media and supplemented with Hb (Fig. **2**). These results show that *FrpB1* is Hb regulated.

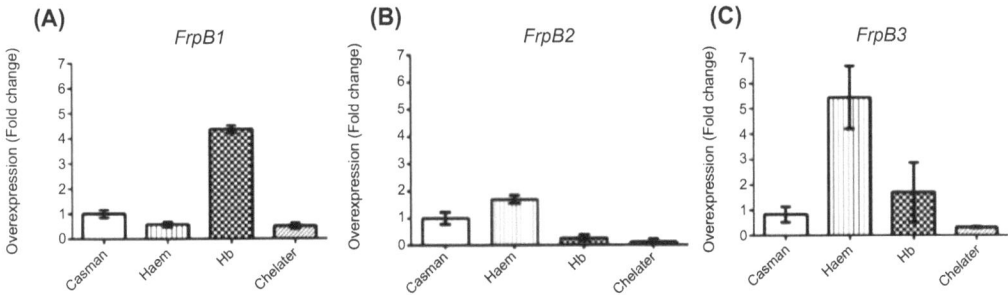

Fig. (2). *H. pylori* expresses the *FrpB1, FrpB2* and *FrpB3* genes, differentially when the culture media is supplemented with haem, Hb or under iron starvation. *H. pylori* was cultivated in Casman medium under iron starvation, and supplemented with Hb, haem or iron. Then, the mRNA was purified and the samples were quantified using real-time PCR. Error bars show the dispersion of the data. *FrpB1* is increased when Hb is added as an iron source (panel A). *FrpB2* is increased with haem (panel B), while *FrpB3* is increased with haem and free iron source (panel C).

FrpB1, FrpB2 AND FrpB3 PROTEINS HAVE THE DOMAINS INVOLVED IN HB-BINDING

Hb-receptors are proteins localized in the bacterial outer membrane. They have the ability to bind and transport Hb into the cell through a Top-dependent mechanism by using eight residues of amino acid (two motifs) FRAP and NPNL [18 - 21] for instance ChuA protein of *E. coli* has FRAP and NPNL motifs to bind Hb. In the majority of the Hb-receptors reported, they are separated by a sequence of approximately ten to twenty amino acids (Fig. **3**). Amino acid sequences of FrpB1 (Q9ZKX4), FrpB2 (Q9ZKT4) and FrpB3 (Q9ZJA8) of *H. pylori* have these motifs and show some changes however, multiple amino acid sequences from different bacteria have revealed at least one change of these FRAP and NPNL motifs [19, 22] without affecting their Hb-binding properties [22].

```
ChuA   LFGSYAQAFRAPTMGE---MYNDSKHFSIGRFYTNYWVPNPNLRPETNETQEYG-------FGLR---
FrpB3  LKVSYAYVTKGALPGDDVLMRDPTVIY-----------QRNLRPSIGQNVEFNVDYNSKYFNVRGAA
FrpB1  LKITYSQVTRGVMPGDGVYMRQNDLRY-----------AKNIKPEVGSNAEFNIDYSSQYFSGRAA-
FrpB2  FRLSYAYVTRGPMPGGLVWMRQDNLRY-----------NRNLKPEIGQNAEFNTEYSSQYFDFRAA-
              ****                            ****
```

Fig. (3). Multiple sequence alignment of FRAP and NPNL motifs necessary for Hb-binding. A section of the sequence of the ChuA protein of *E. coli* and the FrpB proteins of *H. pylori* are shown. FRAP and NPNL motifs necessary for haem or Hb-binding are shown with asterisks. Amino acid sequences were loaded onto the ClustalW serverhttps://www.ebi.ac.uk/Tools/msa/muscle/ and the JalWiev 10.2. Amino acid sequence of ChuA (Q7DB97) (Hb-binding receptor of *E. coli* was used as a template). Amino acid residues in grey are conserved in all the sequences, while amino acid residues in black only are conserved in two or three sequences.

3D STRUCTURES OF FrpB1, FrpB2 AND FrpB3 ARE TYPICAL OF MEMBRANE RECEPTOR PROTEINS

The 3D-structure of FrpB proteins shows the required motifs for Hb-binding. In Fig. (**4**), amino acid sequences of FrpB1, 2 and 3 were modelled by the Chimera 1.12 software. 3D analysis revealed the typical barrel structure, formed by β-sheets corresponding to membrane proteins (white structure). In black, FRAP and NPNL motifs are shown, they are necessary for haem- or Hb-binding. ChuA protein of *E. coli* has the same structure and the same FRAP and NPNL motifs. Inside of FrpB proteins, there is a structure that forms a smaller plug domain inside the hydrophilic barrel that has been suggested to allow the passing of iron source through the membrane. In fact, it is similar to the ChuA protein of *E. coli*. The FRAP and NPNL motifs involved in Hb-binding [22] are highlighted. These results show that the three FrpB proteins have a similar structure to ChuA [23, 24].

Previous works have demonstrated that the *FrpB1* gene has the sequence fur (TAATAATnATTATTA) and it is repressed by iron using Fur system. The ferric uptake regulator (Fur) senses intracellular iron availability and plays a central role in maintaining iron homeostasis, additionally, this system can also diminish the intracellular iron. Nevertheless, it has not been reported for the *FrpB3* gene. *In silico* analysis of the region upstream of *FrpB3* has not revealed a probable fur sequence either [25]. All of this could explain why the source (Hb, haem or iron starvation) increse the expression of *FrpB1, FrpB2* or *FrpB3* differentially. Although all three proteins have the typical barrel structure, only *FrpB1* is fur regulated.

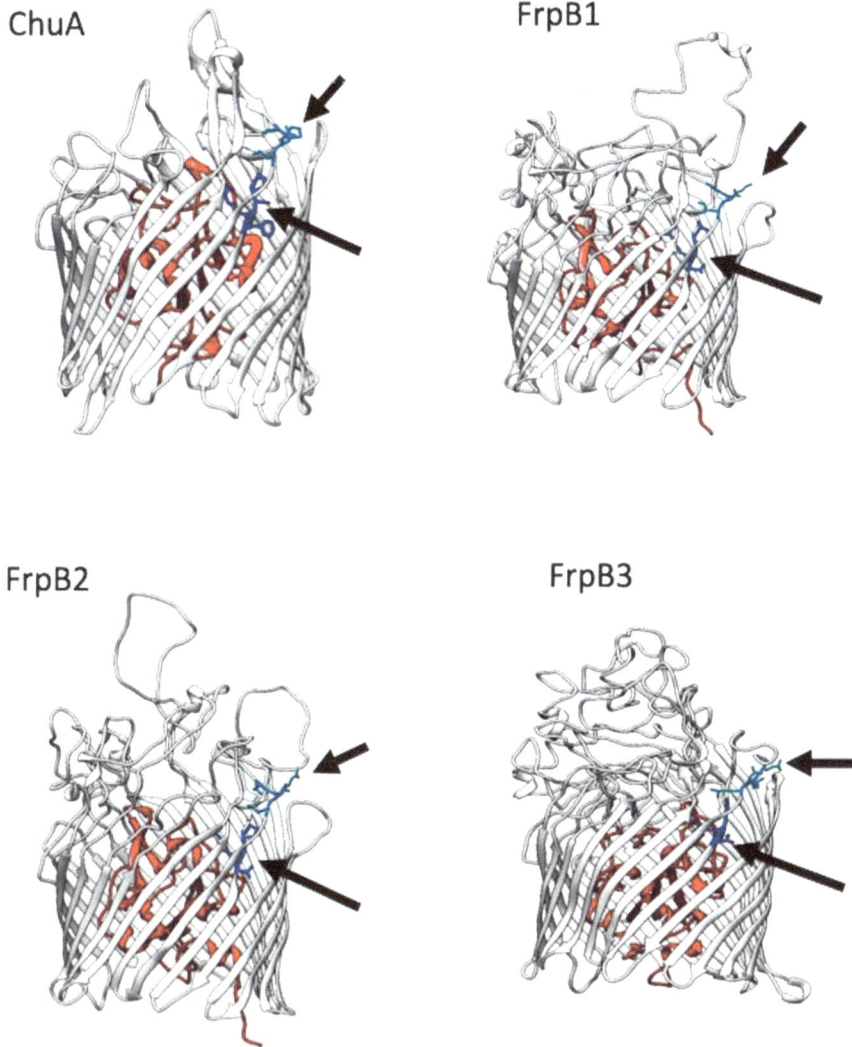

Fig. (4). 3D structure modeling of the FrpB proteins. FrpB1, 2 and 3 from *H. pylori* showed 3D structures. Motifs FRAP (small arrow, cian color) and NPNL (big arrow, blue color). These motifs are observed in several HB-binding proteins reported and they are necessary for Hb-binding. Plug structure is showed in red color. Amino acid sequences of FrpB1, 2 and 3 were used to construct the model by the Chimera 1.12 program. ChuA protein from *E. coli* was used as a template.

DISCUSSION

H. pylori is a gram-negative bacteria. This human pathogen needs iron in order to survive. In the human host, there are several iron sources such as Tf, Lf, Hb, or haem [7]. To obtain iron, this pathogen has developed a mechanism consisting in the expression of outer membrane proteins that bind Hb or haem [21]. Those proteins bind the iron source directly and several proteins have been investigated. For instance, FrpB is a protein family composed of three proteins: FrpB1, FrpB2 and FrpB3 [16]. FrpB1 and FrpB2 bind Hb, but FrpB2 binds haem as well. FrpB3 was previously characterized and it was found that it binds haem. Therefore, these results suggest that *FrpB* genes are probably regulated by the Fur iron system, which acts as a ferrous-dependent transcriptional repressor. There are bacteria that express proteins regulated by the Fur iron system, for instance, *PeuA* in *vibrio* [26], *pfeR*, *pvdS*, *tonB* and *fumC* in *Pseudomonas aeruginosa* [27], *HasA* in *Serratia marcescens* [4], TbpA and TbpB in *Neisseria gonorrhoeae* [28]. Additionally, *in silico* analyses using the Ferric uptake regulation protein (P0A9A9 FUR_ECOLI) from *E. coli* as a template, showed that in the proteome of *H. pylori* there is a Ferric uptake regulation protein (Q9ZM26 FUR_HELPJ). Surprisingly, the *H. pylori* genome has the box core sequence Fur [25]. All of this explains why Hb, haem and iron starvation increase the expression of the *FrpB1, FrpB2* or *FrpB3* genes differentially. 3D modelling shows that the FrpB1, FrpB2 or FrpB3 proteins have a structure of a barrel typical of Hb-binding membrane receptors [24], this structure is necessary to allow the passage of haem through the membrane (Fig. 5). Barrel structure has been observed in Hb-binding receptors such as Has of *Serratia marcescens* [20], CopB of *Moraxella catarrhalis* [29], HmbR of *Neisseria meningitidis* [8]. 3D structures of FrpB proteins also show the motifs FRAP and NPNL necessary for Hb-binding. These motifs have been observed in receptors of some bacteria, for instance, *Photobacterium damselae* [30], HupO of *Vibrio fluvialis* [31], BhuR of *Bordetella avium* [23], HemR of *Yersinia enterocolitica* [18], HmuR of *Porphyromonas gingivalis* [19, 32] and ChuA of *Escherichia coli* [5] and they share the same function. Although FrpB3 is expressed under iron sufficiency [33, 15], it can be classified as an iron-regulated protein because it has the FRAP and NPNL motifs. On the other hand, the expression of each FrpB protein depends on the iron source and each gene has a different expression pattern, for this reason, it is believed that each gene is sensitive to a specific source of iron.

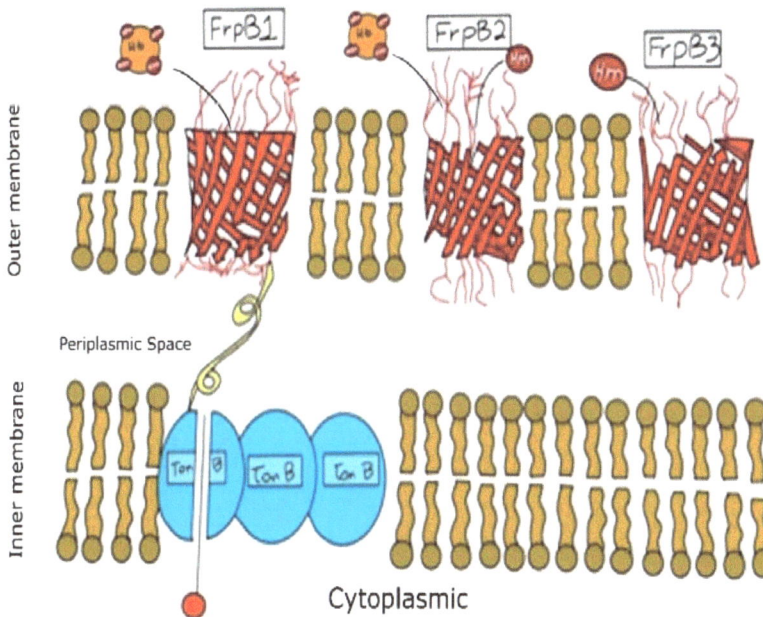

Fig. (5). *H. pylori* expresses FrpB1, FrpB2 and FrpB3 in the outer membrane (they are shown in red color). Their expression depends on the iron source availability. FrpB1 binds Hb, FrpB2 binds haem and FrpB3 also binds haem. However, any FrpB protein can bind another iron source. The TonB system is shown in blue, this system provides energy to introduce the iron source to the cytoplasmic space. Hb is shown in orange, while haem is shown in red.

This chapter describes the principal insights that attempt to explain how the expression of a family of outer membrane proteins is regulated by the iron, haem or Hb. *H. pylori* is a bacterium that requires a high concentration of iron because it has been reported that it can cause anemia when it is infecting humans [10 - 12]. This can explain why *H. pylori* has several genes, which express many proteins involved in iron acquisition such as FrpB1, FrpB2 or FrpB3 [16]. All these results attempt to explain why *H. pylori* is a pathogen equipped with mechanisms involved in iron acquisition. Maybe the iron helps to tolerate the hostile conditions present in the stomach, having crucial roles when this bacterium is invading and infecting [34]. Given the microbiome research and the large unexplored area of non-invasive imaging of microbiota a concise treatment of bacterial, ferromagnetic metal ion regulation may have huge implications in clinical modalities like magnetic resonance imaging (MRI) to detect infection caused by this pathogen, due to the higher metabolic activity of this iron [35].

CONCLUSION

This chapter describes the FrpB family of *H. pylori* formed by 3 proteins FrpB1, FrpB2 and FrpB3. Their respective genes are regulated by the iron source differentially. *FrpB1* is regulated by Hb while *FrpB2* and *FrpB3* are regulated by haem, in addition FrpB3 could also be regulated by Hb. 3D structure developed the motifs FRAP and NPNL necessary for Hb-binding however some differences were observed, which could explain the sensitivity to some iron sources. *H. pylori* is a human pathogen equipped with a family of protein to use Hb or haem as iron source in the human to invade tissues such as stomachs.

CONSENT FOR PUBLICATION

Not applicable.

CONFLICT OF INTEREST

The authors confirm that the content of this chapter has no conflict of interest.

ACKNOWLEDGEMENTS

José de Jesús Olivares Trejo thanks CONACYT for sabbatical scholarship (Convocatoria Estancia Sabática Nacional 2019-1).

REFERENCES

[1]   Andrews SC, Robinsón AK, Rodríguez-Quiñones F. Bacterial iron homeostasis. FEMS Microbiol Rev 2003; 27(2-3): 215-37.
       [http://dx.doi.org/10.1016/S0168-6445(03)00055-X] [PMID: 12829269]

[2]   Wandersman C, Delepelaire P. Bacterial iron sources: from siderophores to hemophores. Annu Rev Microbiol 2004; 58: 611-47.
       [http://dx.doi.org/10.1146/annurev.micro.58.030603.123811] [PMID: 15487950]

[3]   Genco CA, Dixon DW. Emerging strategies in microbial haem capture. Mol Microbiol 2001; 39(1): 1-11.
       [http://dx.doi.org/10.1046/j.1365-2958.2001.02231.x] [PMID: 11123683]

[4]   Sapriel G, Wandersman C, Delepelaire P. The SecB chaperone is bifunctional in *Serratia marcescens*: SecB is involved in the Sec pathway and required for HasA secretion by the ABC transporter. J Bacteriol 2003; 185(1): 80-8.
       [http://dx.doi.org/10.1128/JB.185.1.80-88.2003] [PMID: 12486043]

[5]   Torres AG, Payne SM. Haem iron-transport system in enterohaemorrhagic *Escherichia coli* O157:H7. Mol Microbiol 1997; 23(4): 825-33.
       [http://dx.doi.org/10.1046/j.1365-2958.1997.2641628.x] [PMID: 9157252]

[6]   Smalley JW, Olczak T. Heme acquisition mechanisms of *Porphyromonas gingivalis* - strategies used in a polymicrobial community in a heme-limited host environment. Mol Oral Microbiol 2017; 32(1): 1-23.
       [http://dx.doi.org/10.1111/omi.12149] [PMID: 26662717]

[7]   Smith AD, Wilks A. Extracellular heme uptake and the challenges of bacterial cell membranes. Curr

Top Membr 2012; 69: 359-92.
[http://dx.doi.org/10.1016/B978-0-12-394390-3.00013-6] [PMID: 23046657]

[8]   Stojiljkovic I, Srinivasan N. *Neisseria meningitidis* tonB, exbB, and exbD genes: Ton-dependent utilization of protein-bound iron in Neisseriae. J Bacteriol 1997; 179(3): 805-12.
[http://dx.doi.org/10.1128/JB.179.3.805-812.1997] [PMID: 9006036]

[9]   Kusters JG, van Vliet AH, Kuipers EJ. Pathogenesis of *Helicobacter pylori* infection. Clin Microbiol Rev 2006; 19(3): 449-90.
[http://dx.doi.org/10.1128/CMR.00054-05] [PMID: 16847081]

[10]   Beckett AC, Piazuelo MB, Noto JM, *et al.* Dietary Composition influences incidence of *Helicobacter pylori*-induced iron deficiency anemia and gastric ulceration. Infect Immun 2016; 84(12): 3338-49.
[http://dx.doi.org/10.1128/IAI.00479-16] [PMID: 27620719]

[11]   Flores SE, Aitchison A, Day AS, Keenan JI. *Helicobacter pylori* infection perturbs iron homeostasis in gastric epithelial cells. PLoS One 2017; 12(9)e0184026
[http://dx.doi.org/10.1371/journal.pone.0184026] [PMID: 28873091]

[12]   Elloumi H, Sabbah M, Debbiche A, *et al.* Systematic gastric biopsy in iron deficiency anaemia. Arab J Gastroenterol 2017; 18(4): 224-7.
[http://dx.doi.org/10.1016/j.ajg.2017.11.005] [PMID: 29273468]

[13]   Kao CY, Sheu BS, Wu JJ. *Helicobacter pylori* infection: An overview of bacterial virulence factors and pathogenesis. Biomed J 2016; 39(1): 14-23.
[http://dx.doi.org/10.1016/j.bj.2015.06.002] [PMID: 27105595]

[14]   Worst DJ, Otto BR, de Graaff J. Iron-repressible outer membrane proteins of *Helicobacter pylori* involved in heme uptake. Infect Immun 1995; 63(10): 4161-5.
[http://dx.doi.org/10.1128/IAI.63.10.4161-4165.1995] [PMID: 7558334]

[15]   González-López MA, Olivares-Trejo JJ. The gene FrpB2 of *Helicobacter pylori* encodes an hemoglobin-binding protein involved in iron acquisition. Biometals 2009; 22(6): 889-94.
[http://dx.doi.org/10.1007/s10534-009-9240-5] [PMID: 19357969]

[16]   Alm RA, Bina J, Andrews BM, Doig P, Hancock RE, Trust TJ. Comparative genomics of *Helicobacter pylori*: analysis of the outer membrane protein families. Infect Immun 2000; 68(7): 4155-68.
[http://dx.doi.org/10.1128/IAI.68.7.4155-4168.2000] [PMID: 10858232]

[17]   Carrizo-Chávez MA, Cruz-Castañeda A, Olivares-Trejo J de J. The *FrpB1* gene of *Helicobacter pylori* is regulated by iron and encodes a membrane protein capable of binding haem and haemoglobin. FEBS Lett 2012; 586(6): 875-9.
[http://dx.doi.org/10.1016/j.febslet.2012.02.015] [PMID: 22449974]

[18]   Bracken CS, Baer MT, Abdur-Rashid A, Helms W, Stojiljkovic I. Use of heme-protein complexes by the *Yersinia enterocolitica* HemR receptor: histidine residues are essential for receptor function. J Bacteriol 1999; 181(19): 6063-72.
[http://dx.doi.org/10.1128/JB.181.19.6063-6072.1999] [PMID: 10498719]

[19]   Simpson W, Olczak T, Genco CA. Characterization and expression of HmuR, a TonB-dependent hemoglobin receptor of *Porphyromonas gingivalis*. J Bacteriol 2000; 182(20): 5737-48.
[http://dx.doi.org/10.1128/JB.182.20.5737-5748.2000] [PMID: 11004172]

[20]   Benevides-Matos N, Biville F. The Hem and Has haem uptake systems in *Serratia marcescens*. Microbiology 2010; 156(Pt 6): 1749-57.
[http://dx.doi.org/10.1099/mic.0.034405-0] [PMID: 20299406]

[21]   Braun V, Hantke K. Recent insights into iron import by bacteria. Curr Opin Chem Biol 2011; 15(2): 328-34.
[http://dx.doi.org/10.1016/j.cbpa.2011.01.005] [PMID: 21277822]

[22]   Liu X, Olczak T, Guo HC, Dixon DW, Genco CA. Identification of amino acid residues involved in

heme binding and hemoprotein utilization in the *Porphyromonas gingivalis* heme receptor HmuR. Infect Immun 2006; 74(2): 1222-32.
[http://dx.doi.org/10.1128/IAI.74.2.1222-1232.2006] [PMID: 16428772]

[23]   Murphy ER, Sacco RE, Dickenson A, *et al.* BhuR, a virulence-associated outer membrane protein of bordetella avium, is required for the acquisition of iron from heme and hemoproteins. Infect Immun 2002; 70(10): 5390-403.

[24]   Fairman JW, Noinaj N, Buchanan SK. The structural biology of β-barrel membrane proteins: a summary of recent reports. Curr Opin Struct Biol 2011; 21(4): 523-31.
[http://dx.doi.org/10.1016/j.sbi.2011.05.005] [PMID: 21719274]

[25]   Pich OQ, Carpenter BM, Gilbreath JJ, Merrell DS. Detailed analysis of *Helicobacter pylori* Fur-regulated promoters reveals a Fur box core sequence and novel Fur-regulated genes. Mol Microbiol 2012; 84(5): 921-41.
[http://dx.doi.org/10.1111/j.1365-2958.2012.08066.x] [PMID: 22507395]

[26]   Crosa JH. Signal transduction and transcriptional and posttranscriptional control of iron-regulated genes in bacteria. Microbiol Mol Biol Rev 1997; 61(3): 319-36.
[http://dx.doi.org/10.1128/.61.3.319-336.1997] [PMID: 9293185]

[27]   Ochsner UA, Vasil ML. Gene repression by the ferric uptake regulator in *Pseudomonas aeruginosa*: cycle selection of iron-regulated genes. Proc Natl Acad Sci USA 1996; 93(9): 4409-14.
[http://dx.doi.org/10.1073/pnas.93.9.4409] [PMID: 8633080]

[28]   Kandler JL, Acevedo RV, Dickinson MK, Cash DR, Shafer WM, Cornelissen CN. The genes that encode the gonococcal transferrin binding proteins, TbpB and TbpA, are differentially regulated by MisR under iron-replete and iron-depleted conditions. Mol Microbiol 2016; 102(1): 137-51.
[http://dx.doi.org/10.1111/mmi.13450] [PMID: 27353397]

[29]   Aebi C, Stone B, Beucher M, *et al.* Expression of the CopB outer membrane protein by *Moraxella catarrhalis* is regulated by iron and affects iron acquisition from transferrin and lactoferrin. Infect Immun 1996; 64(6): 2024-30.
[http://dx.doi.org/10.1128/IAI.64.6.2024-2030.1996] [PMID: 8675303]

[30]   Naka H, Hirono I, Aoki T. Molecular cloning and functional analysis of *Photobacterium damselae* subsp. piscicida haem receptor gene. J Fish Dis 2005; 28(2): 81-8.
[http://dx.doi.org/10.1111/j.1365-2761.2004.00601.x] [PMID: 15705153]

[31]   Ahn SH, Han JH, Lee JH, Park KJ, Kong IS. Identification of an iron-regulated hemin-binding outer membrane protein, HupO, in *Vibrio fluvialis*: effects on hemolytic activity and the oxidative stress response. Infect Immun 2005; 73(2): 722-9.
[http://dx.doi.org/10.1128/IAI.73.2.722-729.2005] [PMID: 15664910]

[32]   Olczak T, Simpson W, Liu X, Genco CA. Iron and heme utilization in *Porphyromonas gingivalis*. FEMS Microbiol Rev 2005; 29(1): 119-44.
[http://dx.doi.org/10.1016/j.femsre.2004.09.001] [PMID: 15652979]

[33]   Bumann D, Aksu S, Wendland M, *et al.* Proteome analysis of secreted proteins of the gastric pathogen *Helicobacter pylori*. Infect Immun 2002; 70(7): 3396-403.
[http://dx.doi.org/10.1128/IAI.70.7.3396-3403.2002]

[34]   Senkovich O, Ceaser S, McGee DJ, Testerman TL. Unique host iron utilization mechanisms of *Helicobacter pylori* revealed with iron-deficient chemically defined media. Infect Immun 2010; 78(5): 1841-9.https://dx.doi.org/10.1128%2FIAI.01258-09
[http://dx.doi.org/10.1128/IAI.01258-09] [PMID: 20176792]

[35]   Mclatchie N, Giner-Sorolla R, Derbyshire SWG. 'Imagined guilt' *vs* 'recollected guilt': implications for fMRI. Soc Cogn Affect Neurosci 2016; 11(5): 703-11.
[http://dx.doi.org/10.1093/scan/nsw001] [PMID: 26746179]

CHAPTER 8

Molecular Mechanisms of *Babesia* Invasion: Potential Targets for Vaccine Development

Juan Mosqueda[1,*], **Susana Mejia-López**[1,2] and **Miguel Angel Mercado-Uriostegui**[1,2]

[1] *Immunology and Vaccines Laboratory. Natural Sciences College, Autonomous University of Queretaro; Queretaro, Qro, Mexico*

[2] *Doctorado en Ciencias Biológicas. Natural Sciences College, Autonomous University of Queretaro; Queretaro, Qro, Mexico*

Abstract: *Babesia bovis* and *Babesia bigemina* are protozoan parasites of the Apicomplexa phylum that cause bovine babesiosis, a cattle disease transmitted by ticks of the Rhipicephalus genera. It is a disease of the tropical and subtropical regions, therefore in Mexico, it is present in 51.5% of the national territory. The severe negative impact of cattle ticks and bovine babesiosis on the livestock industry in Mexico and the world persists due to the absence of safe and effective commercial vaccines. Vaccines based on genomics and biotechnological tools promise to be a solution to this problem. With the complete genome sequence of *Babesia bovis* and *Babesia bigemina*, genomic studies of these pathogens are now possible and valuable information is available on the essential characteristics of their composition and their comparison with the other Apicomplexa protozoa of importance in human and animal health, as well as the identification of new genes with vaccination or therapeutic potential. In this chapter, we review the latest knowledge in the cellular and molecular mechanisms that trigger a protective, immune response and the identification of the molecular targets for vaccine development, all of which are a key priority to develop control measures against these pathogens.

Keywords: Bovine babesiosis, Erythrocyte invasion, Molecular targets, Vaccine development.

INTRODUCTION

Bovine babesiosis is a disease of cattle, in the American continent, it is transmitted by *Rhipicephalus microplus and R. annulatus* ticks, and is caused by *Babesia bovis* and *Babesia bigemina*, two protozoan parasites of the Apicomplexa phylum. It is a disease of the tropical and subtropical regions; therefore in

* **Corresponding author Juan Mosqueda:** Immunology and Vaccines Laboratory, C. A. Facultad de Ciencias Naturales, Universidad Autónoma de Querétaro; Carretera a Chichimequillas, Ejido Bolaños, Querétaro Querétaro 76140, México; Tel: +52 4921564376; E-mail: joel.mosqueda@uaq.mx

Mexico, it is present in 51.5% of the national territory [1]. The cost caused by the ticks and the diseases they transmit has not been fully determined. Rodriguez-Vivas [2] estimated the cost associated with *Rhipicephalus microplus* ticks (the main vector of bovine babesiosis) to be 573 million dollars per year, only in Mexico, and not considering the costs associated with the diseases they transmit. The severe negative impact of cattle ticks and bovine babesiosis on the livestock industry in most parts of the world persists and this is due to the absence of safe and effective commercial vaccines in many countries, including Mexico. In some countries like Argentina, Australia, Israel, and South Africa, there are live, attenuated vaccines, which are very effective but have many disadvantages, such as their high production cost, the risk of spreading other diseases, and their potential reversion to virulence. In this chapter, we first review the latest knowledge about the cellular and molecular mechanisms that trigger a protective immune response against *Babesia* infection, then we focus on the molecular targets for vaccine development. Finally, we review the bioinformatics tools that are useful to identify candidate B and T cell epitopes.

The Immune Response Against Babesiosis

The cellular and humoral immune response in cattle infected with *Babesia bigemina* and *B. bovis* follow a typical response to protozoa. In endemic *Babesia* areas, cattle under 10 months old do not show clinical signs of the disease when they are first exposed to the parasite. Young cattle have a higher percentage of mononuclear cells and a greater capacity for nitric oxide production (NO), which has a potent antimicrobial activity [3]. The production of NO is induced by the secretion of INF-γ and TNF-α from mononuclear phagocytes, which have autocrine activity for the production of NO [4].

In a primary infection, macrophages, dendritic cells, and naive B cells recognize *Babesia* antigens as non-self in the spleen. In this organ, antigen processing and presentation by MHC class II molecules is followed by naive Th cell recognition. This is followed by clonal expansion and activation, which leads to Th1 cell polarization. B-cell activation also occurs, and this generates two populations (Fig. **1**). The first population that is generated in greater proportion is composed of short-lived plasma B cells that play the role of effector cells, followed by a reduced population of B lymphocytes that become low-affinity antibody-producing (IgM) cells against the antigens of the pathogen. In two weeks, most antibody-producing cells (IgM) die and a small proportion of long-lived B cells stored in the bone marrow remains; IgM antibody levels decline rapidly after controlling the first infection and IgG levels are still very low. When cattle come again into contact (secondary infection) with *Babesia*, the memory B cells quickly begin clonal expansion and the number of effector cells is also exponentially increased, the production of IgG antibodies increases significantly as well as the affinity of these antibodies for the antigen, as affinity maturation is taking place [5, 6].

In subsequent infections, the immune response is generated in 3-5 days so that the disease is fully controlled. After this stage, the effector cells and antibody-producing cells begin to die, and a small population of B cells remains for a long time as memory cells that respond quickly to a subsequent reinfection years later. IgG levels decrease slowly and can remain in circulating blood for years without losing their function. In some cases, memory B cells can generate cross protection, since some antigens are highly conserved among different species of the same genus of protozoa [7, 8].

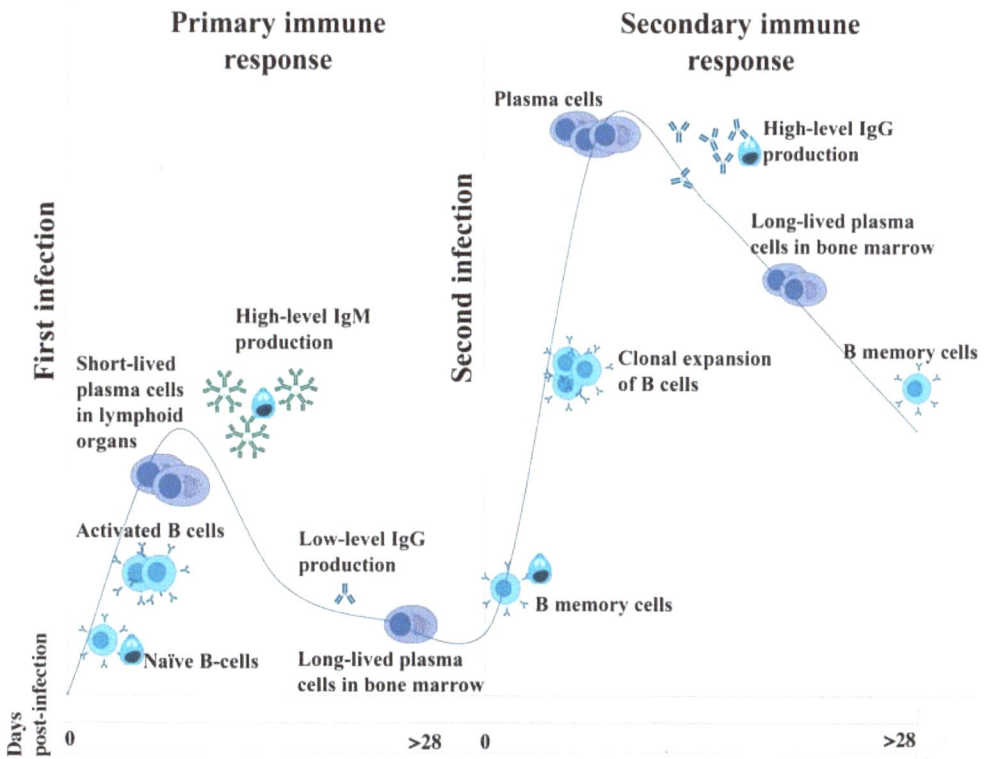

Fig. (1). Immune response to *Babesia* parasites. Primary immune response occurs after first contact with *Babesia* antigens inducing primary clonal expansion of B cells and low affinity IgM and IgG antibodies. A secondary exposure to the same antigens induces a fast and strong immune response characterized by high affinity IgG antibodies.

DEVELOPMENT OF VACCINES AGAINST *BABESIA*

Bovine babesiosis is endemic in tropical and subtropical regions, and cattle under 10 months old, do not develop clinical signs when they are infected with the parasite, so when they reach adulthood, they have a protective immunity against the parasite. However, cattle raised in tick-free areas, and over a year old, are highly susceptible to the disease when they are exposed to the parasite for the first time; they develop an acute infection and, in some cases, if not treated on time, the disease causes high morbidity and death [9]. Vaccination is a strategy for the prevention of bovine babesiosis in these animals.

Live Vaccines

Live vaccines are composed of bovine erythrocytes infected with attenuated *Babesia* parasites. These parasites are obtained from the splenectomized cattle or from *in vitro* cultures. Parasite attenuation is achieved by infecting splenectomized cattle in serial passages until the parasites lose their virulence. Infected bovine blood is obtained from these cattle after 17-20 passages and is used to prepare the doses. Subsequently, the bovines are vaccinated with a dose of erythrocytes infected with the attenuated parasites [10].

Live attenuated vaccines are characterized by rounds of parasite multiplication in the host erythrocytes for some days, without causing the disease. Importantly, the presence of parasite antigens promotes the activation of a Th1 immune response in which immune cells secrete INF-γ and induce the production of specific IgG2 antibodies [11]. Vaccination confers strong immune protection for several years [12]. Successful control of the disease has been achieved in some countries through the use of live vaccines, however, the adverse effects of this type of vaccines are as follows:

- Loss of immunoprotection of the strains used for the vaccine, which is due to the phenotypic variants that arise between the *Babesia* strains, so it is necessary to isolate new strains [13].
- High production cost, including highly strict quality controls for its elaboration, and a cold chain for vaccine maintenance [14].
- Use of antibabesial drugs after vaccination in order to protect adult cattle from the effects of a poorly attenuated live vaccine [15].
- Risk of contamination with other pathogens like *Anaplasma marginale*, viruses, and even prions [10].
- Reversion to virulence, when the attenuated strains still contain a low proportion of virulent parasites [13].

Exoantigens

Vaccines based on exoantigens, are preparations of supernatants from *Babesia* cultures. Exoantigens are secreted proteins that are released into the media culture during the invasion process. These exoantigens are collected from the in vitro culture supernatant and are used as vaccine antigens. Exoantigen-based vaccines can induce protection against heterologous infections from different *Babesia* strains. However, exoantigens generate a poor cell-mediated immune response [16].

Recombinant Proteins and Proteins as Vaccine Agents

The development of a recombinant vaccine was undertaken due to the necessity to have a stable, easy-to-produce, immunizing agent with immunoprotective and reproducible activity [17]. All of these are characteristics that live attenuated vaccines cannot provide.

The first recombinant antigens against *Babesia* were 12D3, 11C5 and 21B4 proteins obtained from parasite extracts and separated by chromatography. Wright *et al.* [7], first immunized cattle with 12D3 and 11C5 subunits, subsequently challenged the cattle with a virulent strain of *B. bovis*, a decrease in parasitemia was observed in vaccinated cattle after the eighth day post-infection. Subsequently, the use of recombinant proteins involved in the invasion of *Babesia* merozoites to the erythrocyte was proposed. Among the most studied antigens involved in this process are described below and in Fig. (**2**).

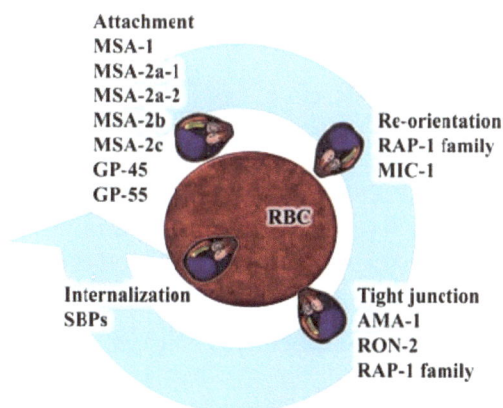

Fig. (2). Invasion mechanism of *Babesia bovis* and B. bigemina. It shows the antigens involved in the different steps of the invasion process characterized in these species.

Variable Merozoite Surface Antigens (VMSAs)

Some of the first merozoite surface proteins that were proposed as vaccine candidates were the Variable Merozoite Surface Antigens (VMSA). They are glycoproteins that belong to the VMSA superfamily. The VMSA family of proteins includes MSA-1 and MSA-2. The MSA-1 protein contains a single-copy gene, while MSA-2 is a family of four genes (MSA-2a1, a2, b, and c). These proteins are expressed on the surface of *Babesia bovis* merozoites and sporozoites and they are involved in adhesion to the erythrocyte during the invasion process [18, 19]. Bovines immunized with a recombinant MSA-1 protein (rMSA-1) produced antibodies that inhibited in erythrocyte invasion by merozoites *in vitro*. Immunized animals were infected with a virulent strain of *B. bovis*, however, no decrease in parasitemia was observed during the post-infection period and it was concluded that bovine antibodies against rMSA-1 did not induce total immune protection against bovine babesiosis [20]. Subsequently, it was shown that MSA-1 is a highly variable surface protein among *B. bovis* strains [21, 22].

The MSA-2 family includes MSA-2a1, MSA-2a2, MSA-2b and MSA2c. These are surface antigens expressed on the surface of merozoites and sporozoites [19]. It has been shown that the MSA-2c protein has a higher degree of conservation among different strains of *B. bovis* at the geographical level (Mexico-Australia), which is a characteristic that supports its inclusion as a vaccine candidate [23]. Moreover, MSA2c has been shown to contain B epitopes by *in-silico* predictions and antibodies generated against those epitopes or the whole protein has the ability to neutralize red blood cell invasion [24, 25, 19]. Unfortunately, except for MSA-2c, most of the MSA-2 members are hypervariable antigens, which makes them poor vaccine candidates [26].

Rhoptry-Associated Protein 1 (RAP-1)

Rhoptries are small, tear-shaped organelles at the apical end of infective stages of Apicomplexa parasites, and they are involved in invasion mechanisms. The Rhoptry-Associated Protein 1 (RAP-1) is a protein contained in the rhoptries of the merozoite and sporozoite stages, and it is secreted during erythrocyte invasion. Its proposed function is to modify the erythrocyte membrane during its invasion. RAP-1 is encoded by a gene that has two copies, which were generated by a duplication event [27].

RAP-1 has conserved B epitopes between different strains of *B. bovis* from several geographical areas and it has been reported that RAP-1 contains conserved T-cell epitopes as well; for this reason, it has been proposed that a RAP-1 is a vaccine candidate against *B. bovis* [28 - 30]. Purified native RAP-1 induces partial immunity in cattle as it reduces the percentage of parasites after challenge, but no difference in antibody production was observed between a control group and a group immunized with the protein [31, 32].

The amino terminal region of RAP-1 contains cysteine residues and it is structurally conserved among different *Babesia* species, while the carboxyl terminal region contains tandem repeats of 23 amino acids [29]. An analysis of the amino and carboxy terminal regions of RAP-1 showed that both regions stimulated clones of CD4+ T-cells from cattle exposed to *B. bovis*, indicating the presence of T-cell epitopes. Th cells (CD4+) stimulated with amino terminal regions of RAP-1 proliferated to a greater extent than cells stimulated with the carboxyl terminal region [29].

Based on these results, a recombinant protein (RAP-1 NT) was developed. When cattle were immunized with RAP-1 NT, they showed an increase in CD4+ T cell proliferation and INF-γ production, as well as an increase of IgG2 antibodies, all of which indicators of a Th1 response. However, when the immunized cattle were challenged with a pathogenic strain of *B. bovis*, the animals had clinical signs and were not protected against the disease. Additionally, the antibodies did not neutralize merozoite invasion *in vitro*. In this work, they concluded that immunization with a single protein is not sufficient to induce protection because there could be more than one mechanism of infection and more than one protein involved in this process [33].

Apical Membrane Antigen (AMA-1)

AMA-1 is a microneme protein present in all parasite members of the Apicomplexa phylum [34]. AMA-1 is formed by three regions, an extracellular amino-terminal region, a transmembrane region and an intracellular carboxy-terminal region. The amino terminal region has three domains; I, II, and III [35], and it has been shown that domain III interacts with other protein complexes (RON) in the formation of a structure called tight junction, that promotes the invagination of the host cell [36, 37]. Antibodies generated against amino terminal peptides from *B. bovis* AMA-1 inhibited bovine erythrocytes invasion by *B. bovis* merozoites *in vitro* up to 65% [38]. Furthermore, *B. bovis* AMA-1 peptides obtained by *in-silico* predictions of conserved, B-cell epitopes, are recognized by sera from naturally infected animals, suggesting recognition of those epitopes by the immune system [39].

Rhoptry Neck Protein (RON-2)

RON-2 is a protein secreted by the rhoptries. In parasites of the phylum Apicomplexa, the interaction between AMA-1 and RON-2 is necessary for the formation of a close junction and the beginning of the invasion process. In *B.*

bovis, RON-2 is encoded by a single-copy gene and has been reported to be highly conserved between strains [40]. RON-2 contains a CLAG domain that allows cytoadherence to the surface of erythrocytes during the invasion process and subsequently it attaches to AMA-1 in domain III.

Synthetic peptides from *B. bovis* RON-2 were recognized by antibodies present in the sera of naturally infected animals, using an indirect ELISA and immunofluorescence (IFAT). Additionally, antibodies were generated by immunizing cattle with those peptides and they blocked the erythrocyte invasion by *B. bovis* merozoite *in vitro* [40]. All of these, indicate that *B. bovis* RON2 conserved epitopes, can be considered as vaccine candidates.

Micronemal Protein-1 (MIC-1)

MIC proteins are adhesion proteins secreted by the micronemes, which are small, round organelles of Apicomplexa protozoa. During the initial steps of the invasion process, MIC-1 recognizes the surface of erythrocytes through sialic acid-binding Micronemal Adhesive Repeat (MAR) domains, then more MIC-1 proteins are secreted and are used for anchoring other MIC proteins to the parasite membrane [41]. Subsequently after recognition of the erythrocyte by the parasite, the apical orientation and invasion processes begin.

The *B. bigemina* MIC-1 protein is encoded by a single copy gene that is orthologous to the *B. bovis* gene. These sequences are similar to those in other Apicomplexa protozoa, for example *Toxoplasma gondii*. Additionally, MIC-1 in *Babesia bigemina* has been proposed as a vaccine candidate, not only because it contains the MAR domains, but because it also contains conserved, B-cell epitopes that induce the generation of antibodies that block erythrocyte invasion by merozoite *in vitro* [42].

Spherical Body Protein 4 (SBP-4)

The spherical bodies are big, round organelles of some Apicomplexa parasites, which are specialized in the storage of proteins involved in the development of protozoa inside the host cell. There are at least four proteins characterized from these organelles in *Babesia* spp.: SPB-1, SPB-2, SPB-3 and SPB-4. Particularly, SBP-4 is expressed in the intra-erythrocytic stages during the development of the parasite. The SBP-4 protein has been reported in *B. orientalis*, *B. bovis* and *B. bigemina* [43]. It has not been reported in other Apicomplexa protozoa [44]. This characteristic is favorable for using this protein as a vaccine agent, but also for the development of diagnostic tests [45].

Hapless 2 (HAP-2)

Hapless 2 protein was identified in male gametocytes of the plant *Arapbidopsis thaliana*. It was subsequently identified in algae, insects and protozoa including *Plasmodium* spp. In *Plasmodium berguei*, HAP-2 is necessary for the fusion of gamete membranes, but not for adhesion between the male and female gametes [46, 47].

The *hap-2* gene of *B. bigemina* has similarity with *hap-2* of *P. berguei* and in both cases, HAP-2 is not expressed in asexual stages, but it is only expressed in gametes. It has been shown in *in vitro assays*, that antibodies against HAP-2 block the formation of *B. bigemina* zygotes, thus, supporting the incorporation of HAP-2 in a transmission-blocking vaccine, impeding the transmission of *Babesia* parasites to ticks [48].

Next Generation Vaccines

The reported setbacks for the development of recombinant vaccines, based on a single antigen and the limitations in the production of live vaccines, have led to propose the development of new strategies for the development of vaccines against babesiosis. A new strategy is the use of two or more immunogenic antigens combined. The development of bovine babesiosis vaccines based on multi-antigenic and multi-epitopic recombinant protein constructs has currently been proposed. This strategy is based on the identification and incorporation of specific immunogenic regions that contain T and B-cell epitopes [49], and these regions are expressed together on a single chimeric antigen.

Jaramillo *et al*. [50], proposed a vaccination strategy using a chimeric protein, which was designed based on regions that have B and T epitopes of RAP-1, HSP-20, and MSA-2c proteins from *B. bovis*. Mice immunized with this chimeric antigen produced antibodies and their specific T cells were stimulated against the RAP-1, MSA-2c and HSP20 antigens, concluding that the chimeric protein has B and T -cell epitopes that are necessary to achieve a cellular and humoral immune response. However, a group of cattle, vaccinated with a chimeric gene, failed to achieve immunological protection when challenged with a virulent strain, suggesting that other antigens should be included [51].

Another immunization strategy is the development of genetically modified live vaccines with deletions of specific genes. A transgenic strain of *B. bovis* deficient in the 6-CysA and 6-CysB genes was developed. These genes are expressed on the surface of the parasite membrane of sexual stages, which develop within the tick midgut and may be involved in the sexual fusion of the gametes for zygote formation. Genetically modified organisms could be used as vaccine candidates to block the transmission of *Babesia* parasites to ticks [52].

The use of nanotechnology for vaccines against *Babesia* has been proposed for two reasons: (i) as immunomodulators to help polarize an immune response, or (ii) as transporters for molecules like chimeric proteins or antibodies. The first point is related to the use of nanoparticles (Np) of polymeric origin, such as chitosan or PLGA (Poly-lactic-co-glycolic acid), which have shown to increase cellular responses when administered intramuscularly or subcutaneously [53]. PLGA-Np have been tested as adjuvants for a wide range of antigens, including hydrophobic antigens [54, 55], hepatitis B virus antigens [56], *Bacillus anthracis* [57], tetanus toxoid protein [55] and ovalbumin [58].

The nanoparticles are also used as vehicle systems for the administration of antigens and to extend the exposure time of antigens to the immune system. Some vaccines that include aluminum nanoparticles as vehicles are the tetanus, diphtheria and influenza vaccines [59]. Gold nanoparticles are some of the most studied Np as vaccine vehicles due to their modifiable surface. Gold nanoparticles can be joined to different molecules like functional groups on their surface that function as ligands. Gold nanoparticles can be used to administer peptides and as a transport platform because they increase their size and the exposure time of peptides compared to direct administration [60].

The functionalization of gold nanoparticles is possible with ligands that allow the binding of other molecules as co-stimulants or adjuvants. It has been shown that the conjugation of gold nanoparticles with CpG sequences can direct the immune response towards dendritic cells, increasing the presentation of a specific antigen, inducing specific T-cell responses [58].

In *Babesia*, CpG sequences have been shown to induce a mitogenic effect on specific B cells. This could be because CpG sequences contain a high frequency of CG dinucleotides that are also present in the open reading frame of the RAP-1 protein. Dinucleotides could be involved in modulating the host immune response during *Babesia* infection [61, 62], and these sequences can be used as co-stimulators in nanotechnology-based vaccines against babesiosis.

Prediction of B-cell Epitopes as the First Step in the Development of Next Generation Vaccines

After all the failed attempts for the development of a vaccine that confers total protection against *Babesia*, the existence of conserved peptide sequences in proteins involved in the invasion mechanism has been confirmed. Bioinformatics has been a key tool for the search of conserved peptide sequences that could function as vaccine targets. Peptides from different *Babesia* parasite proteins involved in the erythrocyte invasion process, such as AMA-1 [39], MIC-1 [42], RON-2 [63, 40], RAP-1, SBP-4, MSA-2c, among others, have been reported [1].

The first step for the identification of B-cell epitopes, is to obtain and sequence the selected genes of *Babesia* from strains in different geographical regions of the world.

To achieve this, blood samples are taken from infected cattle from different geographic regions where babesiosis is present. The DNA is then extracted and used to amplify the gene encoding the protein of interest. It is essential to clone the gene sequence into a cloning vector using competent bacterial cells and to purify it for sequencing. The designing of primers is important for the specific amplification of the region of interest. The NCBI Blast tool that allows comparing the similarity of the primers with the sequences available in the data base can be used to avoid the amplification of other unwanted sequences. Raw sequences obtained by Sanger sequencing require a curing treatment in order to be translated into protein sequences [64].

Current sequencers can generate erroneous readings at the beginning and at the end of the sequencing process, these errors can be reduced or increased depending on the process of purification and integrity of the DNA and the efficiency of the PCR reaction. Programs such as the ORFinder (https://www.bioinformatics.org/sms2/orf_find.html), that allows the analysis of DNA sequences and shows the different ORFs in the sequence, thus finding the start and stop codons, can be used for the identification of the open reader frame (ORF) of sequenced PCR products [65]. By doing this, the size of the sequence is gradually reduced by eliminating regions that are not essential for the prediction of the peptides.

Some genes have introns and exons, in these cases, it is necessary to remove non-coding regions (introns) from the coding sequence. The Genscan program (http://hollywood.mit.edu/GENSCAN.html) can be used to perform this function, however, the algorithms used to development this program, are based on vertebrate, maize and Arabidopsis ORFs [66, 64]. After curing the DNA sequences by removing introns, the translation of the DNA to protein sequence is performed. There are several tools for the translation of DNA into protein, for example: Translate (https://web.expasy.org/translate/), sequence translation (https://www.ebi.ac.uk/Tools/st/), the BLASTx of the NCBI translates a sequence and it can search for similar sequences in the database [67, 64].

Prediction of Transmembrane Helices

The prediction of transmembrane helices is of great help for identifying extracellular regions of proteins so that, antibodies against these target regions can be efficiently generated. The TMHMM Server v. 2.0 (http://www.cbs.dtu.dk/services/TMHMM/) allows making these predictions using the N-best algorithm, which also allows finding the orientation and location of transmembrane helices in the sequences. This program should not be used with proteins that are not associated with the cell membrane, such as cytoplasmic proteins [68].

Signal Peptide Prediction

Some proteins have a signal peptide, which is a small peptide that is cleaved from the protein sequence at the time it passes through the Golgi apparatus. This process must be simulated when processing the sequence *in-silico*. The SignalP-5.0 server (http://www.cbs.dtu.dk/services/SignalP/), predicts the signal of peptides in all domains based on an algorithm of deep neural networks that allows the identification of signal peptides with high accuracy [69].

B-cell Epitopes Prediction

The programs for predicting B-cell epitopes use different algorithms, therefore, it is recommended to use at least three different programs with different prediction algorithms.

ABCPred (http://crdd.osdd.net/raghava/abcpred/) is a widely used tool for the prediction of B-cell epitopes. ABCPred uses a recurrent learning algorithm based on neural networks with a database of 700 confirmed B-cell epitopes and 700 random epitopes. This algorithm allows to predict B-cell epitopes with 65.93% accuracy using recurrent neural networks [70].

BEPIPred (http://www.cbs.dtu.dk/services/BepiPred/cite.php) is a tool based on a trained algorithm on epitopes annotated from antibody-antigen interactions. This algorithm uses a database of predicted peptides based on 3D protein crystallography and a large collection of peptides from the IEDB database. This program combines amino acid propensity scales and a Hidden Markov Model (HMM) to improve the prediction results [71].

BCPREDS (http://ailab.ist.psu.edu/bcpred/index.html) allows the analysis of protein sequences for the prediction of B-cell epitopes by three different algorithms. The first prediction method is through the amino acid pair (AAP) scale; it has been shown that this scale has a better performance in predicting amino acid propensity than other scales with different algorithms when combined with a support vector machine (SVM) classifier, reaching 71% reliability in prediction [72]. The second method is BCPred. This method allows predicting linear peptides using Kernel sub-sequence with 75.8% prediction reliability. This method is based on the same neural network algorithm that ABCPred uses, however, BCPred's predictions with this algorithm can be too optimistic [73]. The third prediction method is FBCPred, based on predicting flexible length linear B-cell epitopes. This method can epitopes of any length, unlike AAP and BCPred that have fixed lengths of 12, 14, 16, 18, 20, and 22 amino acids [74].

BCEPred (http://crdd.osdd.net/raghava/bcepred/) is a program that has 1029 experimentally tested Immunodominant and immunogenic B-cell epitopes and 1029 random peptides. The sequences in this database were obtained through WISS-PROT. It allows the measurement of different B-cell epitopes in proteins, such as hydrophobicity, flexibility, accessibility, transmembrane helices rotation, antigenicity, residue exposure, and polarity simultaneously. The database covers a wide range of B-cell epitopes of viruses, bacteria, fungi, and protozoa. BCEPred uses different prediction algorithms, including the Parker's method, which allows measurement of the hydrophobicity of the peptides by means of a hydrophobicity scale consisting of the retention times of the peptides by reverse phase HPLC [75]. The Karplus method allows measuring the flexibility of the sequences. The 3Karplus scale measures flexibility, based on a calculation of the mobility of the segments of 31 known proteins, based on the B-factors of these proteins [76]. The Emini method allows measuring the accessibility of a protein using the formula $Sn = (dn + 4 + i) (0.37) - 6$; Sn is the surface probability, dn is the fractional surface probability value on a scale from 1 to 6. A sequence with a six amino acid peptide with Sn equal to one and the probabilities greater than 1.0 indicates a greater probability that this peptide is on the surface of the protein [77]. The Pellequer method identifies antigenic regions in protein sequences with the turn scale, using a structural database of 87 proteins reaching 70% accuracy in predicting known epitopes [78]. The Kolaskar method is used to predict the antigen propensity of peptides in protein sequences. This scale allows the identification of peptides in protein sequences. The analysis uses a database of confirmed antigenic sites in an experimental way, if the program detects a cysteine, a valine or a leucine residue in the antigenic determinant and if they are found on the surface of the protein, they are very likely immunogenic regions. This method has the ability to predict antigenic determinants in sequences of seven amino acids with 70% reliability for prediction of antigenic propensity [79]. The exposed surface scale and polarity scale are used to predict exposed regions and their polarity. These models analyze segments of seven amino acids to identify epitope regions. The polarity scale provides information about the surface domains, loops, hydrophobic domains, nucleation sites and spatial positions of the protein molecules of interest [80].

Assessment of the Specificity and Conservation of the Epitope Sequence.

Once the peptides are selected, a pBLAST must be performed to confirm *in-silico*, that these peptides are conserved in different strains of the pathogen from different geographical regions [64]. It is necessary to perform a pBLAST analysis in the species in which the peptides will be used as vaccine agents, in order to prevent their immune system from detecting them as their own or to generate an unwanted, autoimmune response. Experimentally, the recognition of predicted peptides must be confirmed with the use of bioinformatics tools. The peptides can be evaluated by indirect ELISA, indirect immunofluorescence and western-blotting using sera from cattle that were exposed to the disease [40, 42]. Due to their small size, peptides are not good candidates to be used as vaccine agents for the following reasons; the size of these peptides may be between <1 and 3 kDa; protein molecules of this size do not have the necessary immunogenicity to generate a good immune response. There are different options to increase the immunogenicity, for instance, the synthesis of peptides conjugated with BSA (Bovine Serum Albumin). This serum protein has 59 lysine residues and a molecular weight of 59 KDa. This protein has 30-35 linker sites. Keyhole limpet hemocyanin (KLH) is a protein isolated from *Megathura crenulata* and has a molecular weight that ranges from 0.45 to 130 KDa. Ovalbumin (OVA) is the second most used conjugate after the BSA. However, the problem with these systems is the generation of cellular and humoral responses against the proteins to which the peptides are conjugated [81].

Peptide immunogenicity of Multiple Antigenic Peptides (MAPs)

Synthesis of peptides in lysine dendrimers is an option that reduces the nonspecific response of the immune system against the proteins to which the peptides are conjugated, while increasing the size of the molecule, therefore increasing its immunogenicity. This system is called Multiple Antigenic Peptide (MAP). The limitation of the use of peptides in a MAP format is that, the larger the size of the matrix and the sequence of the peptides, the higher the increase in price. The milligram of a chemically synthesized peptide in MAP varies between US$ 15 to 30 (April 2020), depending on whether they are synthesized in a linear way, in a MAP dendrimer of two, four, eight or sixteen peptides per matrix. Purity also increases the cost, the higher the purity of the peptides, the better immune responses are achieved.

Adjuvant Use

The administration of the peptides as vaccine candidates requires the use of an adjuvant that facilitates the process of entry into B-cells to initiate a good immune response that remains longer within the animal to increase the time of exposure to the antigen. The use of a single peptide against *Babesia* parasites does not generate total protection against the disease, but the use of several peptides from different proteins involved in the process of erythrocyte invasion can improve the results by blocking different parts of this process [40, 42].

SUMMARY

Babesiosis is a very important disease in human and animal health. Control of the disease through vaccination is only possible in some countries through the use of live vaccines. Recombinant vaccines are not available primarily due to the antigenic variation of molecular targets. The invasion mechanism of *Babesia* parasites is similar to that of other Apicomplexa species, therefore, proteins encoded by homologous genes involved in invasion mechanisms, or in the fusion of sexual stages, can be evaluated as candidates to be included in a multi-antigen vaccine. Immunogenicity, cell surface exposure, induction of an adequate cellular immune response, and the ability to induce neutralizing antibodies are important features to consider. Through the use of bioinformatics, molecular biology, immunology and nanotechnology, a vaccine against this disease can be a reality.

CONSENT FOR PUBLICATION

Not applicable.

CONFLICT OF INTEREST

The authors confirm that the content of this chapter has no conflict of interest.

ACKNOWLEDGEMENT

The research was funded by FONDEC-UAQ (PN 2017/7256). Susana Mejía-López and Miguel Ángel Mercado-Uriostegui received a fellowship from Becas Nacionales CONACyT-México.

REFERENCES

[1]   Mosqueda J, Olvera-Ramirez A, Aguilar-Tipacamu G, Canto GJ. Current advances in detection and treatment of babesiosis. Curr Med Chem 2012; 19(10): 1504-18.
[http://dx.doi.org/10.2174/092986712799828355] [PMID: 22360483]

[2]   Rodríguez-Vivas R, Grisi L, Pérez de León A, *et al.* Potential economic impact assessment for cattle parasites in Mexico. Rev Mex Cienc Pecu 2017; 8(1): 61.
[http://dx.doi.org/10.22319/rmcp.v8i1.4305]

[3]   Goff WL, Johnson WC, Parish SM, *et al.* IL-4 and IL-10 inhibition of IFN-γ- and TNF-α-dependent nitric oxide production from bovine mononuclear phagocytes exposed to *Babesia bovis* merozoites. Vet Immunol Immunopathol 2002; 84(3-4): 237-51.
[http://dx.doi.org/10.1016/S0165-2427(01)00413-5] [PMID: 11777537]

[4]   Goff WL, Johnson WC, Parish SM, Barrington GM, Tuo W, Valdez RA. The age-related immunity in

cattle to *Babesia bovis* infection involves the rapid induction of interleukin-12, interferon-gamma and inducible nitric oxide synthase mRNA expression in the spleen. Parasite Immunol 2001; 23(9): 463-71.
[http://dx.doi.org/10.1046/j.1365-3024.2001.00402.x] [PMID: 11589775]

[5]   Estes DM, Brown WC. Type 1 and type 2 responses in regulation of Ig isotype expression in cattle. Vet Immunol Immunopathol 2002; 90(1-2): 1-10.
[http://dx.doi.org/10.1016/S0165-2427(02)00201-5] [PMID: 12406650]

[6]   Brown WC, McElwain TF, Palmer GH, Chantler SE, Estes DM. Bovine CD4(+) T-lymphocyte clones specific for rhoptry-associated protein 1 of *Babesia bigemina* stimulate enhanced immunoglobulin G1 (IgG1) and IgG2 synthesis. Infect Immun 1999; 67(1): 155-64.
[http://dx.doi.org/10.1128/IAI.67.1.155-164.1999] [PMID: 9864210]

[7]   Wright IG, Goodger BV, Leatch G, Aylward JH, Rode-Bramanis K, Waltisbuhl DJ. Protection of *Babesia bigemina*-immune animals against subsequent challenge with virulent *Babesia bovis*. Infect Immun 1987; 55(2): 364-8.
[http://dx.doi.org/10.1128/IAI.55.2.364-368.1987] [PMID: 3542832]

[8]   Smith RD, Molinar E, Larios F, Monroy J, Trigo F, Ristic M. *Bovine babesiosis*: pathogenicity and heterologous species immunity of tick-borne *Babesia bovis* and B bigemina infections. Am J Vet Res 1980; 41(12): 1957-65.
[PMID: 7212429]

[9]   Florin-Christensen M. suarez C, Rodriguez A, Flores D, Schnittger L. Vaccines against bovine babesiosis: where we are now and possible roads ahead. Parasitology 2014; 141(12): 1563-92.
[http://dx.doi.org/10.1017/S0031182014000961]

[10]   Callow LL, Dalgliesh RJ, de Vos AJ. Development of effective living vaccines against bovine babesiosis--the longest field trial? Int J Parasitol 1997; 27(7): 747-67.
[http://dx.doi.org/10.1016/S0020-7519(97)00034-9] [PMID: 9279577]

[11]   Combrink MP, Troskie PC, Du Plessis F, Latif AA. Serological responses to *Babesia bovis* vaccination in cattle previously infected with *Babesia bigemina*. Vet Parasitol 2010; 170(1-2): 30-6.
[http://dx.doi.org/10.1016/j.vetpar.2010.02.008] [PMID: 20207488]

[12]   Mahoney DF, Kerr JD, Goodger BV, Wright IG. The immune response of cattle to *Babesia bovis* (syn. *B. argentina*). Studies on the nature and specificity of protection. Int J Parasitol 1979; 9(4): 297-306.
[http://dx.doi.org/10.1016/0020-7519(79)90078-X] [PMID: 489236]

[13]   Bock RE, de Vos AJ, Kingston TG, Shiels IA, Dalgliesh RJ. Investigations of breakdowns in protection provided by living *Babesia bovis* vaccine. Vet Parasitol 1992; 43(1-2): 45-56.
[http://dx.doi.org/10.1016/0304-4017(92)90047-D] [PMID: 1496802]

[14]   de Waal DT, Combrink MP. Live vaccines against bovine babesiosis. Vet Parasitol 2006; 138(1-2): 88-96.
[http://dx.doi.org/10.1016/j.vetpar.2006.01.042] [PMID: 16504404]

[15]   Kuttler KL, Johnson LW. Chemoprophylactic activity of imidocarb, diminazene and oxytetracycline against *Babesia bovis* and B. bigemina. Vet Parasitol 1986; 21(2): 107-18.
[http://dx.doi.org/10.1016/0304-4017(86)90151-2] [PMID: 3739203]

[16]   Patarroyo JH, Prates AA, Tavares CA, Mafra CL, Vargas MI. Exoantigens of an attenuated strain of *Babesia bovis* used as a vaccine against bovine babesiosis. Vet Parasitol 1995; 59(3-4): 189-99.
[http://dx.doi.org/10.1016/0304-4017(94)00756-3] [PMID: 8533277]

[17]   Wright IG, Casu R, Commins MA, *et al.* The development of a recombinant *Babesia* vaccine. Vet Parasitol 1992; 44(1-2): 3-13.
[http://dx.doi.org/10.1016/0304-4017(92)90138-Y] [PMID: 1441189]

[18]   Suarez CE, Florin-Christensen M, Hines SA, Palmer GH, Brown WC, McElwain TF. Characterization of allelic variation in the *Babesia bovis* merozoite surface antigen 1 (MSA-1) locus and identification

of a cross-reactive inhibition-sensitive MSA-1 epitope. Infect Immun 2000; 68(12): 6865-70.
[http://dx.doi.org/10.1128/IAI.68.12.6865-6870.2000] [PMID: 11083806]

[19] Mosqueda J, McElwain TF, Palmer GH. *Babesia bovis* merozoite surface antigen 2 proteins are
      expressed on the merozoite and sporozoite surface, and specific antibodies inhibit attachment and
      invasion of erythrocytes. Infect Immun 2002; 70(11): 6448-55.
      [http://dx.doi.org/10.1128/IAI.70.11.6448-6455.2002] [PMID: 12379726]

[20] Hines SA, Palmer GH, Jasmer DP, Goff WL, McElwain TF. Immunization of cattle with recombinant
      Babesia bovis merozoite surface antigen-1. Infect Immun 1995; 63(1): 349-52.
      [http://dx.doi.org/10.1128/IAI.63.1.349-352.1995] [PMID: 7806376]

[21] Tattiyapong M, Sivakumar T, Takemae H, *et al.* Genetic diversity and antigenicity variation of
      Babesia bovis merozoite surface antigen-1 (MSA-1) in Thailand. Infect Genet Evol 2016; 41: 255-61.
      [http://dx.doi.org/10.1016/j.meegid.2016.04.021] [PMID: 27101782]

[22] Borgonio V, Mosqueda J, Genis AD, *et al.* msa-1 and msa-2c gene analysis and common epitopes
      assessment in Mexican *Babesia bovis* isolates. Ann N Y Acad Sci 2008; 1149(1): 145-8.
      [http://dx.doi.org/10.1196/annals.1428.035] [PMID: 19120194]

[23] Florin-Christensen M, Suarez CE, Hines SA, Palmer GH, Brown WC, McElwain TF. The *Babesia
      bovis* merozoite surface antigen 2 locus contains four tandemly arranged and expressed genes
      encoding immunologically distinct proteins. Infect Immun 2002; 70(7): 3566-75.
      [http://dx.doi.org/10.1128/IAI.70.7.3566-3575.2002] [PMID: 12065497]

[24] Dominguez M, Echaide I, Echaide ST, *et al. In silico* predicted conserved B-cell epitopes in the
      merozoite surface antigen-2 family of *B. bovis* are neutralization sensitive. Vet Parasitol 2010; 167(2-
      4): 216-26.
      [http://dx.doi.org/10.1016/j.vetpar.2009.09.023] [PMID: 19850413]

[25] Wilkowsky SE, Farber M, Echaide I, *et al. Babesia bovis* merozoite surface protein-2c (MSA-2c)
      contains highly immunogenic, conserved B-cell epitopes that elicit neutralization-sensitive antibodies
      in cattle. Mol Biochem Parasitol 2003; 127(2): 133-41.
      [http://dx.doi.org/10.1016/S0166-6851(02)00329-8] [PMID: 12672522]

[26] Genis AD, Mosqueda JJ, Borgonio VM, *et al.* Phylogenetic analysis of Mexican *Babesia bovis* isolates
      using msa and ssrRNA gene sequences. Ann N Y Acad Sci 2008; 1149(1): 121-5.
      [http://dx.doi.org/10.1196/annals.1428.070] [PMID: 19120189]

[27] Suarez CE, Palmer GH, Hötzel I, McElwain TF. Structure, sequence, and transcriptional analysis of
      the *Babesia bovis* rap-1 multigene locus. Mol Biochem Parasitol 1998; 93(2): 215-24.
      [PMID: 9662706]

[28] Mosqueda J, McElwain TF, Stiller D, Palmer GH. *Babesia bovis* merozoite surface antigen 1 and
      rhoptry-associated protein 1 are expressed in sporozoites, and specific antibodies inhibit sporozoite
      attachment to erythrocytes. Infect Immun 2002; 70(3): 1599-603.
      [http://dx.doi.org/10.1128/IAI.70.3.1599-1603.2002] [PMID: 11854249]

[29] Norimine J, Suarez CE, McElwain TF, Florin-Christensen M, Brown WC. Immunodominant epitopes
      in *Babesia bovis* rhoptry-associated protein 1 that elicit memory CD4(+)-T-lymphocyte responses in
      B. bovis-immune individuals are located in the amino-terminal domain. Infect Immun 2002; 70(4):
      2039-48.
      [http://dx.doi.org/10.1128/IAI.70.4.2039-2048.2002] [PMID: 11895969]

[30] Suarez CE, Palmer GH, Hines SA, McElwain TF. Immunogenic B-cell epitopes of *Babesia bovis*
      rhoptry-associated protein 1 are distinct from sequences conserved between species. Infect Immun
      1993; 61(8): 3511-7.
      [http://dx.doi.org/10.1128/IAI.61.8.3511-3517.1993] [PMID: 7687587]

[31] Yokoyama N, Suthisak B, Hirata H, *et al.* Cellular localization of *Babesia bovis* merozoite rhoptry-
      associated protein 1 and its erythrocyte-binding activity. Infect Immun 2002; 70(10): 5822-6.
      [http://dx.doi.org/10.1128/IAI.70.10.5822-5826.2002] [PMID: 12228313]

[32]   Brown WC, McElwain TF, Ruef BJ, *et al. Babesia bovis* rhoptry-associated protein 1 is immunodominant for T helper cells of immune cattle and contains T-cell epitopes conserved among geographically distant *B. bovis* strains. Infect Immun 1996; 64(8): 3341-50.
[http://dx.doi.org/10.1128/IAI.64.8.3341-3350.1996] [PMID: 8757873]

[33]   Norimine J, Mosqueda J, Suarez C, *et al.* Stimulation of T-helper cell gamma interferon and immunoglobulin G responses specific for *Babesia bovis* rhoptry-associated protein 1 (RAP-1) or a RAP-1 protein lacking the carboxy-terminal repeat region is insufficient to provide protective immunity against virulent *B. bovis* challenge. Infect Immun 2003; 71(9): 5021-32.
[http://dx.doi.org/10.1128/IAI.71.9.5021-5032.2003] [PMID: 12933845]

[34]   Narum DL, Thomas AW. Differential localization of full-length and processed forms of PF83/AMA-1 an apical membrane antigen of *Plasmodium falciparum* merozoites. Mol Biochem Parasitol 1994; 67(1): 59-68.
[http://dx.doi.org/10.1016/0166-6851(94)90096-5] [PMID: 7838184]

[35]   Howell SA, Well I, Fleck SL, Kettleborough C, Collins CR, Blackman MJ. A single malaria merozoite serine protease mediates shedding of multiple surface proteins by juxtamembrane cleavage. J Biol Chem 2003; 278(26): 23890-8.
[http://dx.doi.org/10.1074/jbc.M302160200] [PMID: 12686561]

[36]   Besteiro S, Dubremetz JF, Lebrun M. The moving junction of apicomplexan parasites: a key structure for invasion. Cell Microbiol 2011; 13(6): 797-805.
[http://dx.doi.org/10.1111/j.1462-5822.2011.01597.x] [PMID: 21535344]

[37]   Crawford J, Tonkin ML, Grujic O, Boulanger MJ. Structural characterization of apical membrane antigen 1 (AMA1) from Toxoplasma gondii. J Biol Chem 2010; 285(20): 15644-52.
[http://dx.doi.org/10.1074/jbc.M109.092619] [PMID: 20304917]

[38]   Gaffar FR, Yatsuda AP, Franssen FF, de Vries E. Erythrocyte invasion by *Babesia bovis* merozoites is inhibited by polyclonal antisera directed against peptides derived from a homologue of *Plasmodium falciparum* apical membrane antigen 1. Infect Immun 2004; 72(5): 2947-55.
[http://dx.doi.org/10.1128/IAI.72.5.2947-2955.2004] [PMID: 15102807]

[39]   Barreda D, Hidalgo Ruiz M, Hernandez Ortiz R, Ramos J, Galindo Velasco E, Mosqueda J. Identification of conserved peptides containing B-cell epitopes of *Babesia bovis* AMA-1 and their potential as diagnostics candidates Transbound Emerg Dis 2020; 67(2): 60-8.

[40]   Hidalgo-Ruiz M, Suarez CE, Mercado-Uriostegui MA, *et al. Babesia bovis* RON2 contains conserved B-cell epitopes that induce an invasion-blocking humoral immune response in immunized cattle. Parasit Vectors 2018; 11(1): 575.
[http://dx.doi.org/10.1186/s13071-018-3164-2] [PMID: 30390674]

[41]   Silva MG, Ueti MW, Norimine J, *et al. Babesia bovis* expresses a neutralization-sensitive antigen that contains a microneme adhesive repeat (MAR) domain. Parasitol Int 2010; 59(2): 294-7.
[http://dx.doi.org/10.1016/j.parint.2010.03.004] [PMID: 20304092]

[42]   Hernández-Silva DJ, Valdez-Espinoza UM, Mercado-Uriostegui MA, *et al.* Immunomolecular characterization of MIC-1, a novel antigen in *Babesia bigemina*, which contains conserved and immunodominant b-cell epitopes that induce neutralizing antibodies. Vet Sci 2018; 5(2): 32.
[http://dx.doi.org/10.3390/vetsci5020032] [PMID: 29570654]

[43]   Guo J, Li M, Sun Y, *et al.* Characterization of a novel secretory spherical body protein in *Babesia orientalis* and *Babesia orientalis*-infected erythrocytes. Parasit Vectors 2018; 11(1): 433.
[http://dx.doi.org/10.1186/s13071-018-3018-y] [PMID: 30045776]

[44]   Terkawi MA, Seuseu FJ, Eko-Wibowo P, *et al.* Secretion of a new spherical body protein of *Babesia bovis* into the cytoplasm of infected erythrocytes. Mol Biochem Parasitol 2011; 178(1-2): 40-5.
[http://dx.doi.org/10.1016/j.molbiopara.2011.02.006] [PMID: 21406202]

[45]   Cruz-Reséndiz A, Aguilar-Tipacamú G, Alpirez F, Valdiviczo-López B, Mcndoza-Nazar P, Ruiz-

Sesma B, *et al.* Expresión recombinante de la Proteína de los Cuerpos Esféricos 4 (SBP-4) de Babesia bigemina. Que hacer científico en Chiapas 2016; 11(2).

[46]   Liu Y, Tewari R, Ning J, *et al.* The conserved plant sterility gene HAP2 functions after attachment of fusogenic membranes in *Chlamydomonas* and *Plasmodium* gametes. Genes Dev 2008; 22(8): 1051-68.
[http://dx.doi.org/10.1101/gad.1656508] [PMID: 18367645]

[47]   von Besser K, Frank AC, Johnson MA, Preuss D. Arabidopsis HAP2 (GCS1) is a sperm-specific gene required for pollen tube guidance and fertilization. Development 2006; 133(23): 4761-9.
[http://dx.doi.org/10.1242/dev.02683] [PMID: 17079265]

[48]   Camacho-Nuez M, Hernández-Silva DJ, Castañeda-Ortiz EJ, *et al.* Hap2, a novel gene in *Babesia bigemina* is expressed in tick stages, and specific antibodies block zygote formation. Parasit Vectors 2017; 10(1): 568.
[http://dx.doi.org/10.1186/s13071-017-2510-0] [PMID: 29132437]

[49]   Mosqueda J, Falcón Neri A, Ramos Aragón J, Canto Alarcón G, Camacho-Nuez M. Estrategias genómicas y moleculares para el control de la babesiosis bovina. Rev Mex Cienc Pecu 2012; 3 (Suppl. 1): 51-9.

[50]   Jaramillo Ortiz JM, Del Médico Zajac MP, Zanetti FA, *et al.* Vaccine strategies against *Babesia bovis* based on prime-boost immunizations in mice with modified vaccinia Ankara vector and recombinant proteins. Vaccine 2014; 32(36): 4625-32.
[http://dx.doi.org/10.1016/j.vaccine.2014.06.075] [PMID: 24968152]

[51]   Jaramillo Ortiz JM, Paoletta MS, Gravisaco MJ, *et al.* Immunisation of cattle against *Babesia bovis* combining a multi-epitope modified vaccinia Ankara virus and a recombinant protein induce strong Th1 cell responses but fails to trigger neutralising antibodies required for protection. Ticks Tick Borne Dis 2019; 10(6): 101270.
[http://dx.doi.org/10.1016/j.ttbdis.2019.101270] [PMID: 31445874]

[52]   Alzan HF, Cooke BM, Suarez CE. Transgenic *Babesia bovis* lacking 6-Cys sexual-stage genes as the foundation for non-transmissible live vaccines against bovine babesiosis. Ticks Tick Borne Dis 2019; 10(3): 722-8.
[http://dx.doi.org/10.1016/j.ttbdis.2019.01.006] [PMID: 30711475]

[53]   Guy B. The perfect mix: recent progress in adjuvant research. Nat Rev Microbiol 2007; 5(7): 505-17.
[http://dx.doi.org/10.1038/nrmicro1681] [PMID: 17558426]

[54]   Shen H, Ackerman AL, Cody V, *et al.* Enhanced and prolonged cross-presentation following endosomal escape of exogenous antigens encapsulated in biodegradable nanoparticles. Immunology 2006; 117(1): 78-88.
[http://dx.doi.org/10.1111/j.1365-2567.2005.02268.x] [PMID: 16423043]

[55]   Diwan M, Tafaghodi M, Samuel J. Enhancement of immune responses by co-delivery of a CpG oligodeoxynucleotide and tetanus toxoid in biodegradable nanospheres. J Control Release 2002; 85(1-3): 247-62.
[http://dx.doi.org/10.1016/S0168-3659(02)00275-4] [PMID: 12480329]

[56]   Thomas C, Rawat A, Hope-Weeks L, Ahsan F. Aerosolized PLA and PLGA nanoparticles enhance humoral, mucosal and cytokine responses to hepatitis B vaccine. Mol Pharm 2011; 8(2): 405-15.
[http://dx.doi.org/10.1021/mp100255c] [PMID: 21189035]

[57]   Manish M, Rahi A, Kaur M, Bhatnagar R, Singh S. A single-dose PLGA encapsulated protective antigen domain 4 nanoformulation protects mice against *Bacillus anthracis* spore challenge. PLoS One 2013; 8(4): e61885.
[http://dx.doi.org/10.1371/journal.pone.0061885] [PMID: 23637922]

[58]   Demento SL, Cui W, Criscione JM, *et al.* Role of sustained antigen release from nanoparticle vaccines in shaping the T cell memory phenotype. Biomaterials 2012; 33(19): 4957-64.
[http://dx.doi.org/10.1016/j.biomaterials.2012.03.041] [PMID: 22484047]

[59]   Bansal V, Kumar M, Dalela M, Brahmne HG, Singh II. Evaluation of synergistic effect of biodegradable polymeric nanoparticles and aluminum based adjuvant for improving vaccine efficacy. Int J Pharm 2014; 471(1-2): 377-84.
       [http://dx.doi.org/10.1016/j.ijpharm.2014.05.061] [PMID: 24939616]

[60]   Oh E, Susumu K, Mäkinen A, Deschamps J, Huston A, Medintz I. colloidal stability of gold nanoparticles coated with Multithiol-Poly(ethylene glycol) ligands: Importance of structural constraints of the sulfur anchoring groups. J Phys Chem C 2013; 117(37): 18947-56.
       [http://dx.doi.org/10.1021/jp405265u]

[61]   Brown WC, Corral RS. Stimulation of B lymphocytes, macrophages, and dendritic cells by protozoan DNA. Microbes Infect 2002; 4(9): 969-74.
       [http://dx.doi.org/10.1016/S1286-4579(02)01623-4] [PMID: 12106790]

[62]   Brown WC, Estes DM, Chantler SE, Kegerreis KA, Suarez CE. DNA and a CpG oligonucleotide derived from *Babesia bovis* are mitogenic for bovine B cells. Infect Immun 1998; 66(11): 5423-32.
       [http://dx.doi.org/10.1128/IAI.66.11.5423-5432.1998] [PMID: 9784553]

[63]   Mosqueda J, Hidalgo-Ruiz M, Calvo-Olvera DA, *et al.* RON2, a novel gene in *Babesia bigemina,* contains conserved, immunodominant B-cell epitopes that induce antibodies that block merozoite invasion. Parasitology 2019; 146(13): 1646-54.
       [http://dx.doi.org/10.1017/S0031182019001161] [PMID: 31452491]

[64]   Altschul SF, Gish W, Miller W, Myers EW, Lipman DJ. Basic local alignment search tool. J Mol Biol 1990; 215(3): 403-10.
       [http://dx.doi.org/10.1016/S0022-2836(05)80360-2] [PMID: 2231712]

[65]   Stothard P. The sequence manipulation suite: JavaScript programs for analyzing and formatting protein and DNA sequences. Biotechniques 2000; 28(6): 1102-1104, 1104.
       [http://dx.doi.org/10.2144/00286ir01] [PMID: 10868275]

[66]   Burge C, Karlin S. Prediction of complete gene structures in human genomic DNA. J Mol Biol 1997; 268(1): 78-94.
       [http://dx.doi.org/10.1006/jmbi.1997.0951] [PMID: 9149143]

[67]   Gasteiger E, Gattiker A, Hoogland C, Ivanyi I, Appel RD, Bairoch A. ExPASy: The proteomics server for in-depth protein knowledge and analysis. Nucleic Acids Res 2003; 31(13): 3784-8.
       [http://dx.doi.org/10.1093/nar/gkg563] [PMID: 12824418]

[68]   Möller S, Croning MD, Apweiler R. Evaluation of methods for the prediction of membrane spanning regions. Bioinformatics 2001; 17(7): 646-53.
       [http://dx.doi.org/10.1093/bioinformatics/17.7.646] [PMID: 11448883]

[69]   Almagro Armenteros JJ, Tsirigos KD, Sønderby CK, *et al.* SignalP 5.0 improves signal peptide predictions using deep neural networks. Nat Biotechnol 2019; 37(4): 420-3.
       [http://dx.doi.org/10.1038/s41587-019-0036-z] [PMID: 30778233]

[70]   Saha S, Raghava GP. Prediction of continuous B-cell epitopes in an antigen using recurrent neural network. Proteins 2006; 65(1): 40-8.
       [http://dx.doi.org/10.1002/prot.21078] [PMID: 16894596]

[71]   Jespersen MC, Peters B, Nielsen M, Marcatili P. BepiPred-2.0: improving sequence-based B-cell epitope prediction using conformational epitopes. Nucleic Acids Res 2017; 45(W1): W24-9.
       [http://dx.doi.org/10.1093/nar/gkx346] [PMID: 28472356]

[72]   Chen J, Liu H, Yang J, Chou KC. Prediction of linear B-cell epitopes using amino acid pair antigenicity scale. Amino Acids 2007; 33(3): 423-8.
       [http://dx.doi.org/10.1007/s00726-006-0485-9] [PMID: 17252308]

[73]   El-Manzalawy Y, Dobbs D, Honavar V. Predicting linear B-cell epitopes using string kernels. J Mol Recognit 2008; 21(4): 243-55.
       [http://dx.doi.org/10.1002/jmr.893] [PMID: 18496882]

[74]   Proceedings of the CSB 2008 Conference. Stanford. 2008; pp. 26-9.

[75]   Parker JM, Guo D, Hodges RS. New hydrophilicity scale derived from high-performance liquid chromatography peptide retention data: correlation of predicted surface residues with antigenicity and X-ray-derived accessible sites. Biochemistry 1986; 25(19): 5425-32.
[http://dx.doi.org/10.1021/bi00367a013] [PMID: 2430611]

[76]   Karplus P, Schulz G. Prediction of chain flexibility in proteins. Naturwissenschaften 1985; 72(4): 212-3.
[http://dx.doi.org/10.1007/BF01195768]

[77]   Emini EA, Hughes JV, Perlow DS, Boger J. Induction of hepatitis A virus-neutralizing antibody by a virus-specific synthetic peptide. J Virol 1985; 55(3): 836-9.
[http://dx.doi.org/10.1128/JVI.55.3.836-839.1985] [PMID: 2991600]

[78]   Pellequer JL, Westhof E, Van Regenmortel MH. Correlation between the location of antigenic sites and the prediction of turns in proteins. Immunol Lett 1993; 36(1): 83-99.
[http://dx.doi.org/10.1016/0165-2478(93)90072-A] [PMID: 7688347]

[79]   Kolaskar AS, Tongaonkar PC. A semi-empirical method for prediction of antigenic determinants on protein antigens. FEBS Lett 1990; 276(1-2): 172-4.
[http://dx.doi.org/10.1016/0014-5793(90)80535-Q] [PMID: 1702393]

[80]   Ponnuswamy PK, Prabhakaran M, Manavalan P. Hydrophobic packing and spatial arrangement of amino acid residues in globular proteins. Biochim Biophys Acta 1980; 623(2): 301-16.
[http://dx.doi.org/10.1016/0005-2795(80)90258-5] [PMID: 7397216]

[81]   Lee BS, Huang JS, Jayathilaka LP, Lee J, Gupta S. Antibody production with synthetic peptides. In: Schwartzbach S, Skalli O, Schikorski T, Eds. High-Resolution Imaging of Cellular Proteins. Methods in Molecular Biology, vol. 1474. New York: Humana Press 2016; 25-47.

SUBJECT INDEX

A

Acid phosphatase 107

Acinetobacter baumannii infection 111

Adaptive immune 63, 75, 101, 127, 128, 133, 134, 135, 136
  activation 101
  immune response (AIR) 63, 75, 127, 128, 133, 134, 135, 136

Adaptive immunity 65, 111, 127
  stimulated 111

Adenohypophysis 129

Agents 4, 6, 25, 26, 27, 31, 32, 35, 45, 100, 114, 138
  antiinfective 4, 6
  anti-TB 26
  antituberculosis 27, 31
  antiviral 32
  immunostimulatory 35
  intracellular parasitic 138
  therapeutic 100, 114

Airway epithelial cells (AECs) 74, 75, 76, 77, 78, 79, 80, 81, 82

Allicin 25, 33, 37, 38, 39, 40, 45
  bioavailability 39

Allium sativum 37

All trans-retinoic acid (ATRA) 108, 115

Alveolar 67, 74, 75, 76, 78, 79, 80, 82, 83, 84, 85, 86, 88, 110, 113
  epithelial cells 67, 84
  macrophages (AMs) 74, 75, 76, 78, 79, 80, 82, 83, 84, 85, 86, 88, 110, 113
  neutrophils 85

Amino acids 38, 57, 153, 167, 173
  non-proteinogenic 38

AMP-activated protein kinase 101, 112
  pathway 112

Androgen receptors (AR) 134

Anemia 150, 151, 157

Antibabesial drugs 164

Antibiotics 1, 7, 8, 12, 13, 14, 15, 30, 110, 114
  cycloserine 8
  potent macrolide 114

synergy 14
  third-generation 1

Antigen-presenting cells (APCs) 66, 88, 132, 133, 136

Antigens 75, 86, 128, 162, 163, 165, 166, 169, 170, 175
  hydrophobic 170
  hypervariable 166

Antimicrobial molecules induced by 61, 65
  autophagy 65
  vitamin 61, 65

Antimicrobial 61, 66
  oxygen and nitrogen radicals 66
  pathways 61

Antimicrobial peptides 1, 2, 13, 14, 15, 45, 56, 57, 59, 64, 67, 74, 76, 77, 110
  induction 45, 110

Anti-oxidant potency 36

Anti-retroviral therapy (ART) 91

Anti-TB drugs 25, 26, 27, 30, 32, 33, 43, 44, 45

Ascorbic acid 30

Aspergillus fumigatus 61

ATP 27, 29
  hydrolysis 29
  synthesis 27

Autophagosomelysosome fusion 65, 105
  blocking 105

Autophagy 33, 34, 56, 65, 91, 100, 101, 102, 103, 104, 105, 106, 107, 108, 109, 110, 111, 112, 113, 114, 116
  activating 114
  avoiding 106
  host-induced 112
  induced 33, 109, 110
  machinery 100, 101
  maturation process 65
  modulation 114
  noncanonical 106
  pathway 104
  proteins 65, 116
  receptors 104
  tuberculosis-associated 104

www.ingramcontent.com/pod-product-compliance
Lightning Source LLC
Chambersburg PA
CBHW041659210326
41598CB00007B/464